The Treatment
of Schizophrenia

The Treatment
of Schizophrenia

A HOLISTIC APPROACH

Based on the Readings of Edgar Cayce

David McMillin, M.A.

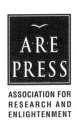

ASSOCIATION FOR
RESEARCH AND
ENLIGHTENMENT

A.R.E. Press • Virginia Beach • Virginia

Copyright © 1991
by David McMillin
1st Printing, June 1991 by Lifeline Press
Reprinted August 1997 by A.R.E. Press

Printed in the U.S.A.

A.R.E. Press
Sixty-Eighth & Atlantic Avenue
P.O. Box 656
Virginia Beach, VA 23451-0656

Library of Congress Cataloging-in-Publication Data
McMillin, David.
The treatment of schizophrenia : a holistic approach based on
the readings of Edgar Cayce / David McMillin, M.A.
     p. cm.
Originally published: Virginia Beach, Va. : Lifeline Press, © 1991.
Includes bibliographical references.
ISBN 0-87604-384-8 (pbk.)
1. Schizophrenia—Treatment—Miscellanea. 2. Cayce, Edgar,
1877-1945. Edgar Cayce readings. I. Title.
[RC514.M397 1997]
616.89'8206—dc21   97-8463

Cover design by Richard Boyle

Edgar Cayce Readings © 1971, 1993, 1994, 1995, 1996
by the Edgar Cayce Foundation.
All rights reserved.

CONTENTS

Introduction

◆———

ALTHOUGH THE WORK of Edgar Cayce is generally known among persons interested in transpersonal studies, much of the public, including the mental health community, is not acquainted with this body of information. This introduction will provide some biographical information about Edgar Cayce and a brief discussion of his career as a "psychic diagnostician" for those readers unfamiliar with the subject. Cayce's life will be viewed from a broader perspective—as a seer reiterating the "perennial philosophy." The introduction will conclude with a statement of purpose and a brief overview.

Cayce's Life and Work

Edgar Cayce was born on March 18, 1877, on a farm near Hopkinsville, Kentucky. His childhood was marked by paranormal experiences such as seeing and speaking to recently deceased relatives and sleeping with his head on textbooks to memorize school lessons. His abilities as a psychic diagnostician surfaced during his early twenties when he developed a gradual paralysis of the throat and medical doctors were unable to provide relief. As a last resort, he allowed a friend to hypnotize him so that he could reestablish the altered state of consciousness that he had utilized as a child to memorize his school books. From this trance state, he was able to diagnosis his condition and prescribe treatments which remedied his problem.

Cayce was hesitant to use his ability to help others. He felt responsible for the information and was concerned that the suggested treatments might have deleterious effects. Consequently, many of the early beneficiaries of his services were desperate cases, often given up by medical doctors. Working within the medical establishment, in partnership with various physicians who utilized his gift, Cayce felt assured that his unusual ability would do no harm. After several years as a professional photographer and part-time psychic, Cayce became convinced of the validity of his psychic gift. In service to humanity, he devoted the rest of his life to giving readings for those who sought his help.

Cayce refused to "cash in" on this ability. He preferred to offer his services on a donation basis. Consequently, many readings were provided free or for nominal donations. Cayce suffered financial hardship for most of his life and apparently accepted monetary austerity as his karma for having squandered resources in a previous life.

As an indication of Cayce's interest in providing help to persons suffering from physical illness, the bulk of the readings (over 9,000) were given in response to health issues. The remainder cover virtually every field of human endeavor, from religion and philosophy to business and international affairs. The readings that address mental health are particularly relevant to the present work and cover the entire field including psychosis, depression, anxiety, dementia, personality disorders, developmental disorders, etc. Treatises on learning and memory, the nature of personality, perception, psychosocial development, consciousness, the meaning of sleep, etc., are interspersed throughout the readings and provide intriguing perspectives on these concepts. Apart from the content of Cayce's readings, the trance process itself is a fascinating aspect of Cayce's work. Harmon Bro provides a glimpse into the trance procedure and the physical context of the readings:

What took place in the morning and afternoon trance sessions, in the months that followed when I heard and took notes on some six hundred of Cayce's readings, was a profound shock. Nothing could adequately prepare one for the amount of swift helpfulness that flowed from the unconscious man. His outward procedures were simple enough. Cayce sat on his plain green studio couch in his cheerful windowed study, across the room from his desk and little portable typewriter. He prayed, then lay down and step by step went unconscious. He spoke in measured address about each person or need to which his wife, sitting beside him, quietly directed his attention. After an hour or more of discourse and questions which his secretary recorded in shorthand, he came swiftly back to consciousness, remembering nothing of what he had said, and got up to resume the activities of his busy correspondence and office. It was all done in broad daylight and simplicity, as naturally as if he were still taking portraits in a photographic studio. But the plainness of the process did not take away the jolt of seeing him accomplish day after day what our culture said was impossible. (Bro, 1990, p. 58)

Although many of the early readings were not recorded, over 14,000 were stenographically transcribed and have been preserved by the Association for Research and Enlightenment (A.R.E.) in Virginia Beach, Virginia. Recognizing the need for confidentiality, each reading is assigned a number corresponding to the person or group requesting information. The identifying number is followed by another number designating the sequence of the reading. For example, a reading cited as 182-6 indicates that this reading is the sixth in a series of readings for an individual or group designated as 182. Throughout this text, additional background information is provided for the numerous citations from the readings. When available, the sex and age of the recipient and the date of the reading are included. This is important because age and gender differences have been documented in schizophrenia. Also, the date of the reading can be helpful to those interested in the evolution of Cayce's psychic ability.

Naturally, the question as to the source of the trance information was put to the sleeping Cayce. Many such examples are scattered throughout the readings. Two excerpts are cited here to provide an introduction to the dynamics of the psychic process.

254-2   3/19/19

In this state the conscious mind is under subjugation of the subconscious or soul mind. The information obtained and given by this body is obtained through the power of mind over mind, or power of mind over physical matter, or obtained by the suggestion as given to the active part of the subconscious mind. It obtains its information from that which it has gathered, either from other subconscious minds—put in touch with the power of the suggestion of the mind controlling the speaking faculties of this body, or from minds that have passed into the Beyond, which leave their impressions and are brought in touch by the power of the suggestion. What is known to one subconscious mind or soul is known to another, whether conscious of the fact or not. The subjugation of the conscious mind putting the subconscious in action in this manner or in one of the other of the manners as described, this body obtains its information when in the subconscious state.

Q. Is this information always correct?

A. Correct insofar as the suggestion is in the proper channel or in accord with the action of subconscious or soul matter.

254-30   4/13/26

Then, consider also that which has been given, that through the subconscious or superconscious forces of the entity the manifestations may take place; or from the superconscious or subconscious forces of entities that may have passed into that designated as the spiritual realm. Through these, or through the universal consciousness or cosmic consciousness from the very abilities of the entity Edgar Cayce to wholly subjugate the physical consciousness as to allow the use of physical or mental or spiritual influences in the realms about the entity.

Then, that which wavers or hinders or repels or blocks the activity through this channel when in such a state may be from these causes; namely:

The unwillingness of the body-consciousness to submit to the suggestion as pertaining to information desired at that particular time. Or the activity of the physical in such a manner as to require the influence or supervision of the superconsciousness in the body, or ill health, at such a period. Or the mental attitude of those about the body that are not in accord with the type, class or character of information sought at that particular time. Or there may be the many variations of the combination of these, influencing one to another, as to the type, class or real activity of the entity or soul that seeks the information.

Note that the psychic process described in these excerpts was a cooperative venture. The attitudes and actions of the persons involved (i.e., the individual directing the session by giving suggestions and asking questions, the individual(s) seeking the information, staff persons in the room during the readings, etc.) had a direct effect on the accuracy and helpfulness of the reading. Also note the intrapsychic cooperation involved—the interface among conscious, unconscious, and superconscious processes reflecting the underlying unity of body, mind, and spirit.

One further comment about the nature and source of Cayce's trance information—the readings stated that Edgar Cayce's unconscious mind could communicate with the unconscious minds of those seeking help. In one trance session, when Cayce was asked, "Who is giving this information?" he simply replied, "Self" (2713-3). In a similar case, he answered, "From the body itself! and *for* the body itself physically" (5654-1). Apparently, Cayce's dissociative faculty relied heavily upon the unconscious mind of those seeking assistance. The ability of unconscious minds to communicate is an interesting phenomenological question in regard to the purported source of the information. But the therapeutic ramifications of such a process are more than merely speculative. If the unconscious mind of an afflicted individual is knowledgeable about the illness, could this aspect of the self be recruited into the healing process? The readings consistently stated that such was the case and insisted that "all healing comes from within." In cases of major mental illness such as schizophrenia, the inner response was considered essential; therapeutic modalities such as suggestive therapeutics and therapeutic milieu were regularly suggested to access this inner resource.

Although there are many books available which discuss the life of Edgar Cayce, three biographies provide direct access to the salient points of Cayce's life. *There Is a River* by Thomas Sugrue (1942) was the first extensive account of Cayce's life and contributed greatly to public recognition of his work. The philosophy chapter near the end of the book is a concise statement of the perennial philosophy propounded by Cayce and is suggested for those interested in this aspect of the readings. *Edgar Cayce—The Sleeping Prophet* by Jess Stearn (1967) is a highly readable work by a popular, contemporary author. *A Seer Out of Season: The Life of Edgar Cayce* by Harmon Bro (1990) is a scholarly and often poetic work, and is undoubtedly the most realistic of the biographies. Bro provides a rare glimpse into the humanity and foibles of Cayce while simultaneously portraying the larger context of Cayce's life.

The Perennial Philosophy of the Cayce Readings

Although biographical information and glimpses into his hypnotic technique provide a silhouette of the man, a greater appreciation of the life and work of Edgar Cayce is possible only when one utilizes a broader perspective. The significance of Cayce's contribution is most evident in the context of historical traditions, and Harmon Bro provides insight into this historical/cultural dimension of Cayce's work. Bro worked with Cayce for a short while before Cayce's death in 1945. In due course he wrote a doctoral dissertation on Cayce's work along with numerous other books on the subject including the aforementioned biography.

After carefully defining and differentiating various categories (i.e., shaman, oracle, diviner, and medium), Bro eliminates such titles for Cayce. Although there were distinct similarities between Cayce and some of the biblical prophets, Bro feels that Cayce could most appropriately be regarded as a seer—a seer out of season:

> All in all, he seemed to belong among those who could manifest only one or two of the prophets' typically many-sided gifts. Where some figures in the long history of religions, including the tribal medicine man or magician, appeared to specialize in direct healing, Cayce's was essentially a cognitive gift, dependent on the activity of others to change bodies or human affairs. The category of seer seemed most fitting for one with authentic visions and a genuine relation to the divine, yet in effect a stunted prophet . . . I would in time find parallels to important features of Cayce in such seers as the Moslem kahin, the Hindu rishi, the Sumerian baru, the Japanese urandi, the Egyptian honu, the Buddhist arhat, the Peruvian piage, and figures from Roman and Celtic history . . . But Cayce in modern America, with no recognizable tradition for his gift and

work, and no community of faith to support him, was a seer out of cultural time or season. (Bro, 1990, pp. 129-132)

Bro's recognition of the broader ramifications of Cayce's work provides a context for understanding the readings. If Edgar Cayce is to be regarded as a seer, the information that flowed through him can be viewed as representing the "perennial philosophy."

But there is a much more sophisticated view of the relation of humanity and Divinity, a view held by the great majority of the truly gifted theologians, philosophers, sages, and even scientists of various times. Known in general as the "perennial philosophy" (a name coined by Leibnitz), it forms the esoteric core of Hinduism, Buddhism, Taoism, Sufism, and Christian mysticism, as well as being embraced, in whole or part, by individual intellects ranging from Spinoza to Albert Einstein, Schopenhauer to Jung, William James to Plato. Further, in its purest form it is not at all anti-science but, in a special sense, trans-science or even ante-science, so that it can happily coexist with, and certainly complement, the hard data of the pure sciences. This is why, I believe, that so many of the truly brilliant scientists have always flirted with, or totally embraced, the perennial philosophy, as witness Einstein, Schrodinger, Eddington, David Bohm, Sir James Jeans, even Isaac Newton. (Wilber, 1981, pp. 3-4)

Aldous Huxley (1944) advocates a similar perspective of the perennial philosophy which emphasizes the "tripartite" quality of human nature. Significantly, the tripartite "body/mind/spirit" interface is a major theme in the Cayce readings and provides the foundation for the "holistic" perspective advocated in this book.

The Perennial Philosophy is primarily concerned with the one, divine Reality substantial to the manifold world of things and lives and minds (p. viii). In other words, there is a hierarchy of the real (p. 33). But all of these men, even La Rochefoucauld, even Machiavelli, were aware of certain facts which twentieth-century psychologists have chosen to ignore—the fact that human nature is tripartite, consisting of a spirit as well as of a mind and body; the fact that we live on the borderline between two worlds, the temporal and the eternal, the physical-vital-human and the divine ... (p. 115) Man's final end, the purpose of his existence, is to love, know and be united with the immanent and transcendent Godhead (p. 38).

Recognition of Cayce's work as representative of the perennial philosophy—as an extension of a tradition of ideas and practices which underlie most of the world's major religions and philosophies—is essential for a full appreciation of Cayce's contribution. From this perspective, he cannot simply be dismissed as a religious fanatic seeking to establish an esoteric cult, a crackpot practicing medical quackery and milking desperate innocents of their resources, or a deluded psychotic experiencing pathological trance states resulting in thousands of incoherent, implausible psychic readings. To the contrary, Cayce's life and work exemplify a long and respected tradition among the great cultures of the world. Although his beliefs have a definite Judeo-Christian orientation, his recognition of the continuity of consciousness, including such Eastern concepts as karma and reincarnation, attest to the scope of his perspective. Just as Huxley recognized that "knowledge is a function of being" (1944, p. vii), Bro suggests that Cayce's life is an example of "love surprised by wisdom."

Cayce belongs somewhere among the stumbling, surprised explorers of new terrain, only partly able to describe what they see, and tempted to doubt their own experiences. His trances disclose (as glances over the shoulder in his unending medical effort) penetrating views of good and evil, worship and ethics, community and disintegration, the earthy and the transcendent, gifts of insight from East and West, and a Christ who is everyone's destiny but nobody's cultural captive. (Bro, 1990, pp. 14-15)

Thus, the psychic readings of Edgar Cayce are not a source of supernal, infallible information. Rather, they represent the efforts of a sincere man seeking to be of service.

The perennial philosophy itself is diverse in its manifestations due to the nature of language and the limits of the conscious mind. "Whenever, for any reason, we wish to think of the world, not as it appears to common sense, but as a continuum, we find that our traditional syntax and vocabulary are quite inadequate ... in all expositions of the Perennial Philosophy, the frequency of paradox, of verbal extravagance, sometimes even of seeming blasphemy" (Huxley, 1944, p. 34). Persons who have studied the Cayce readings will attest to Huxley's observation—the language and style of the readings can be complex and even arduous. The fact that the method employed by Cayce is not generally recognized or accepted in Western culture comes as no surprise. It is primarily the materialistic beliefs underlying the contemporary perspective which makes the perennial philosophy appear incredible. Fortunately, one does not have to be a student of, or believer in, the perennial philosophy to investigate and benefit from information such as the Cayce readings. Interested readers are encouraged to read some of the biographical material about Cayce's life and decide for themselves regarding the plausibility of the Cayce readings.

The Purpose of This Book

The purpose of this book is to make the Cayce readings accessible to mental health professionals and other individuals interested in alternative perspectives on schizophrenia. The comprehensiveness of the readings is a natural product of their holistic philosophy and is a major strength of this approach. The readings address the total picture—the clinical arena of etiology and treatment, the interpersonal and intrapsychic struggles of families attempting to help a member suffering from major mental illness, and more generally, the meaning of debilitating illness (e.g., the cosmic significance of personal misfortune, etc.).

This manuscript can be considered as an extension of two important articles on the application of the Cayce material to the treatment of major mental illness. Both works were presented at a medical symposium at the A.R.E. Clinic in Phoenix, Arizona. James C. Windsor (1969) entitled his paper, "A Holistic Theory of Mental Illness," and provided an excellent review of the Cayce material in relation to the whole spectrum of mental illness. Charles T. Cayce (1978) focused on the treatment of schizophrenia in his paper, "Concerning a Physical Basis for Mental Illness." These articles provided the impetus for this work and are highly recommended reading. Windsor's paper is particularly significant because it has been heralded as the point at which "the field of holistic medicine began" (McGarey, 1983, p. ix). The association of "holism" with the Cayce readings has become widely recognized, culminating in this reference from an editorial in the *Journal of the American Medical Association:*

> The roots of present-day holism probably go back 100 years to the birth of Edgar Cayce in Hopkinsville, Ky. By the time he died in 1944 [sic], Cayce was well recognized as a mystic who entered sleep trances and dictated a philosophy of life and healing called "readings." His base was established at Virginia Beach, Va., now the headquarters of the Cayce Foundation. Closely associated with that foundation is the Association for Research and Enlightenment, Inc. [A.R.E.], which also runs a medical clinic under physician direction in Arizona. (Callan, 1979, p. 1156)

As Callan has noted, the designation of "holism" has come to include a wide variety of philosophies and modalities. Certainly his observation that holism has, in certain instances, become "fuzzy," "self-centered," and financially opportunistic is well taken. Since "holism" has become associated with so much that is clearly not in keeping with its origin, the term is employed in the title of this work with a reservation—namely, that *holism* be limited to the meaning assigned by Windsor as derived from the Cayce readings: " . . . Cayce saw a person as a whole, with mind, body, and spirit as a single unit, all so closely tied that it was not possible for one aspect to be diseased, either physically or mentally, without the whole person suffering the consequences" (Windsor, 1969, p. 1). An excerpt from the readings may be useful to further delineate the body/mind/spirit interface:

1861-4   M. 33   1/13/40
First—one finds self in a three-dimensional plane of consciousness; all that may be known materially is subject to that dimension.
That as may be comprehended in the mental may reach into a fourth-dimensional plane—as the variation between a book with its dimensions and the contents of same, which may be of a mental reaction entirely.
Yet the spiritual import is the premise, as to what is the ideal, purpose and intent of same—as to the effect the contents of such a book would have upon an individual entity.
Or, one in the material phases of his experience draws men-

tally upon comparisons of things, conditions, experiences, through the mental faculties of the body; and his reaction is still dependent upon the ideal he holds . . . Do not confuse rote, or mental growth, with spiritual import. It is true that the combination of H_2O constantly produces water. It is true that the bow upon the string at a certain tone constantly produces C, or another note, to which the attunement is made to a first cause—as H_2O is to a first cause. But it is not always water that is wanted with hydrogen and oxygen. Neither is it always C that is desired upon the tune or tone of the instruments.

This excerpt provides an illustration of holism by defining the role of the physical, mental, and spiritual dimensions with common examples from chemistry and music. It helps to dispel some of the "fuzziness" of these constructs by defining "mental" and "spiritual" in everyday terms. The spiritual dimension is designated by words such as meaning, purpose, value, intentionality, etc. The spiritual provides guidance and direction—it sets the agenda. Mental processes actively manifest the spiritual agenda in thought and ideas. The physical aspect is represented in strictly physical terms. In the preceding analogy, the physical dimension was represented by material substance such as the binding and ink-covered pages of a book.

However, the readings caution against viewing the tripartite as separate processes. Great emphasis is placed on viewing the three primary aspects as unified and inseparable so long as an individual is alive. Thus, the fundamental unity of body, mind, and spirit represents the foundation of holism. The question naturally arises, "How do body, mind, and spirit interface—what is the basis of this unity?" The short answer is, "Through the nervous systems and endocrine glands in the body." The long answer is a major focus of this book. For the readings consistently maintain that disease, and particularly major mental illnesses such as schizophrenia, results from incoordination of these systems. Hence, treatment necessarily must be directed to the whole person (body, mind, and spirit) in order to reestablish coordination.

As Chapter One will amply demonstrate, schizophrenia has a strong physical (somatic) component. The Cayce readings anticipated many of the findings of contemporary medical science in this regard by providing graphic descriptions of the etiological factors and developmental course of this illness. The readings diverge from current models by insisting that there is more to this condition than physical pathology. Schizophrenia strikes at the integration of body, mind, and spirit. Thus, all three aspects of selfhood must be addressed during treatment.

Note that the title focuses on treatment rather than simply a general consideration of schizophrenia. This emphasis is based upon the readings' preference for applied knowledge. For example, knowledge of etiological factors is important to the extent that it can be employed for effective treatment, not because it may support a particular theoretical position. With this in mind, a therapeutic model will be proposed which lends itself to empirical validation.

This book is offered as an introduction with the intention that it may serve as a useful reference for individuals interested in the further study of the Cayce readings on schizophrenia. It is hoped that the reader will take advantage of the actual readings by examining them first-hand. Individuals who are sympathetic to the transpersonal perspective should find this book helpful, because it deals with the problems of major mental illness from the vantage point of expanded consciousness. Professionals with a more traditional orientation should find the manuscript sufficiently scholarly and focused to be interesting and stimulating.

An attempt has been made to document the information in the readings with citations from the current clinical and research literature. The intention is to provide a solid foundation for the consideration of the ideas presented and should not be viewed as an attempt to prove the material or convert practitioners with a more mainstream perspective. The documentation is also congruent with Cayce's admonition to substantiate any presentation of the material: "DO NOT let any portion of that published be thrown at the public, or make claims that are not able to be verified from EVERY ANGLE!" (254-88)

It is crucial that professionals who are interested in applying this approach have access to information from the readings and the mainstream literature. A comparative study offers the possibility of integration of the best from various perspectives. Hopefully, such integration could lead to more effective treatment options.

However, there are also legal ramifications here. The current high rate of malpractice litigation combined with the increasing number of "alternative" modalities being developed make it advisable for health care professionals interested in progressive treatment models to be familiar with the literature in all areas.

Although the primary emphasis of this book is to present the Cayce perspective in a manner which facilitates application by professionals in clinical and research areas, many others should find this book interesting and readable. With the possible exception of the first chapter, which contains a fairly technical literature review, most of this book should be comprehensible to the motivated nonprofessional. Such a person may be a family member or friend of someone who has been diagnosed as having schizophrenia. Or perhaps individuals carrying the diagnosis may wish to view the problem from an alternative perspective. The final chapter provides a summary of the Cayce approach. Any reader who gets bogged down in an earlier section may wish to skip to Chapter Eight for a simplified overview.

The thesis of this book is that the psychic readings of Edgar Cayce provide a plausible perspective on the etiology and treatment of schizophrenia, and therefore are deserving of serious consideration by progressive mental health professionals. The goal of this book is to serve as a catalyst for the application of the principles and techniques found in the Cayce readings—both in the clinical and research areas. As will be repeated frequently throughout this work, the ideas suggested by Cayce are to be regarded as hypotheses which need to be applied and evaluated. Cayce often cautioned against uncritical acceptance of the ideas presented in the readings, and they are not promoted here as self-authenticating truths.

Application may occur in several areas and at various levels. Chapter Six presents a therapeutic model which may be utilized in two ways: within a private practitioner format or an institutional format. Clinicians and researchers may be stimulated to use some of the suggestions in their respective fields without specific reference to the Edgar Cayce readings. The goal is for the information to be applied for the benefit of those suffering from schizophrenia. If using the citations from more traditional sources will facilitate the application of the information, so be it. That is one of the primary reasons for providing the citations.

Although the clinical and research areas are the primary focus, application may also occur at the interpersonal level within the family structure of those dealing with this problem. Having the Cayce perspective available as an alternative viewpoint on schizophrenia may constructively change how friends and relatives relate to persons suffering from the disorder.

The holistic approach of Edgar Cayce offers the opportunity to view schizophrenia as a potential growth experience for all involved. Make no mistake about it, this approach does not propose a therapeutic panacea. To the contrary, the Cayce approach is in agreement with the psychological and psychiatric literature in attesting to the complexity and severity of schizophrenia. What the Cayce approach does offer is the opportunity to view this problem from a broader perspective with the hope of providing significant relief for those suffering from this devastating disorder.

A Brief Overview

Chapter One provides a brief review of what is known about schizophrenia and recognizes the importance of the scientific literature in this field. Chapter Two can be viewed as the counterpart to the first chapter in that it covers much of the same material from the perspective of the Cayce readings. The compare/contrast format provides a vehicle for examining the congruency between the two sources while focusing on important differences.

Chapter Three consists primarily of case study summaries. Due to the immense volume of information contained in the readings, a means of presenting this information in a condensed, yet intelligible form is required. Hopefully, these summaries will be an effective vehicle for addressing the complexity and magnitude of the information. Naturally, it is recognized that the data contained in these summaries do not constitute empirical fact and are not provided for that purpose. Anecdotal data from case studies are a very limited resource for research purposes. Yet in circumstances such as this, where retrospective analysis is the only available means of accessing data, it is a reasonable means of presenting such information for clinical consideration.

Chapters Four and Five can be regarded as a "therapeutic tandem" embodying the theory and practice of treatment and rehabilitation. The therapeutic principles discussed in Chapter Four represent the philosophy of the readings. They provide the conceptual and spiritual underpinning of the therapeutic process. Chapter Five elaborates the clinical techniques which comprise the holistic model.

Chapter Six is an attempt to translate the therapeutic model into a format familiar to contemporary mental health professionals. The recognition that the "Cayce approach" to rehabilitation requires the participation of professionals at many levels, requires that a workable, responsible framework be established. The possibilities for applying the Cayce material to this problem are unlimited and the model presented in this chapter should be considered as a starting point rather than a finished product.

Chapter Seven discusses the research implications of the Cayce material. The schizophrenia literature is ambiguous with variability being a primary source of confusion. The readings may provide insights into the major sources of variability (i.e., heterogeneity and nonspecificity). Other topics considered in Chapter Seven include validation of the therapeutic model introduced in Chapter Six and various research questions pertaining to therapeutic techniques (e.g., manual medicine, electrotherapy, etc.).

Chapter Eight is a summary of the previous chapters and provides an opportunity to draw some conclusions about the Cayce perspective. The various appendices serve as a repository for selections from the readings on topics commonly cited by Cayce and relevant to the subject of schizophrenia.

In all instances throughout this book, abundant citations from the Cayce readings are provided so that the readings can speak for themselves. The author, of necessity, has served as a translator in many respects, in order that the material can be made accessible to the contemporary mental health field. Readers are encouraged to study the excerpts, and indeed the original readings if so motivated, to develop alternative interpretations and perspectives.

1

A Literature Review of Schizophrenia

◆

SCHIZOPHRENIA IS A devastating illness accounting for about 1/5 of all chronic and severe disability (Jablensky, 1989). This disorder afflicts about 1% of the world's population and consumes between $20-$40 billion annually (North, 1989). Schizophrenia is diagnosed by the presence of psychotic symptoms during the active phase of the disorder (i.e., delusions and hallucinations) and produces characteristic disturbances in mental processes and affect. Typically, the deteriorating course of the illness results in a level of functioning below that previously achieved and involves a distorted sense of self, loss of volition, impaired interpersonal functioning, distorted relationship to the external world, and inappropriate psychomotor behavior (American Psychiatric Association, 1987).

The term schizophrenia is only the most recent label for this form of insanity. Almost a century ago, Kraepelin introduced the concept of dementia praecox:

We designate as dementia praecox the development of a simple, more or less pervasive, state of mental weakness, which manifests itself as an acute or subacute mental disorder. The course of this disease process can exhibit very different patterns . . . This behavior indicates, I believe, that in all likelihood we are dealing with an organic change in the brain. (Kraepelin, in Jablensky, 1989, p. 516)

Kraepelin's seminal description of the schizophrenic disorder (which he labeled dementia praecox) is important for several reasons: (1) it lays the foundation for a physiological basis of the illness, (2) it suggests a hereditary component in the etiology of schizophrenia, (3) it embodies a systems view (more about this later in the section on variability and nonspecificity in schizophrenia), and (4) it is the diagnostic category used by Edgar Cayce in his psychic readings on the subject.

Since Kraepelin's influential definition of dementia praecox as a chronic process resulting from brain tissue degeneration, numerous theorists and researchers have provided supporting models and empirical data to bolster this disease model of schizophrenia. Perhaps the boldest theoretical attempt to integrate biological findings of brain pathology to a general model of schizophrenia was proposed by Crow (1980).

It seems that two syndromes can be distinguished in those diseases currently described as schizophrenic and that each may be associated with a specific pathological process. The first (type I syndrome, equivalent to "acute schizophrenia," and characterized by the positive symptoms—delusions, hallucinations, and thought disorder) is in some way associated with a change in dopaminergic transmission; the second process (the type II syndrome, equivalent to the "defect state," and characterized by the negative symptoms—affective flattening and poverty of speech) is unrelated to dopaminergic transmission but may be associated with intellectual impairment and, perhaps, structural changes in the brain. (Crow, 1980, p. 68)

Research supporting this hypothesis indicates that schizophrenics with poor long-term outcome and a preponderance of negative symptoms tend to have enlarged brain ventricles (e. g., Johnstone et al., 1976; Crow, 1980; Andreasen et al., 1982). This has been interpreted as indicating deterioration through some degenerative process. The precise mechanism of atrophy has not been identified.

A genetic component of schizophrenia has been demonstrated by numerous studies (see Murray & Harvey, 1989, for an excellent review) which have examined the link between heredity and schizophrenia. Twin studies have provided the strongest evidence of this link. Adoption studies have substantiated the congenital origins of schizophrenia by separating out aspects of the physical and cultural environments of subjects. However, it is important to remember that even among the closest genetic relatives (e.g., identical twins) the maximum risk is only about 50% for the identical cotwin of a schizophrenic. Thus schizophrenia, as it is currently defined, is not strictly a hereditary disorder but is associated with a significant genetic factor in some cases.

The biological dimension of schizophrenia was further emphasized when the antipsychotic effects of certain drugs were discovered in the 1950s. These medications revolutionized the treatment of schizophrenia by providing a means of relieving some of the worst symptoms of the disorder (delusions and hallucinations).

The antipsychotic drugs also instigated a new era of research into the biochemistry of schizophrenia. This research has focused on the neurotransmitters within the brain which are most clearly affected by the antipsychotic drugs and the brain systems which utilize these neurotransmitters.

The leading theory in this field posits that the symptoms of schizophrenia result from a dysfunction in dopamine transmission within the brain (dopamine is one of the major neurotransmitters in the brain). The "dopamine hypothesis" of schizophrenia is based upon three factors: (1) neuroleptic pharmacotherapy appears to produce a reduction in central nervous system (CNS) dopaminergic activity which is roughly proportional to its ability to relieve acute symptoms; (2) schizophrenics seem to be sensitive to drugs which increase CNS dopaminergic outflow; and (3) prolonged exposure of nonschizophrenic persons to high levels of amphetamine can produce a psychosis similar to paranoid schizophrenia (Alpert & Friedhoff, 1980).

This hypothesis has come under increasing criticism in recent years due to a lack of direct supporting evidence and a number of anomalies which appear to contradict the notion of hyperdopaminergia as the sole pathology in schizophrenia (e.g., Csernansky,

Holman, & Hollister, 1983). Alpert and Friedhoff (1980) have provided an excellent review of this evidence and conclude, "Dopamine appears important but cannot be viewed as a simple pathogen." (p. 387)

Although antipsychotic medications have proven to be the most effective treatment option for schizophrenia, reviews of course and outcome consistently reveal patterns of variable response and high relapse. Hogarty (1984) reviewed 12 studies (N = 814) and found that about 40% of the patients relapsed within one year. Drug compliance seems to have not been a major factor since patients in studies receiving depot neuroleptics had similar relapse rates. Even with drug compliance, Herz (1986) has described schizophrenia as "an illness characterized by exacerbation and remissions" (p. 46).

Because a sizable number of patients are either resistant to drug therapy or relapse periodically in spite of it, mental health practitioners have evolved psychosocial and educational strategies to supplement treatment with medications. Hogarty (1984) has provided an excellent review of these approaches and suggests that the combination of drugs and psychosocial interventions produce the lowest rate of relapse to date. Even with these integrated therapies, rehabilitation of schizophrenics is still problematic. "Despite our best efforts, a subsample of patients continue either to relapse or to adjust poorly to these modern drug and psychosocial programs. Increasingly, we have observed that such patients have been greatly distressed during their aftercare experience." (Hogarty, 1984, p. 40)

Variability and Nonspecificity in Schizophrenia

Variability refers to a tradition of diverse and contradictory findings prevalent in the study of schizophrenia. Bellak and Strauss (1979) expressed the frustration that is produced by variability in schizophrenia:

> The sense of frustration is most especially related to the fact that excellent investigators, in seemingly well-controlled studies, find contradictory results. A splendid demonstration of that problem was recently given by Matthysee, who devoted nearly one half of a lecture to present data that support the dopamine hypothesis and the second part to data that invalidate the same hypothesis. He, too, then arrived at an opinion we have expressed in various ways at different times . . . The

divergence of data may suggest that the manifest form of the schizophrenic syndrome is arrived at by different pathogenic pathways. (Bellak & Strauss, 1979, p. 441)

Schizophrenia is diagnosed by the presence of symptoms, and there exists no objective, noninterview-based measure with which to diagnose the syndrome. While variance due to innaccurate diagnosis has been blamed for inconsistent findings, there is a growing tendency to view schizophrenia as a group of related illnesses rather than a single disease.

Most investigators concur that the illness we usually call by a single name—"schizophrenia"—is probably a heterogeneous group of disorders that share the common features of psychotic symptoms, partial response to neuroleptics, and a relatively poor outcome. Patients who share these common features are, however, clinically quite diverse. Further, research investigations have repeatedly demonstrated that the most consistent finding one can obtain is a very large variance in any variable that may be measured in schizophrenia, ranging from cognitive to neurochemical . . . The diversity in schizophrenia suggests that the disorders grouped under this general term may in fact represent several different specific diseases that may differ in important ways, such as involvement of different neurotransmitter systems, different brain regions, or different etiological agents. (Andreasen, 1985, p. 380)

To further complicate matters, research and clinical experience in schizophrenia points to the importance of nonspecificity in the syndrome. Nonspecificity may be defined as the tendency for various symptoms and indices of pathophysiology to be shared by the major mental illnesses.

Heimann (1985) points out that the extensive orienting response literature in schizophrenia is burdened by nonspecificity. This research suggests that schizophrenics have abnormal autonomic nervous system (ANS) response to nonsignal tones whereby sample patient populations usually produce two equal groups of "responders" and "nonresponders." Division into these discrete psychophysiological groups have been found to correlate with symptom clusters and therapeutic outcome (Ohman, 1981). Heimann's research has demonstrated that similar electrodermal patterns exist among depressed populations. In particular, about half of the patient samples diagnosed as schizophrenic and depressed produce no orienting reflex to nonsignal stimuli. This pattern has been significantly correlated to clinical features of emotional withdrawal, disturbed thought processes, increased exhibition of mannerisms, slowed bodily movements, increased somatic complaints, and depressed mood. Heimann notes, "The inhibition of the orienting reflex indicates that the patient, whether schizophrenic or depressed, has access to pathophysiological mechanisms of emotional withdrawal and information rejection, which he uses when the pathological process has caused a disturbance in the homeostatic equilibrium of information uptake and information processing" (p. 86).

In an extensive review of the differential diagnosis of schizophrenia and manic-depressive illness, Pope and Lipinski (1978) point out the nonspecificity of "schizophrenic symptoms" in relation to affective disorders:

> We conclude that most so-called schizophrenic symptoms, taken alone and in cross section, have remarkably little, if any, demonstrated validity in determining diagnosis, prognosis, or treatment response in psychosis. In the United States, particularly, overreliance on such symptoms alone results in overdiagnosis of schizophrenia and underdiagnosis of affective illnesses, particularly mania. This compromises both clinical treatment and research. (Pope & Lipinski, 1978, p. 811)

Schizoaffective disorder represents American psychiatry's attempt to deal with this aspect of nonspecificity. "The term *Schizoaffective Disorder* has been used in many different ways since it was first introduced as a subtype of Schizophrenia, and represents one of the most confusing and controversial concepts in psychiatric nosology." (American Psychiatric Association, 1987, p. 208) Lieberman's exasperation at this quandary illustrates the nosological dilemma of schizoaffective disorder:

> DSM-I, DSM-II, and ICD-9 have steadfastly included it under schizophrenia. But several authors . . . contend that it more closely resembles manic-depressive illness, at least in its initial phase. Still other authors . . . have categorized schizoaffective illness as somewhere-in-between, describing it as a

hybrid state, the midpoint on a continuum, or a third psychosis distinct unto itself. The complexities are raised to a higher power still, when one considers that schizophrenia and, more recently, affective disorders are being redefined as spectrums rather than homogeneous unitary entities. Add to this the geographical and temporal diagnostic variances that occur, and we are finally forced to confront ourselves less eloquently with the question, "What does it all mean?" (Lieberman, 1979, p. 438)

Reports of ventricular enlargement in bipolar affective disorder (Pearlson & Veroff, 1981; Nasrallah, McCalley-Whitters & Jacoby, 1982) and schizophrenia, schizoaffective, and bipolar affective disorder (Rieder et al., 1983) provide examples of nonspecificity in neuropathological studies.

Response to medication is another important example of nonspecifity. Antipsychotic drugs relieve the florid symptoms of psychosis in a variety of diagnostic categories, thus their therapeutic action cannot be specifically linked to schizophrenia. Furthermore, these drugs are not specific in their mode of action since they affect a wide variety of neurotransmitters and body systems (Lickey & Gordon, 1983).

The idea of nonspecificity can be traced back to the writings of Kraepelin. He compared the manifestations of disease to:

... the different stops of an organ, which are set according to the extent of pathological changes and which now give the expressions of the disorder their own special coloring, regardless of which influences triggered their play. The disorders thus generated are therefore not characteristic of a particular circumstance or perhaps only inasmuch as it is known to prefer this or that stop, or even restrict itself to just one. (Kraepelin, 1920, in Heimann, 1985, p. 83)

The "organ stops" imagined by Kraepelin can be conceptualized as referring to the various systems of the body. In this analogy, the brain systems which utilize the neurotransmitter dopamine can be regarded as some of the principal "stops" in schizophrenia.

The noted variability and nonspecificity associated with this illness has encouraged some researchers to look for other "stops" (i.e., systems) which may also be involved. Broadening the scope of investigation can be described as a "systems approach" because an analysis of the various aspects of the disorder more closely resembles a dynamic process rather than a static disease entity. Systems theory is a multifactorial approach which diminishes the relevance of the construct of causality. Both the ordering of the factors and the extent to which they interact is important (Milsum, 1985). In theoretical terms, causal relations should not be regarded as simple and linear. In practical terms, this means that many researchers and clinicians have not been content to view schizophrenia as simply a disease of dopamine neurotransmission in the brain, but have been flexible and have proceeded systematically.

Our own view of the monoamine hypothesis of schizophrenia is that in schizophrenia there is a secondary alteration in brain monominergic systems. The etiology of this alteration could be either genetic or produced by environmental insults. In this view, the primary problem usually does not reside in the dopaminergic system. Rather, stress may impinge on the vulnerable system, causing increased release of monamines (in particular, dopamine). This production of excess dopamine may be responsible for the hallucinations, delusions, formal thought disorder (marked incoherence, derailment, tangentiality, or illogicality), and bizarre or disorganized behavior of schizophrenia. The defect symptoms of schizophrenia, alogia, affective flattening, anhedonia, asociality, avolition, and apathy may be produced either by direct insult to the brain or through repeated acute episodes. (Wyatt et al., 1988, p. 14)

Research has produced an abundance of data implicating a wide variety of systems including endocrine, immune, neuromuscular, cardiovascular, and autonomic nervous systems (Meltzer, 1976, 1987; Harris, 1988; Nielsen et al., 1988). Autonomic nervous system (ANS) involvement is particularly significant in terms of the amount of research accumulated and the serious implications of ANS dysfunction. A brief review of the ANS literature in schizophrenia can serve as an example of how "peripheral" systems are important to the understanding of schizophrenia.

Autonomic Nervous System Involvement in Schizophrenia

Empirical research has consistently provided evidence of ANS abnormalities among various schizophrenic populations. Generally speaking, this body of research has been interpreted as representing a hyperaroused ANS in schizophrenia (e.g., Depue & Fowles, 1973). Peripheral indicators of autonomic arousal such as heart rate, sweat secretion, and spontaneous skin conductance responses are increased (Albus et al., 1982).

Antipsychotic drugs tend to return schizophrenics' electrodermal activity to the normal range, suggesting that ANS arousal may be associated with the schizophrenic process. This viewpoint is supported by research in which the B-adrenergic antagonist, propranolol, has produced clinical improvement in patients who had marginal response to medication treatment (Yorkston et al., 1977). In these cases, propranolol may have inhibited hyperaroused adrenergic receptors within the sympathetic branch of the ANS.

Traditionally, the ANS has been considered a convenient and nonintrusive index of central nervous system (CNS) functioning. The work of Gruzelier and Venables (1972, 1973) is a good example of this approach. They measured skin conductance orienting response (SCOR) and noted that about 50% of their schizophrenic subjects did not produce any SCORs ("nonresponders") and the other 50% produced SCORs but did not habituate to the orienting response ("responders").

This research was interpreted by Mednick as suggesting a hyperaroused ANS in schizophrenics. Mednick was perhaps the first proponent of significant ANS involvement in the etiology of schizophrenia. His learning-theory approach views schizophrenics as having a genetic predisposition for an ANS which is easily aroused (Mednick, 1958). The social consequences of this inherited tendency is avoidance which results in withdrawal and social isolation. Likewise, arousing cognitions would be supplanted by extraneous thoughts which would lessen autonomic activity. The reinforcing qualities of social withdrawal and irrelevant cognitions with regard to inherited ANS hyperactivity could account for the wide range of symptoms associated with schizophrenia.

Bernstein's research (1987) with "orienting response" (OR) points to "a discrepancy between autonomic and EEG-alpha reactivity in schizophrenia."

My own multichannel studies have shown a lack of concordance between autonomic and EEG response in schizophrenia. On the basis of power spectral analyses, our background
EEG data confirmed the findings of others—reduced alpha
power, slowed dominant alpha frequency, and increased beta
power . . . In phasic response, however, we have found no impairment in the 4-29 Hz bandwidth studied, despite the deficit
in autonomic response. Since our work shows that phasic EEG
response in this bandwidth primarily involves the alpha band,
our studies point essentially to a discrepancy between autonomic and EEG-alpha reactivity in schizophrenia. It would be
important to map any such CNS-ANS dissociations. (Bernstein, 1987, p. 632)

Bernstein's work suggests that central and autonomic OR may be
integrated in normal individuals, but disintegrated in many schizophrenic patients. Since the CNS OR appears to function properly,
Bernstein wonders if the problem could be a "withdrawal of conver-
gent autonomic OR" (p. 632). This notion of incoordination between
the CNS and ANS is an important concept to keep in mind and will
be discussed later (Chapters Two and Five) in the context of the
Cayce readings and the osteopathic literature which implicate abnormal ANS response in schizophrenia.
    Other researchers have noted ANS abnormalities among schizo-
phrenics and concluded that these abnormalities may be significant
to the etiology and course of the disorder. Rubin (1976) views the
ANS abnormalities among schizophrenics as resulting from an imbalance between the sympathetic and parasympathetic branches
of the ANS. He cites evidence of abnormal cardiovascular reactions,
responses of blood sugar to stress, and temperature regulation on
exposure to cold as representing aberrant ANS responses in schizophrenia. He suggests that some of the beneficial effects of medications result from their ability to improve cholinergic and adrenergic
imbalances within the ANS. He recommends that attention be focused on determining which system is out of balance in each patient so that the most effective medication can be prescribed for
each individual. Rubin recognizes the role of environmental stress
in the activation of the ANS and proposes that an ANS imbalance
could become accentuated by stress.
    In a recent study focusing on ANS imbalance in schizophrenia,
Nielsen et al. (1988) found evidence of altered balance in schizophre-

nia. Thirty-eight schizophrenics and eleven healthy controls were tested for heart-rate and blood pressure response in supine and standing positions. Results of the study "indicated a dysfunction in the autonomic nervous system per se and the previous interpretations of attentional orienting responses in schizophrenia is questioned. Medication with neuroleptics seems to partly normalize the autonomic reactivity rather than being the cause of autonomic dysfunction" (p. 193). The authors interpreted their data as indicating an increased activity in the sympathetic division and an increased reactivity in the parasympathetic division among schizophrenics.

Svensson has reviewed the literature and commented that "the new data seem to allow a better understanding of how autonomic vulnerability or visceral dysfunction may precipitate or aggravate mental symptoms and disorder" (1987, p. 1). Svensson considers the interaction between the locus coeruleus (LC) and the ANS to be crucial in the understanding of schizophrenia. He cites evidence that the LC serves as a mediator between the peripheral systems (i.e., ANS and visceral organs) and the brain. In his opinion, the LC also monitors external stimuli and regulates attention. Svensson believes that attention deficit in schizophrenia may result from LC preferential attending to aberrant internal stimuli resulting from ANS and visceral arousal. He cites the well-documented excess of cerebrospinal fluid (CSF) noradrenaline (NA) and plasma NA among schizophrenics as evidence of LC and sympathetic arousal. This arousal is stressful and can lead to a "vicious circle of stress at a primary, physiological level. Thus, a psychomatically induced peripheral vegetative disorder or dysfunction may secondarily, via peripheral signaling into the LC system in brain, add to the mental stress of the individual and in this sense make the accommodation with external, environmental stimuli and demands even more difficult" (p. 4). His emphasis on ANS dysfunction, excessive NA levels in CSF and plasma, and the vicious circle of stress associated with schizophrenia is consonant with other researchers who have considered the role of these factors.

The Role of Stress

Stress has assumed an increasingly important role as a nonspecific factor in clinical and research approaches to schizophrenia. Two categories of stress have been identified as contributing to the exacerbation of psychotic symptoms.

Stressful *life events* have been shown to be associated with schizophrenic episodes (Brown & Birley, 1968; Leff et al., 1983). Since the illness itself is likely to encourage stressful life events, researchers have classified life events into categories based upon their relationship to the illness. The first category is comprised of events resulting directly from the illness, the second category contains events possibly caused by the illness, and the third category is composed of life events that are judged to be independent of the illness. The last two categories provide the data for research and are called "possibly independent" and "independent," respectively. Leff (1985) reviewed this research and concluded that stressful life events, independent of the illness, play a significant role in the occurrence of schizophrenic episodes. Other researchers have failed to replicate these findings but believe that stressful life events may be important in "genetic" or familial schizophrenia (Gruen & Baron, 1984).

Expressed emotion (EE) is a second form of stress which has been researched heavily during the last two decades. Brown et al. (1962) first reported this phenomenon. Schizophrenic men released from psychiatric hospitals in England relapsed more often if they returned home to live with parents or spouses than if they found independent lodging (e.g., hostels, apartments, etc.). Follow-up interviews revealed that the quality of the emotional relationship between patients and relatives was an important factor in the rate of relapse. Analysis of interpersonal styles suggested that critical comments or overinvolvement by relatives was associated with increased risk of relapse. This finding has been replicated in the United States (Vaughn & Leff, 1976) and has been generally accepted as valid (Goldstein, 1987).

An important study of the relationship between stress and psychophysiological measures was conducted by Tarrier et al. (1979). A group of schizophrenic subjects and healthy controls (n = 42) were measured for spontaneous electrodermal activity and diastolic blood pressure while alone with the experimenter and also in the presence of a close relative of the subject. Schizophrenic subjects with relatives previously judged to be high EE showed significantly higher elevations of both psychophysiological measures. Since the experiment was duplicated in home and laboratory settings, the ecological validity of the design is noteworthy. Data gathered in the laboratory differed from home data and did not produce a significant result. The authors conclude that the laboratory is not an appropriate setting for measuring schizophrenic patients' reactivity to their social environment. They view their study as supporting the "concept of arousal used previously to explain the provocation of schizophrenic relapses by these social situations" (p. 315).

From a theoretical perspective, stress has been incorporated into a number of models. Probably the strongest candidate is the diathesis/stress model (Zubin & Spring, 1977). This theory postulates that "each of us is endowed with a degree of vulnerability that under suitable circumstances will express itself in an episode of schizophrenic illness" (p. 109). This vulnerability may result from a variety of factors such as genetics, traumas, specific diseases, perinatal complications, family experiences, adolescent peer interactions, and other life events. Stress is a nonspecific construct which may be produced by maturational changes, ingestion of toxic substances, inadequate nutrition, infection, interpersonal difficulties, etc. The degree to which a factor is stressful to an individual depends upon that individual's ability to moderate the imbalance produced by that factor. This is referred to as coping ability. A person vulnerable to schizophrenia will experience psychotic episodes when stress exceeds the ability to cope. Since the amount of stress will usually vary over time, schizophrenia tends to manifest an episodic course.

Although this model, in its original form, did not specify the exact physiological nature of vulnerability, recent versions of this approach are more specific. Notably, Nuechterlein and Dawson (1984) view information-processing deficits, autonomic reactivity anomalies, and social competence (coping) limitations as the prime vulnerability factors. Stressful life events and prevailing levels of social environment (EE) are regarded as the main stressors. The value of this revised model is its potential for integrating empirical research on cognitive deficits, ANS abnormalities, and social stressors (life events and EE).

In summary, stress can be considered an important nonspecific variable which must be addressed in a therapeutic model. In particular, relapse rates have been closely correlated with stressful environments. Stress-reduction strategies, including stress management education and somatic interventions should be given a high priority in schizophrenia rehabilitation.

Pregnancy and Birth Complications

Numerous studies have investigated the role of pregnancy and birth complications (PBCs) in the etiology of schizophrenia. Mednick and Schulsinger (1965) noted the prevalence of PBCs in a high risk population and these findings have been interpreted as supporting a diathesis/stress model:

> PBCs may trigger genetically predisposed deviations in autonomic responsivity which may in turn be an important component in the development of severe psychopathology. The PBCs seem to damage the homeostatic control of physiological stress response mechanisms . . . These data were used to investigate the plausibility of an old idea in psychiatry known as the diathesis/stress hypothesis . . . Our data seem to confirm this hypothesis, while also extending it in important ways. First, it appears possible that the mechanism actually involved is a biological predisposition which may be indexed by ANS functioning. Second, one type of critical stressor which exacerbates this predisposition may be events pertaining to traumatic birth or difficult pregnancy. (Parnas, Mednick, Moffit & Crapuche, 1981, p. 263)

Whereas Mednick and associates used a longitudinal format which concentrated on high risk populations, other researchers have utilized retrospective approaches which focused on the prevalence of PBCs in adults currently diagnosed as schizophrenic (e.g., Pollack et al., 1966; Woerner et al., 1973; McNeil & Kau, 1978). Lewis and Murray (1987) reviewed this literature and concluded that while obstetric complications (OC) may function within a diathesis/stress model, stronger effects could be expected in patients with low genetic risk. They tested this hypothesis in a sample which included familial schizophrenics (N = 32, history of inpatient psychiatric admission or suicide in a first-degree relative), nonfamilial schizophrenics (N = 136) and neurotic patients (N = 177). OCs were significantly more common among nonfamilial schizophrenics with the frequency of OCs in the familial group being similar to that of neurotic patients. Because OCs have been associated with CT scan abnormalities in psychiatric patients (e.g., Turner et al., 1986; Pearlson et al., 1985), the researchers decided to investigate this relationship in their sample. "Radiologists' reports were abnormal in

42% of those with definite OC compared with 20% of those with an equivocal OC and only 13% of those with no known OC (x2 = 12.5, P < 0.001)." (p. 416) "Our interpretation of the available evidence is that ventricular enlargement is most common in those schizophrenic patients without a family history of psychiatric disorder, thus implying that it is environmental origin." (p. 417)

Another promising area of research related to pregnancy and birth complications is the seasonality of schizophrenic births. In 1929, Tramer reported that more schizophrenics are born during the winter and early spring than during other seasons (Tramer, 1929). Since Tramer's initial report, over 40 articles on schizophrenic birth seasonality have appeared (see review by Bradbury & Miller, 1985) implicating numerous possible etiological factors (e. g., viral infection, malnutrition, vitamin deficiency, prenatal or obstetrical complications, ambient temperatures, etc.). Socioeconomic factors may contribute to this phenomenon since women and newborn infants of lower socioeconomic status are disproportionately exposed to almost all of these etiological factors (Bierman et al., 1965; Pasamanick & Knobloch, 1971; Frederick & Adelstein, 1978; Eisner et al., 1979). Gallagher, McFalls, and Jones (1983) report a prevalence of seasonality effect among black schizophrenics which may also be related to socioeconomic status. For an excellent discussion of this subject (and the possibility that season of birth may be a factor in bipolar disorder—shades of nonspecificity!) see Boyd, Pulver, and Stewart (1986).

The seasonality hypothesis has been contested, most notably by Lewis (1989), on the basis of age-incidence effects. This highly technical criticism suggests that seasonality is an artifact resulting from errors in the design and interpretation of seasonal studies. As the controversy still rages (see *Schizophrenia Bulletin*, 1990, Vol. 16, No. 1), one may regard the seasonality issue as representative of schizophrenic research in general—a field where claim and counterclaim are the norm, and where dramatic breakthroughs are hounded by failures of replication and alternative interpretations. As with so much of this literature, the most sensible approach is to recognize that each argument has something to offer:

> In our view, the primary weaknesses of the Lewis article is that it seems to assume that the age-incidence and seasonality hypotheses are mutually exclusive. The rule that there can be only one winner applies in sports, but not in science. We

have no difficulty believing that age incidence exists and needs to be controlled. But, even after it has been controlled in various ways, the majority of the evidence . . . supports the proposition that winter births are disproportionately frequent in schizophrenic adults. (Watson, 1990, p. 9)

Watson's flexibility is both exemplary and necessary. Anyone wishing to understand schizophrenia must utilize all available resources by remaining open-minded to all reasonable perspectives.

The primary importance of the season of birth literature is its potential for identifying a distinct subgroup within the larger heterogeneous population of persons suffering from schizophrenia. Of course this also applies to other areas of PBC research and has major implications for the prognosis and treatment of these incipient subgroups.

In summary, there is ample evidence suggesting that PBCs are significant etiological factors which may contribute to the heterogeneity of schizophrenia. The possibility that such factors may be gender related will be discussed in the following section.

Gender Differences

The recognition of gender differences in schizophrenia goes back to the writings of Kraepelin (1919) who described dementia praecox as a disorder of young men. Recent investigations have expanded upon this insight in virtually all areas of research. "Schizophrenic men have an earlier age of onset, a poorer premorbid history, more negative symptoms, differential neurocognitive functioning, a poorer course, a poorer response to neuroleptics, a lower family morbidity risk for schizophrenia, and differential structural and functional brain abnormalities . . . " (Goldstein & Tsuang, 1990, p. 179). Schizophrenic women, while experiencing superior premorbid social, sexual, and marital adjustment, often present with more depression, self-destructive behaviors, and troubled interpersonal relationships (McGlashan & Bardenstein, 1990).

In attempting to understand the meaning of these findings, researchers have generally focused on the hormonal differences between the sexes and psychosocial factors which could provide an etiological basis for these consistent clinical effects. From a psychosocial perspective, gender differences may reflect differential patterns of familial interactions (Seeman & Hauser, 1984; Goldstein &

Kreisman, 1988). Males are typically burdened with increased cultural expectations at a period of their lives (18-25 years of age) when onset of symptoms is particularly stressful. Parents may blame themselves for their son's breakdown which further exacerbates the situation. On the other hand, later onset of symptoms in females may occur after the woman has left home and established her own family, thus focusing attribution on nonfamilial factors.

Biological factors, which are thought to be involved in the production of psychopathology and are known to be closely related to gender differences, are currently receiving considerable attention. Chief among these factors is the steroid hormone, estrogen. Schizophrenic women often have psychotic exacerbations when estrogen is low (i.e., during premenstruation, postpartum, and at menopause) and better functioning during pregnancy when estrogen is relatively high (Wyatt et al., 1988). Longitudinal studies of medication levels in male and female patients has led Seeman (1983) to suggest that estrogen acts as a natural neuroleptic.

In contrast, males may be disadvantaged by hormonal patterns (testosterone secretion) which produce less mature brains at birth and a greater vulnerability to insult (Seeman & Lang, 1990). This increased vulnerability of males may be enhanced by developmental processes: " . . . puberty, a time of sudden, dramatic hormonal and neurochemical change, is a risk period for the development of schizophrenia which, in females, is made safer by the protective effects of estrogens" (Seeman & Lang, 1990, p. 188).

Other biological anomalies have been associated with gender differences in schizophrenia including regional cerebral blood flow (Gur & Gur, 1990), brain event-related potentials (Josiassen et al., 1990), MRI brain scans (Nasralleh et al., 1990), and brain morphology (Lewine et al., 1990). Kopala and Clark (1990) provide an intriguing discussion of olfactory agnosia in schizophrenia, a gender-related phenomenon: "These findings indicate that the deficit in olfactory identification is confined to male patients with schizophrenia . . . Our own findings of an olfactory agnosia in male patients with schizophrenia, as well as the literature cited, suggest that there may be an abnormality in the sex hormone system in a subsample of males with schizophrenia" (pp. 257 & 259).

The scope and persistency of gender differences in schizophrenia have led some researchers to postulate the existence of etiological subtypes based on gender: " . . . men are at higher risk for a subtype of schizophrenia in which nonfamilial factors are significant" (Goldstein et al., 1990, p. 272). This subtype is apparently particularly vulnerable to environmental insults (e. g., PBCs) and may represent the subtype described by Kraepelin (i.e., dementia praecox as an illness affecting young men). Goldstein et al. caution against simplistic formulations, however: "Rather, our results suggest that schizophrenic men and women may have similar subtypes; however, the *prevalence* of the subtypes among men and women significantly differ" (p. 272).

Somatic Factors Associated with Schizophrenia

Research suggests that persons diagnosed as schizophrenic may be at increased risk for breast cancer and cardiovascular disease while at reduced risk for developing rheumatoid arthritis, osteoarthritis, and lung cancer (Mohamed et al., 1982; Harris, 1988). Whether these patterns of disease are related to organic factors associated with schizophrenia or are the result of lifestyle choices is unclear.

Kidney dysfunction has been proposed as an etiological factor in schizophrenia and hemodialysis suggested as a useful treatment. At least eighteen studies have been conducted since Thoelen et al. (1960) reported significant improvement in 3 of 5 patients who underwent hemodialysis. Wagemaker and Cade (1978, 1979) reported the highest improvement rates (16 of 25) with Scheiber et al. (1983) reporting improvement in 6 of 11 patients.

These reports of clinical efficacy have been countered by several double-blind studies which failed to support hemodialysis as an effective treatment for schizophrenia (see van Kammen et al. (1983) for a review of these studies). The study by van Kammen et al. provides a glimpse into the problematic nature of schizophrenic research. Only 8 of the original 13 patients recruited for the study were able to complete the series of treatments. The selection process was biased toward patients with good premorbid functioning (so as to compare to the Wagemaker and Cade study) and all patients were physically healthy (on the whole, schizophrenics tend to have poorer overall health than the general population). The results of the study are questionable because an inappropriate statistic was used to evaluate the data (a parametric statistic [paired t test] with ordinal level data [rating scale]). The limited population (N = 8) was perhaps the greatest handicap for this study and was noted by the researchers:

The number of patients who completed this double-blind

study of dialysis is small. In a homogeneous disorder with a known pathophysiology, failure to observe response in eight patients is a significant finding; schizophrenia is considered to be a heterogeneous disorder. According to Wagemaker and Cade, a response rate of 68% (16 of 25), which would suggest that a type II statistical error would be quite low, would have been expected even in a small sample. (van Kammen et al., 1983, pp. 315-316)

This study is discussed in more detail to provide a glimpse into the difficulties of doing research in this area. Controlled studies are incredibly difficult to do because of ethical issues and logistical problems inherent in the schizophrenic process. Hence, there are no perfect studies from which to draw categorical conclusions. Whether kidney dysfunction is a factor in schizophrenia is difficult to say. Most likely, given the variability of the disorder, there is a small subgroup of schizophrenics for whom uremia poses a significant complication to a wider systemic dysfunction.

Significant numbers of schizophrenics are polydipsic, which means they have abnormally excessive fluid intake. This condition cannot be totally explained as a side effect of antipsychotic medication because it was first noticed in 1933 by Hoskins and Sleeper before the advent of antipsychotic medications. Polydipsia can lead to hyponatremia (water intoxication) in extreme cases and produce confusion, seizures, coma, and eventually death. Although the actual number of hypnotremic schizophrenic patients is small, there is some evidence that individuals in this subgroup have poor response to neuroleptics and show ventricular enlargement on CT scans (Wyatt, 1988).

In a discussion of the possible role of cholinergic hyperactivity in schizophrenia, Tandon and Greden (1989) point out the range of somatic symptoms associated with schizophrenia:

> While schizophrenia always has been considered to have predominantly psychiatric symptoms, a wide variety of somatic manifestations has been reported, particularly in the older literature. Some of the bodily symptoms of schizophrenia described by Kraepelin include diminished sensitivity to pain, increased secretion of saliva with low-normal specific gravity (suggestive of cholinergic origin), low body temperature with reduced diurnal fluctuations, polydipsia, vasomotor

changes, increased muscle irritability with a variety of abnormal movements, sluggish pupillary reflexes, and an absence of the normal pupillary dilatation in response to psychological stimuli and pain. While analgesia, polydipsia and "water intoxication," pupillary abnormalities suggestive of excessive central parasympathetic outflow, and assorted motor disorders continue to be described in schizophrenia, their prevalence, and the presence and prevalence of other bodily symptoms enumerated by Kraepelin, have not been studied ... (Tandon & Greden, 1989, p. 747)

It should be noted that these somatic symptoms were noted before the advent of antipsychotic drugs. While the meaning of such extensive somatic symptoms remains unclear and may be related to an underlying brain abnormality in schizophrenia, one cannot dismiss the possibility that somatic symptoms may be produced by somatic dysfunctions associated with the disorder. The relevance of this point will become increasingly evident in subsequent chapters.

Summary

The literature on schizophrenia can be summarized as follows:

1. Schizophrenia can best be considered as a complex disorder involving a variety of important systems (biological, psychological, and sociological).

2. Variability and nonspecificity associated with schizophrenia suggest that it is a group of related illnesses with various etiologies rather than a single disease entity. Heterogeneity is the watchword in this literature, with nonspecificity manifesting most often as an overlap with the mood disorders.

3. Although brain systems utilizing the neurotransmitter dopamine are probably involved in most cases, there also appears to be significant involvement of other neurotransmitters and peripheral systems (most notably ANS and endocrine). With this in mind, neurotransmitter dysfunction can be regarded as an effect produced by a variety of potential etiological factors (hence the intrinsic heterogeneity of schizophrenia).

4. There is a strong genetic component associated with schizophrenia but this factor is best considered as hereditary vulnerability rather than a sufficient condition per se (i.e., the diathesis/stress model).

5. Social environment plays an important role, particularly in terms of stress and the probability of relapse.

6. Other environmental factors (particularly those related to pregnancy and birth complications) are significant contributors to the incidence of schizophrenia.

7. Brain degeneration probably occurs in some persons suffering from schizophrenia, particularly among persons exhibiting a chronic course.

8. Gender differences are important factors in the schizophrenic process and may be prime sources of heterogeneity.

9. Although antipsychotic medications produce extensive side effects resulting in numerous somatic symptoms, evidence accrued before the introduction of these drugs suggests that there are inherent somatic symptoms associated with schizophrenia.

10. A multidisciplinary, "biopsychosocial" approach (integrating somatic, psychosocial, and psychoeducational interventions) provides the most successful strategy currently available for the treatment of schizophrenia.

In the chapters which follow, it will become evident that the current literature on schizophrenia is congruent with the perspective developed by Edgar Cayce earlier in this century through his psychic readings. In many respects, the "holistic" approach advocated by Cayce anticipated the "biopsychosocial" models being utilized today.

2

Cayce's Perspective

Holism

IN ANALYZING BODY, mind, soul, all phases of an entity's experience must be taken into consideration. In analyzing the mind and its reactions, oft individuals who would psychoanalyze or who would interpret the reactions that individual entities take, leave out those premises of soul, mind, body. (4083-1)

This excerpt from the Edgar Cayce readings exemplifies the holistic philosophy expounded in the readings and provides the basis for a comprehensive approach to the treatment of schizophrenia. Reading 4083-1 was addressed to an individual from a generation heavily influenced by the ideas of Freud (the reading was given in 1944). However, its message is still relevant, particularly to contemporary mental health professionals and researchers mesmerized by the biochemistry of the brain.

While it is easy to make glib pronouncements about the relevance of holism and the need for a broader perspective, defining specifically what holism entails is not so simple. The holistic perspective utilizes a triune model (body, mind, and spirit) to describe the complex interactions which underlie the phenomenal experience of daily life. This experience can go painfully wrong in certain instances—most notably, in cases of major mental illness. The uniqueness of the Cayce readings, in this respect, lies in the depth and specificity with which the readings elaborate the interface of the triune aspects of selfhood.

As will be the format throughout this book, ample excerpts from the Cayce readings will be quoted in this chapter to allow readers the opportunity to develop their own interpretations. Here are several excerpts which are particularly explicit in describing the interface of mind, body, and spirit. These selections are useful because they address several issues relevant to a discussion of schizophrenia.

2114-1   F. 30   2/24/40
. . . it is well to consider the entity as a whole . . . the entity finds itself made up, as it were, of body, mind and soul . . . There are centers in the physical body through which all phases of the entity's being coordinate with one another; as in the physical functioning there are the pulsations, the heart beat, the lungs, the liver, and all the organs of the body. They each have a function to perform. They each are dependent upon the other, yet they function according to those directions of the mental self—or the nervous systems.

Yet, while the brain and the cords through which the nerves function are the channels, these are not the mental consciousness; though it is through the nerve plasm that the nervous systems carry impulses to the various forces of the system . . .

These naturally, in their various phases, find centers in some portion of the physical or anatomical system through which greater expression is given than in others.

263-13   F. 29   12/16/40
Let it be understood as to how each phase of consciousness or experience affects the other; that is, the associations or connections between the spiritual and the mental body, the spiritual and the physical body, and between the mental and the physical and mental and spiritual . . .

Then, there are centers, areas, conditions in which there

evidently must be that contact between the physical, the mental and the spiritual.

The spiritual contact is through the glandular forces of creative energies . . . Hence we find these become subject not only to the intent and purpose of the individual entity or soul upon entrance, but are constantly under the influences of all the centers of the mind and the body through which the impulses pass in finding a means or manner of expression in the mental or brain self . . .

Thus we find the connection, the association of the spiritual being with the mental self, at those centers from which the reflexes react to all of the organs, all of the emotions, all of the activities of a physical body.

826-11   M. 36   1/11/38

Thy brain is not thy mind, it is that which is used by thy mind!

1468-5   F. 48   8/5/38

As is understood by the body, there is the physical, the mental, the spiritual. All are one, but with their attributes have their activity through the one or the individual entity or body.

The spiritual arises from the centers in the . . . glandular forces that are as hidden energies, or the very nature of the creative or reproductive forces.

There are the abilities of each center, each gland, each atom to reproduce itself within the body—which is the very nature of glandular reaction.

566-7   F. 6   12/12/36

All portions of the nervous system of the physical body, of the physical functioning, are affected by those activities of secretions through glandular forces of the body.

These excerpts contain several major themes which constitute the foundation of the Cayce perspective on mental health:

1)   Mind, body, and spirit interface at definite centers within the physical anatomy.

2)   The mind (or "mental consciousness") is not synonymous with the brain. The mind "uses" the brain and the "cords through

which the nerves function." Thus, the mind/body interface is maintained through the functioning of the nervous systems.

3)   The spiritual interface with the body is maintained through the glands which reflect the nature of the "Creative Force" or God. The essence of glandular functioning is creative (re-creative, as in rebuilding the body and procreative, as in reproduction of the species).

4)   In order to function normally, the nervous systems require a constant supply of numerous chemical substances (e.g., neurotransmitters, "nerve plasm," etc.).

5)   Glandular functioning provides the raw materials essential for neurotransmission and trophic processes within nerve cells.

6)   While it may be helpful at times to think of mind, body, and spirit as if they were separate aspects of the self, one must keep in mind that this is a distortion of the basic wholeness of the entity (i.e., "All are one"). The spirit/mind/body interface is so inherent that dysfunction in one aspect usually affects the whole being. Therefore, holism recognizes this dynamic interaction as expressed through multiple etiological factors, complex pathophysiological processes, diverse symptomatology, and nonspecific treatment modalities.

7)   Since spirit, mind, and body interface within the anatomical structure, somatic dysfunction (produced by such diverse factors as heredity, environmental insult, and systemic imbalances, etc.) may disrupt this interconnection resulting in the symptomology commonly referred to as schizophrenia.

Point 7 is crucial to the thesis of this book and requires further elaboration. Many of the "centers" where mind, spirit, and body interface are outside the cranial encasement and quite vulnerable to insult. In general terms, the autonomic nervous system (ANS) and endocrine glands can be considered as the primary interfaces which are often involved in schizophrenia. In most of the cases of psychosis which Edgar Cayce diagnosed as dementia praecox (the diagnostic precursor of schizophrenia), these two systems were significantly involved and interacted with the central nervous system (CNS) to produce mental symptoms.

Neurotransmission in Schizophrenia

While a multitude of factors have been implicated in the etiology of schizophrenia, contemporary research has focused on faulty neurotransmission in the brain. The "dopamine hypothesis" is the leading contender in this field, although other neurotransmitters are also very likely involved (see discussion in Chapter One). Consequently, any model addressing the treatment of schizophrenia must address the reality of dysfunctional neurotransmission in the brain. On this point the Cayce readings are quite clear—schizophrenia (or as the readings preferred, dementia praecox) invariably involves disturbed brain biochemistry which is directly linked to psychotic symptomology.

The readings were given during an era in which knowledge about the biochemistry of the nervous systems was extremely vague (e.g., none of the major neurotransmitters had been identified). Considering the general ignorance of that period, the Cayce readings were quite lucid in their descriptions of the neuropathology of psychosis. The main difference between Cayce's perspective and contemporary models (e.g., the "dopamine hypothesis") is the context of abnormal neurotransmission. Modern psychiatry appears content to focus on the brain as *the* center of pathology, whereas the readings view brain biochemistry as a single aspect (albeit an essential one) of a larger spectrum which constitutes the whole self. Even if one rejects the readings' contention that the whole self involves nonphysical aspects (i.e., mind and body), one must concede that brain neurotransmission does not exist in isolation. It is extremely dependent upon and affected by the rest of the body. The readings note brain dysfunction in virtually every case of schizophrenia. Just as consistently, however, the readings cite significant somatic dysfunction (such as spinal injury) or glandular disturbances which are regarded as the primary etiological factors. In other words, faulty brain neurotransmission is considered to be more of an effect, rather than a cause. As an example, a fairly common etiological pattern cited in the readings is: hereditary vulnerability + somatic dysfunction → brain dysfunction → psychotic symptoms. The high incidence of somatic complaints and physical abnormalities documented in schizophrenia (see Chapter One) could be considered as important clues to the systemic processes which precede and maintain eventual brain dysfunction.

There are inherent treatment implications in such a perspective. Instead of focusing on the brain, many of the interventions suggested in the readings are directed toward the peripheral systems— most often the spinal column, emunctory system, glands, and assimilative system. In keeping with a holistic emphasis, the readings also recommended treatments aimed at the mental and spiritual dimensions—particularly at the physical interfaces of body-mind-spirit. The recognition that these interfaces necessarily function through biochemical processes is assumed (remember that mind and spirit manifest through "nerve plasm" and glandular secretions). The difference between Cayce's approach and modern psychiatry is that the readings prefer to allow the body to correct its own biochemical dysfunctions. Hence, the interventions are directed at restoring the body's innate ability to rebuild and maintain itself. In contrast, psychiatry has generally adopted the strategy of focusing on brain pathology and intervening with powerful neuroleptics which suppress positive symptoms, presumably by directly altering brain chemistry.

The readings cite several patterns of abnormal neurotransmission in schizophrenia. A brief excerpt from reading 386-1 provides an example of one pattern. Here is a glimpse into the readings' view of the biochemistry of schizophrenia:

> 386-1   F. 20   8/9/33
> This, then, is the difference between an unbalanced condition in a mental reaction [nervous breakdown] and that of dementia—which destroys the reaction in the plasm of the nerve as fixed from the blood supply itself; though, unless there are some material changes, this may become the condition that will ensue.

Miss [386] was experiencing a nervous breakdown which the readings warned could lead to dementia praecox. She was experiencing recurrent auditory hallucinations and certain deficit symptoms associated with schizophrenia (see Chapter Three for a case study summary of her condition). Note the progressive nature of the disorder ("this may become the condition [dementia praecox] that will ensue"). She was at about the age (20) when schizophrenic psychosis commonly occurs.

Also of interest is the biochemical dysfunction which was associated with chronic schizophrenia ("dementia—which destroys the reaction in the plasm of the nerve"). Finally, notice that the nerve plasm is "fixed from the blood supply itself," a recognition that the nervous system (and particularly the brain) does not exist in self-sufficient isolation.

Some Definitions

To set the stage for a further consideration of Cayce's perspective, a couple of definitions are in order. The readings frequently referred to the ANS as the "sympathetic nervous system," focusing on the interconnectedness which is the hallmark of that system (i. e., body systems are interrelated, they act in sympathy with each other with the ANS orchestrating these dynamic interactions). This usage is in keeping with Cayce's tendency to utilize the medical language of his day. He also used other terms for the ANS: "vegetative nervous system" was a common synonym for the ANS during Cayce's era and, although infrequently used today, has been medically appropriate for most of this century (*Taber's Cyclopedic Medical Dictionary*, 1970). "Vegetative" is also particularly descriptive of the role of the parasympathetic branch of the ANS. Other terms which the readings occasionally used in conjunction with the "sympathetic system" were "impulse system," "motivative system," and "imaginative system." The association of impulse and motivation with sympathetic functioning is appropriate given its role in the "fight or flight" reaction. Cayce's understanding of this function included the psychological aspects of motivation, an important consideration in the treatment of a disorder such as schizophrenia (where lack of motivation, especially regarding compliance to treatment, is a major concern). An appreciation of this aspect of ANS functioning also makes Cayce's frequent suggestions for therapies designed to normalize ANS activity more comprehensible (e.g., spinal massage, osteopathy, electrotherapy along the spine, etc.).

The use of the term "imaginative system" refers to Cayce's association of the unconscious mind with the ANS (and the conscious mind with the CNS, which he usually called the "cerebrospinal system"). One can easily grasp the sense of the "imaginative system" by observing the effect of visualizing diverse scenarios and monitoring autonomic functioning (e.g., scenes involving pleasure, pain, fright, etc.). Obviously, imagination is closely linked with ANS response.

Incoordination between the ANS and CNS can thus be regarded as a dissociation of conscious and unconscious processes (readers may wish to review the discussion of ANS/CNS incoordination in Chapter One). The situation becomes more complex when one considers that this interface has transpersonal significance. The readings occasionally referred to the sympathetic nervous system as the nervous system of the soul. This relates directly to the previous reference to the existence within the physical body of definite points of interface with mental and spiritual dimensions. Thus, somatic dysfunction (especially spinal injury) was often cited in the readings as leading to the dissociation of the physical, mental, and spiritual bodies. Reading 4125-5 provides a good description of ANS/CNS interactions in a case of psychopathology:

4125-5   F. Adult 12/22/32
For the moment, let's understand what the sympathetic and the cerebrospinal nervous system are within the human body!

In the cerebrospinal centers, here we have the brain, the spinal cord—which enters through all the cerebrospinal system, passing through each vertebra, and the impingements on same often cause much of the distress to the body-physical. This may be represented as the physical organism.

There is lying along each side of the cerebrospinal system a series, or on either side a cord known as the sympathetic nervous system. Not within the structural portions, but connecting with same at definite points; though in many points connecting with same but at definite points.

The activities of these:

The cerebrospinal, the nerve cord itself, acts for the physical attributes of the body through the impulses. The sympathetic is the greater impulsive system.

Now, materially, very little is set up—other than metaphysics—as to what is the functioning proper of the sympathetic system; but, as has been with this body, by destroying within the imaginative system much that had been builded morally and spiritually within self, became such a shock to the whole of the physical body as to produce—from the sympathetic system into the moral fibre of the cerebrospinal system—those conditions that became as has been experienced by the body. Gradually, disassociation of ideas, disassociation of activities became active within the body, so that the body was racked by torments from without and from within; for there came no response either from the definite activity of the cerebrospinal or the sympathetic system, and those centers that suffered were those that have been outlined as the ones needing—even yet—those stimuli occasionally [osteopathic adjustments] that there may be kept coordination in the system.

Now, these have been released—these pressures, and there

is gradually being created by the activities of the low electrical form [electrotherapy] that making for better associations and connections in the system; there is being gradually added by the activities of the thoughts of the body, by the activities in the glands that work both with the sympathetic and cerebrospinal system, that which makes for better coordinating conditions.

Know that the moral fibre, that the spiritual activities of the system, are being set and attuned . . .

From this discussion, one may catch a glimpse of the expansiveness of the readings and the interconnectedness and interdependence of the body's systems. This is especially true of the ANS and endocrine systems, which were not considered to be merely "handmaidens" of the CNS, but were portrayed as crucial interfaces with transpersonal dimensions.

One final distinction is necessary to understand the meaning of schizophrenia as it is used in the chapters which follow and, more generally, its relationship to the Cayce readings. Although Edgar Cayce didn't use the term schizophrenia, many of the persons who came to him suffering from the symptoms of psychosis carried that diagnosis. Cayce's career as psychic diagnostician spanned almost four decades. For much of that time the term dementia praecox was the accepted diagnostic label for persons exhibiting psychotic behaviors with chronic course. Therefore, it is understandable that he used the term dementia praecox instead of schizophrenia. It is also interesting that he didn't use the diagnosis of dementia praecox indiscriminately for all cases of psychosis but reserved it exclusively for those cases which had brain degeneration. He described the process in detail and stated that there was not a single etiology involved. The multiple causes of dementia praecox are documented in Chapters Three and Seven, and descriptions of the process are included in Appendix C.

Cayce's reluctance to use the term schizophrenia may have involved more than diagnostic obsolescence. Dementia praecox was a useful diagnostic category because it affirmed organic degeneration and deteriorating course.

These were clinical and pathological realities which the readings graphically described. On the other hand, schizophrenia (Bleuler, 1911) was conceptualized as a psychological construct inferring splitting of the personality (i.e., splitting of cognition and affect)—a description which, from the readings' perspective, apparently did not fit the etiology or course of the syndrome. Such a vague and insubstantial concept may have been deemed unsuitable for the condition of those seeking Cayce's help. In the single case where Cayce diagnosed "split personality" (case [1969]), the etiology involved karmic influences (reincarnational patterns) and discarnate possession—factors not congruent with Bleuler's concept of schizophrenia.

For better or worse, schizophrenia is the only term in current use which addresses the chronic psychosis previously labeled dementia praecox. The fact that it includes syndromes of less severity (less "organicity") is the source of variability in the field and is unavoidable at this point. Because virtually all the clinical and research literature has adopted the term schizophrenia, it would be impossible to consider the subject in other terms. One has trouble doing a computer search in this area without using schizophrenia as a descriptor or identifier. How could one actually compare studies or discuss findings in terms other than by which they are defined and conceptualized? Fortunately, the psychiatric establishment has recognized the need to refocus the concept and has proceeded to narrow the definition of schizophrenia. Until these psychoses are redefined (or renamed) and variability is resolved, schizophrenia will apparently have to suffice as the term of choice. Throughout this book it will be given preference, with the designation dementia praecox reserved for those instances where continuity of usage is required to preserve the context of the discussion. In other words, the term schizophrenia can be viewed as including the category of dementia praecox in much the same manner as Crow's Type II designation is conceptualized as a subgroup of schizophrenia.

A Systems Approach

Cayce's approach to schizophrenia can be regarded as a "systems" approach. A typical physical reading would often begin with some general remarks about the condition, perhaps indicating etiological factors or a prognosis. The reading would then usually focus on each of the major systems of the body and point out pathology in each area (i.e., circulatory system, nervous system, and the organs). Treatment suggestions and a brief question-and-answer period would often conclude each reading. The initial reading for each person would typically be more comprehensive, while periodic "check readings" would deal with specific treatment issues. It might be helpful to examine an extended excerpt from a reading to get a sense of how Cayce viewed the body's systems and their interactions.

2200-1   M. Adult   1/20/31
   Yes, we have the body here—[2200]. Now, we find there are abnormal conditions with this body. These, as we find, have to do with the nervous forces of the body and the effect that is created in the system from these pressures existent in the body, as well as we find disorders that are produced by applications [medications] that have been made for the disorders.
   These, then, are conditions as we find them with this body, [2200], we are speaking of, present in this room:
   IN THE BLOOD SUPPLY—This we find shows the effect of sedimentary conditions that have been administered for the body, these acting as an effect of bromides in the system, producing the inability of the blood supply to give that full virile force necessary in the full replenishing of the system. This rather the effect of applications, than the conditions that cause the disorder; yet these impoverishments must eventually, unless corrected, bring disorders in the physical functioning that will be hard to cope with, or will be beyond repair; for the deterioration must eventually set in by continued impoverishments.
   IN THE NERVOUS SYSTEMS THEMSELVES do we find the greater disorder or distress. In times back we find was an accident to the body that produces a lesion in the coccyx. Here we find a seat or a cause which has been heretofore overlooked. While lesions have resulted from same in the lower lumbar, in the lower dorsal, and with the combined conditions that have been applied, we find sympathetic lesions in the whole of the cervical region. This produces, through these pressures, those spasmodic conditions to the reaction between the sympathetic and the cerebrospinal system—which has been termed a mental disorder. The reaction is not mental, but a physical—that acts to, or on, the mental—so that the reflexes that come through the sympathetic system are those that prevent a normal impulse from their reaction, causing that pressure, that condition in the lower end of brain proper that makes for the tendency of the body to move, to react in a wondering manner, to make as for responses of those forces in self of first con-

demnation in self, then as of that as to remove those conditions from self. These come through, then as repressions in first the sympathetic nerve system, from the lower lumbar plexus to the sacrals and coccyx, then to those activities in the glands themselves that secrete for the functioning through the pineal, and making for an engorgement and an inactivity or an ungoverning of the supply of impulse, as well as blood supply to the brain itself proper. Not dementia praecox, nor even softening of [nerve] tissue. Unless these conditions are changed in the impulses to the nerve system this deterioration must eventually set in.

IN THE FUNCTIONING OF THE ORGANS THEMSELVES from these variations, we find these are functioning—under the condition—near normal, as do the reflexes at times from the whole system—but to remove or to change the vibratory forces of the body we will find that those pressures should be relieved that exist in the coccyx, the lumbar, the sacral, and coordinating those of the cervical forces that make for proper impulses through the brain forces. This may be done through the removal of the pressure in an osteopathic-adjustment manner, provided those properties are carried in system that will replenish for the nerve energy itself, that will work with and not against a resuscitating or rejuvenating of the system [as many drugs do]. These medicinal properties would be better in the Mayblossom Bitters, that act directly with the nerve system itself. The dosage of this, as we find, would be from three to four teaspoonsful each day.

Each evening we would also, as the body rests, use those vibrations that come from the Radio-Active Appliance, applying it to the base of the brain first, then to the ankle, in each anode—see? Apply the one first to the 1st and 2nd cervical, then to the ankle. First to the right, then to the left. This we would give for thirty minutes each evening.

The manipulations should be given at least three times each week, and one of these an adjustment. As for the diet, keep away from those that are hard of digestion. Those foods that are nearer or more of the nerve building.

Do that, and we will bring—in three to six months—a near normal body.

Keep as much sunshine as possible, and companionship of a nature that makes for the uplifting and brighter side, creating within that mental impression of the whole replenishing and building body that which lives within, that may aid self most . . .

This excerpt illustrates the holistic approach of the readings and includes many of the themes which will be expanded upon throughout this book:

1) Most "mental" illness involves a strong physical dimension.

2) It is essential to think about how systems function and interface with each other.

3) The drugs used to treat mental illness often have deleterious side effects.

4) Brain degeneration (e.g., dementia praecox) can result from chronic impoverishment of the brain.

5) Injury to the spine can produce "lesions" causing other somatic systems to react "sympathetically."

6) Incoordination between the cerebrospinal and autonomic (sympathetic) systems can produce "mental" symptoms.

7) Osteopathic treatments can be useful in treating "mental illness."

8) When medicinal prescriptions are required, medications utilizing "natural" ingredients are preferred.

9) Electrotherapy (in this case the Radio-Active Appliance) can be useful for balancing the body's systems.

10) Diet is an important consideration in the treatment of mental illness.

11) Outdoor activities in the sunshine and fresh air have great therapeutic value.

12) Supportive/uplifting companionship is important for maintaining a therapeutic milieu.

13) Cognitive therapies which produce constructive mental processes are essential (e.g., suggestive therapeutics which utilize the principle "mind is the builder").

14) Pathology affecting the pineal gland is frequently associated with psychotic symptoms.

15) In most cases, a positive prognosis can be expected if the suggestions are carried out patiently and persistently.

Etiological Factors

The Cayce readings are in agreement with the current literature regarding etiological variability in schizophrenia. Each etiological factor will be discussed at length in later chapters. The present discussion will be brief and will merely serve as an introduction to the subject.

Heredity

Several readings cite heredity as an important etiological factor (e.g., 5690, 282, 300, 4179, 4285, etc.). The readings make a distinction between "hereditary innate" and "hereditary tendencies":

5690-1   M. 27   3/6/31
There are physical defects in the cerebrospinal nerve system. There are also the lacking of elements in the physical forces, as produced by conditions—some a lacking of elements in the physical forces, as produced by conditions—some a tendency in innate influences; not as wholly hereditary innate, as much as hereditary tendencies. Then, with the physical defects, these in their combination bring about that as has been called dementia praecox. This an inability of coordination between sympathetic, cerebrospinal, and the general physical body.

Reading 5690-1 provides an excellent example of "diathesis/stress" etiology. The genetic factor was only a tendency and required an environmental stressor (spinal injury) to produce dementia praecox. Note that impoverishment of the brain was involved in the degenerative process.

Reading 4179-1 apparently provides an example of an "innate" genetic factor since no stressor was noted. The reading cites:

179-1   F. Adult   7/11/22
... hereditary forces both through the individual and that which has been moved over from time past . . . through the organs of gestation or through the genetory organs . . . Through this has been brought the reaction which is acting on the nerve forces through the solar plexus center through organs affecting the predisposition as given by generation by spiritual forces as brought from one world to another . . .

This excerpt relates two important points which Cayce often associated with hereditary factors: (1) heredity provides an ideal vehicle for the transference of karmic patterns from one lifetime to another ("moved over from time past" and "forces as brought from one world to another") and (2) these hereditary patterns are often relayed through the glands, which the readings stated were the spiritual contacts within the body. Because the readings often indicate a close relationship between heredity and karma, a brief discussion of karma might prove helpful.

Karma

The Cayce readings share certain concepts with the Eastern religious traditions. Some of the persons receiving readings were told that their problems were "karmic" in nature. Cayce used the term karma to mean "cause and effect" on a cosmic scale. Since karmic problems were often hereditary in nature, they were usually associated with serious and abiding consequences. A few excerpts will hopefully convey the gist of what Cayce meant by the term. A further explanation can be found in Appendix D.

852-12   F. 18   11/15/35
Environs and hereditary influences are much deeper than that which is ordinarily conceded in the psychology of the present day.
For the environs and the hereditary influences are spiritual as well as physical, and are physical because of the spiritual application of the abilities of the entity in relationship to spiritual development.
For the purpose of each soul's experience in the earth is to become one with the Creative Forces that manifest in human experience, if [the soul] will apply [this] in its relationships to its fellow man.
Hence what one is today is because of what one (the individual soul) has done about that the soul knows of the Creative Force or God in its experience, in whatever environ or consciousness it—the soul—may manifest.

3504-1   M. 29   12/12/43
Sources of these are prenatal conditions as well as karmic. These, of course, may be rejected by many. Yet those who re-

ject same do not supply better reasons, do they?

5044-1   M. 9   5/5/44
In interpreting the physical and mental disturbances here, the sources and basis for these are in the karmic conditions of this body. To those responsible for this body: Rather than feeling it is a calamity, know that it is an opportunity to meet not only those things in self, but to help this individual entity or soul in search for its oneness with the Creative Forces, or God.

Pregnancy and Birth Complications

Pregnancy and birth complications (PBCs) were noted in several cases which were later presented as schizophrenia. [4342] and [5014] were said to have suffered lower spinal injury (breech birth). [3997] apparently suffered PBCs "during inception and in the presentation at birth" (exact nature of the trauma unspecified). Occasionally, the readings would refer to problems during gestation (e.g., [3075]) or "prenatal" conditions. Prenatal probably referred to heredity in most cases, however the etiology of case [271] was said to involve "pressures and incoordinations that are shown from prenatal conditions," an expression consistent with PBC. See Chapter Three for an elaboration of these cases.

Childbirth

The birthing process may be a source of etiological vulnerability for mother as well as baby. Case [2744] has a complex etiology which resembles the diathesis/stress model. This woman was said to have a "prenatal" (hereditary?) tendency for poor eliminations (autointoxication) which manifested as skin blemishes at age 25. Two readings were given for this condition, but caution was noted regarding a more serious condition:

2744-1   F. 25   4/4/28
. . . there are those conditions more of which the body should be warned, and precautions should be taken in time concerning conditions apparent for the body [skin blemishes], these are more of the secondary nature . . . these are not the greater conditions to be warned against . . . the age and the conditions are at that point where corrections need to be made

. . . for these other existent conditions will only build that which would bring detrimental effects to the body [dementia praecox].

Reading 2744-1 suggested osteopathic treatments "for the correction of condition in pelvis region." At the time of the first two readings, the woman was not suffering from mental illness and had no history of such problems. Fourteen years later (age 39) she was in a mental institution suffering from "insanity." A reading was given which described her condition:

2744-3 F. 39   5/8/42
. . . there were and are pressures that exist from those happenings at the time of childbirth. This pressure upon the centers—the end of the spine and in the lumbar and sacralileum axis—has produced those tendencies for deterioration of nerve reflexes . . . unless there is the ability to relieve this pressure soon, there may be the necessity to give the body the vibratory metals . . . to prevent softening or deterioration to brain cells [dementia praecox]. It is NOT a condition of brain tumors, though some of these MAY arise unless there is an even circulation of nerve impulse and blood supply builded in the body . . . There should be the consideration of the first information we gave, for the corrections were never made properly.

The etiological pattern of lower spinal injury producing brain degeneration (usually several years after the insult) is a common theme in the readings and will be discussed at length in other sections. Case [3996] had a similar etiology:

3996-1 F. Adult   12/26/24
In the pelvic organs we find the physical condition causing distress on the body. This produced in times back, at the time when there was the condition of pregnancy, and the pressures in the form of a lesion to the pituitary or pineal glands, and reacting through pituitary glands in brain centers.

This woman was in a state hospital at the time of the reading suffering from "hallucinations" and "delusions of a persecutory nature." She would probably meet current criteria for paranoid schizophrenia (her clinical presentation also resembled descriptions commonly observed for women with her age of onset and good premorbid adjustment; see gender differences in Chapter One). See cases [1475] and [1773] for further descriptions of psychosis resulting from childbirth complications.

Stress

The Cayce readings recognized the role of stress in the etiology and course of schizophrenia. Several cases (e. g., [387], [2359], [4097], [4186], [5228]) were cited as developing from "overworry," mental and physical exhaustion, and environmental stress. In certain cases, uremic poisoning and other forms of toxemia resulted from these stressors and were important factors in the progress of the illness. In such cases, there was usually widespread systemic dysfunction which led to dementia praecox. Case [4097] represents a dramatic example of the role of stress:

> 4097-1 M. Adult 9/16/22
> . . . we find the action of the brain itself to be that of dementia praecox—that is, the softening of the tissue used to present the reaction of impressions to the centers as distributed from the action of the sensory system in itself . . . This, as we find, has been produced by the breaking of cell force itself in the blood supply, as we have given here, to the brain force itself . . . flow of blood through the brain, that can absorb from the system those impurities that have been left and caused the hallucinations of the body at the present time . . .
> Q. What produced these conditions, Mr. Cayce?
> A. Extreme nervous tension that overtaxed the system, as received through the sensory forces, until the cells broke here at the 1st cervical.
> Q. When did that happen . . . ?
> A. 29½ moons ago.

Pathological Neurotransmission

As previously noted, Cayce often stated that pathological neurotransmission within the brain produced the symptoms commonly associated with schizophrenia. Although no specific neurotransmitter was cited, the readings did make many references to processes such as "fluids which in the circulation sustain and maintain the reaction fluid in the nerve channels themselves" (271-5) and "plasm in the nerve forces themselves" (386-3). The nerve cell membrane was frequently noted as a factor in faulty neurotransmission, as evidenced by the following excerpts. The case summaries in Chapter Three provide numerous other examples for those readers interested in this subject.

271-8   M. 34   6/12/33

While there may not be said to be at present any greater deteriorative forces active in the membranes, or those disorders that disturb the equilibrium of the reactions in the nerve system through the activity of brain centers, little of a contributory cause to a betterment has been added since last we had the body here.

396-2   F. 20   9/28/33

As we find, the general conditions in the body are improved from that as we have had before. As the general health is improved, and the inclinations are for the physical functionings to become nearer to normal in their activities, it becomes more necessary to consider the activities of the glands that have caused—and do cause yet—disturbances in the coordination of the reactions in the physical forces of the body itself. There is produced the extravaganza in the activity of the mental forces, or the hallucinations appear, from the incoordinating of the cerebrospinal and the sympathetic reactions in the body. Or, there is what is ordinarily known as inflammation of the membrane through which nerve impulses pass, that tends to make for those irritations that produced a washing away—a plethora—in the activity of same in its reaction . . .

When unusual conditions arise, as the activities where there are the supersensitive influences of outside forces upon the body, and these reactions take the form of hallucinations (from the normal reactions), then the quieting of the body through suggestions will be found much better than with the use of influences [drugs] that would deaden the nerve reactions and tend to increase (as time goes on) those influences from without.

Spinal Injury

According to the Cayce readings, somatic dysfunctions associated with the spine (i.e., lesions, subluxations, "pressures") were the most common etiological factor in cases which today would be disposed as schizophrenia. Spinal injuries were associated with such diverse activities as: falling on ice ([1513], [3641]), a bicycle accident ([3223]), an attempted escape from an attacker ([1789]), as well as the previously noted birth and pregnancy complications. Many cases involved childhood injuries which took several years to manifest in psychosis. The osteopathic and chiropractic literatures are replete with information on the etiology and treatment of these disorders and will be discussed at length in Chapters Five, Six, and Seven.

Spinal injury may be viewed as a stressor. In certain cases heredity is involved and the combined reaction of factors produce psychosis. In other cases, spinal injury served as an "acquired vulnerability" which was exacerbated by stressors such as glandular changes (e. g., puberty and menopause), worry, medication effects, and psychosocial stressors. In both of these scenarios, a diathesis/stress model can best describe the etiological pattern. In rare cases, spinal injury alone was sufficient to produce brain dysfunction (particularly when the cervicals were injured).

Medication Effects

Edgar Cayce died in 1945, several years before the advent of the antipsychotic medication. During Cayce's era, bromides were commonly used as central nervous system depressants. They calmed patients and thus suppressed some of the positive symptoms of the disorder. The readings often stated that such drugs hindered the body's natural regenerative potential and thus contributed to the degenerative process (e. g., [1428], [2022], [2200], [3662], [2721], etc.). For a brief discussion of "bromide intoxication" and other "organic" etiological factors which may be associated with mental syndromes, see the DSM-III-R (American Psychiatric Association, 1987, p. 106).

1452-1   F. 38   10/9/37
In the approach then, first as we find, from the very nature of the reactions, medications—as medical reactions, in the

form of any bromides, or those that would make for a degeneration of the feelings to the system—would only allay; but produce those conditions where softening of the reflexes from brain forces to the activities through the system [dementia] would set up in such natures as to become WHOLLY destructive to the physical body and its reactions.

2721-1   F. 18   4/6/42
The administration of sedatives, while keeping down the ravings (because of the pressures upon the nerve system) has destroyed more than it has aided. For, it has added to the inabilities of some of the organs of the physical forces to assimilate or eliminate properly . . .

Psychosocial Factors

Case [300] represents an interesting manifestation of psychosocial factors. This thirty-five-year-old man had been in a state hospital for ten years at the time of the reading. A letter from the man's doctor (1/27/33) states: "His home environment was very uninviting. His mother died early and his father drank himself into an early grave. He lived with his grandmother, whose mental faculty had deteriorated." The reading commented on his early environment:

300-1   M. 35   3/16/33
. . . the case might be better understood; and in particular offer an opportunity or channel for the study of deeper or reincarnated influences, that go for hereditary and environmental influence . . . Then having been an entity, a body (in the present) with those surroundings or environs that brought about the warping of the instinct and intelligency of the active forces that coordinate with the imaginative and the material influences, we find an incoordination between the mental images as builded by the body [an incoordination between CNS and ANS was noted] . . .

This excerpt contains some fascinating insights into the role of karma and reincarnation, as presented in the Cayce readings. Not only was karma and heredity a factor in this case, but the detrimental home environment itself was apparently chosen by the incoming entity as an opportunity for growth. This transpersonal aspect of Cayce's perspective coincides with the "perennial philosophy" of many of the world's religions in affirming the continuity of consciousness as represented by reincarnation. Another reading (1233-1) focused on the role of heredity and environment by stating, "You have inherited most from yourself, not from family. The family is only a river through which it [the soul] flows!" Interestingly, the treatment suggestions for case [300] were followed and the man apparently had an excellent recovery.

Institutional effects such as neglect and abuse were significant etiological factors in several readings. One has only to imagine the conditions in many of the large state institutions of Cayce's era to realize that such circumstances created tremendous stress on patients. Although these effects cannot be considered as primary etiological factors, neither can they be totally discounted.

1789-1   F. 32   1/13/39
In giving that as may be helpful then, for the physical and the mental welfare of the body—something might be given as to the sources or the causes of the present condition [spinal injury], to say nothing of the horrible effect the environs have upon the body, and that through which this entity or soul has passed in its present environment . . . in [the entity's] present environs, there have been only moments of rationality; and then NO one to respond brought greater and still greater depression to the better self.

Glandular Dysfunction

Glandular dysfunction was the second most common etiological factor cited by the readings (see Figure 3.4 in Appendix A). The endocrine glands were emphasized, with the gonads, pineal, and adrenals receiving most of the attention. The pituitary and thyroid were occasionally mentioned. Failure of the glands to secrete fluids required by the nervous systems was a common pathophysiological pattern. Although glands could become impaired by numerous processes, heredity and lower spinal injury were the two most frequent etiological factors mentioned in the readings. In case [1338] glandular changes resulting from menopause were cited as producing psychosis which may have been dementia praecox:

1338-1   F. 38   2/12/37
As we find with this body here, [1338], there are the mental disturbances that arise from softening of tissue, and this has been since the changes that have come about in the physical reactions of the body . . .
Q. What caused this condition?
A. As given, those periods when changes came about—or the menopause (if it must be given a term) began; there were not the proper precautions taken as to the conditions as set about in the system during those changes. And the effect came upon the coordination between the impulses and brain and nerve tissue.

Case [1475] provides an example of glandular dysfunction resulting from pregnancy:

1475-1   F. 30   11/12/37
Q. What specifically has caused this condition?
A. As we find, the great strain upon the body in childbearing WITHOUT the proper consideration of even keeping an equal balance in the salts and elements of the body; thus depleting the circulation, taking from the system the influences necessary for proper glandular rebuilding, thus drawing upon the system to an extent as to cause deterioration rather than the ability to rejuvenate itself . . . For that is the process or the activity of the glands, to secrete that which enables the body, physically throughout, to REPRODUCE itself!

[1475]'s husband remarked immediately after the reading: "She had 3 children within 3 years and was very 'faddish' about her diet throughout the period—not careful at all about building herself up."
These two cases illustrate two important points: (1) female reproductive biology may put women at a differential risk for developing schizophrenia (e. g., childbearing and menopause; see gender differences in Chapter One), and (2) the role of the glands is primarily regenerative. Glandular dysfunction (especially of the reproductive glands) was frequently cited in the readings as leading to brain pathology. This dysfunction could result from inherited factors or spinal injury (particularly to the lower spine where the nerves serving the pelvic region branch out from the cerebrospinal system). The possibility of psychosis resulting from dysfunction of the sexual

glands will be discussed in Chapter Seven (e. g., endogenous steroid psychosis, depletion of brain neurotransmitters, etc.).

The role of the pineal gland in the production of psychotic symptoms was also emphasized in the readings. Anatomically, the pineal refers to an endocrine gland located in the middle of the brain (attached to the roof of the third ventricle). In the esoteric literature (e.g., Hinduism and Buddhism) the pineal has been referred to as the "third eye" and has been associated with psychic abilities. Traditionally, science has largely ignored the pineal and considered it to be a vestigial organ which has become obsolete in evolutionary terms. Recent advances in endocrinology has changed this view and the pineal is now known to be an active gland whose duties are related to various bodily cycles such as sexual development.

Although Cayce does refer to the pineal in this capacity on occasion, he also uses the term to encompass an energy system which deals directly with the "life force" or "kundalini" energy as described in eastern meditative traditions. This system extends along the spine to the brain and serves as a link to the mental and spiritual realms. The readings state that pathology in this system can result in an opening of a person's consciousness to the cosmic realms. Cayce frequently reported that individuals for whom he was giving readings were in touch with other dimensions of reality and that this transpersonal experience was interpreted by others as hallucinations and delusions. Some excerpts from the readings will serve as an introduction to the pineal system and the reader is referred to Appendix B for a thorough treatment of the subject.

2475-1   M. 44   3/27/41
Yes, we have the body, the enquiring mind, [2475] and those conditions, those experiences of the body in the use of Yoga exercise in breathing . . . These exercises are excellent, yet it is necessary that special preparation be made—or that a perfect understanding be had by the body as to what takes place when such exercises are used.

For, BREATH is the basis of the living organism's activity. Thus, such exercises may be beneficial or detrimental in their effect upon a body . . .

There may be brought about an awareness of this by the exercising of the mind, through the manner of directing the breathing.

For, in the body there is that center in which the soul is expressive, creative in its nature—the Leydig center.

By this breathing, this may be made to expand—as it moves along the path that is taken in its first inception, at conception, and opens the seven centers of the body that radiate or are active upon the organisms of the body . . .

As this life-force is expanded, it moves first from the Leydig center through the adrenals, in what may be termed an upward trend, to the pineal and to the centers in control of the emotions—or reflexes through the nerve forces of the body.

Thus an entity puts itself, through such an activity, into association or in conjunction with all it has EVER been or may be. For, it loosens the physical consciousness to the universal consciousness.

To allow self in a universal state to be controlled, or to be dominated, may become harmful. But to know, to feel, to comprehend as to WHOM or as to WHAT is the directing influence when the self-consciousness has been released and the real ego allowed to rise to expression, is to be in that state of the universal consciousness—which is indicated in this body here, Edgar Cayce . . .

Q. Is there at present any danger to any particular body-function, such as sex; or to general health?

A. As we have indicated, without preparation, desires of EVERY nature may become so accentuated as to destroy—or to overexercise as to bring detrimental forces; unless the desire and purpose is acknowledged and set IN the influence of self as to its direction when loosened by the kundaline activities through the body.

4087-1 M. 6 4/15/44

For as we rind this entity has more than once been among those who were gifted with what is sometimes called second sight, or the superactivity of the third eye. Whenever there is the opening, then, of the lyden [Leydig) center and the kundaline forces from along the pineal, we find that there are visions of things to come, of things that are happening . . .

Possession

In several cases where the pathological process had progressed to actual brain degeneration, Cayce stated that the connections between the physical, mental, and spiritual bodies had been so weakened that total separation or dissociation was produced. This condition left the body open to "external influences" (discarnate entities). In these cases, Cayce stated that possession had occurred.

Possession is not a topic usually associated with schizophrenia in the current clinical literature. Thoughout history, however, various forms of insanity have been regarded as manifestations of demonic influence or spirit possession. With the advent of empirical science and the general adoption of a materialistic outlook, the use of possession as a diagnostic entity fell into disuse. It is not surprising however, given Cayce's cosmic perspective, that several individuals who came to him complaining of mental and physical problems were told that they were suffering from possession.

Cayce's definition of possession is quite specific and is best described by the readings.

281-24   6/29/35

Q. In certain types of insanity, is there an etheric body involved? If so, how?

A. Possession.

Let's for the moment use examples that may show what has oft been expressed from here: There is the physical body, there is the mental body, there is the soul body. They are One . . . The mind, through anger, may make the body do that which is contrary to the better influences of same; it way make for a change in its environ, its surrounding, contrary to the laws of environment or hereditary forces that are a portion of the *élan vital* of each manifested body, with the spirit or the soul of the individual.

Then, through pressure upon some portion of the anatomical structure that would make for the disengaging of the natural flow of the mental body through the physical in its relationships to the soul influence, one may be dispossessed of the mind; thus ye say rightly he is "out of his mind."

Or, where there are certain types or characters of disease found in various portions of the body, there is the lack of the necessary *vital* for the resuscitating of the energies that carry on through brain structural forces of a given body. Thus disintegration is produced, and ye call it dementia praecox—by the very smoothing of the indentations necessary for the rotary influence or vital force of the spirit within same to find expression. Thus derangements come.

Such, then, become possessed as of hearing voices, because of their closeness to the borderland. Many of these are termed deranged when they may have more of a closeness to the universal than one who may be standing nearby and commenting; yet they are awry when it comes to being normally balanced or healthy for their activity in a material world.

5221-1 F. 53 6/9/44

. . . the body is a supersensitive individual entity who has allowed itself through study, through opening the centers of the body, to become possessed with reflexes and activities outside of itself . . .

Q. How did I happen to pick this up?

A. . . . the body in its study opened the centers and allowed self to become sensitive to outside influences.

Q. What is it exactly that assails me?

A. Outside influences. Discarnate entities.

281-6 5/12/32

Q. What has caused the severe attacks during the past week?

A. The return of those influences and forces seeking a home.

Q. Why should those entities return to this body after our prayer?

A. They are as material as individuals, why doesn't an entity return home? They are seeking a home, the same as individuals, personalities!

In the Cayce readings, possession refers to the opening up of the body to discarnate entities who seek to express themselves in the material world. It is often associated with dementia praecox since a dissociation between the mental and physical bodies (i. e., degeneration within the nervous systems) may leave the physical open to influence by other entities. Again, it is important to keep in mind that the readings insisted that mind and spirit interface at definite centers within the physical body. Presumably, dissociation of these interfaces could allow the body to be open to access by other entities.

Possession was occasionally associated with other illnesses such as alcoholism and epilepsy. Cayce was not referring to demonic possession and none of the readings indicated involuntary possession (i.e., against the conscious will of the afflicted individual). For a comprehensive discussion of the subject, see Appendix E.

Treatment of Schizophrenia

Chapters Four, Five, and Six deal extensively with the treatments suggested by Cayce. Therefore, only the rudiments will be discussed here. As stated previously, the Cayce approach is holistic and advocates physical, mental, and spiritual interventions. Examples of each include:

SOMATIC THERAPIES—osteopathy, chiropractic, massage, electrotherapy, nutrition, medication, exercise, hot packs, and hydrotherapy

COGNITIVE/BEHAVIORAL THERAPIES—"suggestive therapeutics" (including but not limited to formal hypnosis), behavioral modeling, establishment of routine, thought monitoring, occupational therapy, and biblio/video therapy

SPIRITUAL THERAPIES—therapeutic milieu, companion therapy, prayer, meditation, "fruits of the spirit," and color and music therapy

Although these modalities were blended to suit each individual, the general pattern was quite simple:

1) provide a therapeutic milieu (emphasizing spiritual qualities such as service and altruism); a companion was often suggested in cases where the individual was incapable of following the suggestions consistently or if suicide was a factor
2) apply somatic therapies (such as osteopathy, chiropractic, massage, hydrotherapy, etc.)
3) use electrotherapy (usually the Wet Cell Battery with gold) to regenerate the nervous system (if deterioration was evident)
4) utilize suggestive therapeutics to access the inner resources of each client
5) provide opportunities for growth and development (e.g., recreational, social, vocational, and artistic activities commonly associated with rehabilitation).

Although the treatment plans were often simple, they were never easy. Attempting to reverse the pathological process in schizophrenia is an immense task requiring the spiritual qualities of patience and persistence, gentleness, kindness, and a profound desire to be of service.

A Word of Caution and a Promise of Hope

From the literature review presented in Chapter One and this brief introduction to the Cayce perspective, it is obvious that schizophrenia is an extremely complex disorder. It is crucial that the reader recognize the difficulties involved in treating this disorder and be aware that this book does not, in any way, suggest that the Cayce approach is "full proof" or easy to apply. To the contrary, Cayce often remarked that the suggestions provided in the readings would have to be carried out patiently and persistently if progress was to be achieved. He would then go on to say that if the persons administering the treatments were not dedicated to the healing process and willing to invest the resources required to follow all the suggestions, it would be best that they not begin the treatments.

For those willing to follow the suggestions in the readings, hope was provided. An encouraging theme which runs through the Cayce readings on this subject is the positive prognosis given by Cayce in the majority of the cases. Quite often, three to six months was given as a time frame in which to expect significant results. Readers are encouraged to study the prognoses cited in Chapter Three. In only the most serious cases were longer recuperative time frames indicated.

Readers will also note a couple of cases where the degeneration of the brain was beyond hope and the soul of the entity had departed the body (i.e. [586], [3315], [5344]). Such cases can have a sobering effect on one's expectations, while simultaneously providing motivation for early and persistent intervention. The Cayce readings never indicated that such extreme deterioration was an inevitable result of the schizophrenic process.

The most unfortunate aspect of the Cayce readings in this area is the lack of application of the suggestions. Many of the afflicted individuals were in state hospitals and had no hope of receiving the suggested treatments. Very often, in such cases, only one reading was given because the caretakers were adamantly opposed to information from psychic sources and blocked any attempts at providing Cayce's treatments. In other cases where the suggestions could have been applied at home, the family members were unwilling to provide the treatments in a consistent manner. Expense was often cited as a justification for failure to provide treatment (many of the readings were given during the Great Depression). These cases were often chronic. The individuals involved came to Edgar Cayce as a last resort after years of failed treatment from numerous doctors and hospitals. Cayce's insistence that recovery would require patient and persistent treatment for a minimum of several months was apparently too much to ask of people discouraged by years of suffering with this disorder.

In the few cases where there was consistent application of the suggestions provided in the readings, remarkable results were produced (i.e., [282], [300], [386], [886], [1513], [1789]). The case of [1789] is particularly inspiring when the whole series of readings for this individual is reviewed and the patience and persistence of [1789]'s family is considered. A brief review of these cases is presented in Chapter Three and the complete readings for [1513] and [1789] are available through the Circulating File program at the A.R.E. (Association for Research and Enlightenment, Virginia Beach, Va.).

A letter from Edgar Cayce to the mother of Miss [2721] addresses these issues concisely and reflects the theme of cautious optimism which pervades the readings. Miss [2721] was at the Rochester State Hospital, Rochester, Minnesota, at the time of the reading, suffering from a "well-established dissociation of the schizophrenic type."

Am in hopes you have found the information for Miss [2721] of interest. Of course I realize what it means to raise false hopes in the minds of others. I realize any thing I may say would appear as if I were blowing my own horn, but please know I realize too that it is not of myself the work is done, but only as the Spirit of Truth may work in or through me. We have had several cases of this nature that seemed hopeless, where seeming miracles have happened. There have been a few people sent to the Macon hospital [Still-Hildreth Osteopathic Sanatorium], so the work there will not be entirely new to them. Do hope you will write them and if it is possible or practical, do hope you will give it a try. Have had many where the condition was not such as real help might be given, but where help has been promised [by the readings] through a certain mode of treatment, or by certain places or individuals, when this was done the help promised has come. Am sure, of the many thousands of readings that have been given, this has been true in practically every case. Many have, of course, been persuaded that the suggestions were all wrong and that the help suggested could not come from such a treatment, but where tried, whatever amount of help was offered has come. We will be glad to try and help anywhere along the line with check-up readings from time to time. Do hope we may be the means of help, and may HIS blessings, His Peace come to you. [Correspondence dated 4/9/42, included in the file for reading 2721-1]

Summary

This chapter has served as an introduction to the psychic readings of Edgar Cayce. The perspective of the readings on schizophrenia is congruent with current clinical and research literature in the following respects:

1. The readings viewed schizophrenia as a syndrome with multiple etiologies and considerable variability.
2. The central nervous system was always involved (e.g., pathological neurotransmission in the brain). Other key systems (i.e., endocrine, ANS, visceral organs, musculoskeletal) were also usually involved and required interventions which produced systemic coordination.
3. Heredity was implicated as a contributory factor in the development of schizophrenia.
4. Stress was also cited as contributing to the production of psychotic symptoms.
5. Cayce's description of brain degeneration (dementia praecox) is consistent with research findings which indicate enlarged ventricles in some persons diagnosed as suffering from schizophrenia.
6. Pregnancy and birth complications play a significant role in the etiology of schizophrenia in certain cases.
7. Psychosocial factors are important in the etiology and course of schizophrenia.

Cayce diverges from the current paradigm by insisting that a holistic approach is necessary to fully understand and treat schizophrenia. The reality of body, mind, and spirit must be acknowledged if one is to grasp the significance of this disorder. It is this holistic perspective which makes the readings so pertinent to clinicians who recognize the need for a progressive approach, integrating established procedures with spiritual awareness. Cayce's expansive perspective also incorporates spiritual and metaphysical concepts (e.g., karma, discarnate possession, and the kundalini energy system) which may be involved in psychoses such as schizophrenia.

A major advantage of utilizing the Cayce perspective is the wealth of information in the readings regarding the way in which the body systems interface with each other and nonphysical dimensions—especially the role of the endocrine glands' and the autonomic nervous system. This interconnectedness of body/mind/spirit at definite points within the body is the foundation of the holistic approach advocated in the readings. From a holistic perspective, schizophrenia can be conceptualized as a disruption or incoordination of the essential interconnectedness of body/mind/spirit. The fact that this interconnectedness is substantially biochemical in nature is borne out by the powerful effect of pharmacological interventions.

A major theme in the readings is that the body is capable of self-healing, with the proper assistance. Thus treatment is directed at re-establishing the body's innate ability to maintain itself.

Finally, the approach suggested by Cayce has the potential for helping millions of persons suffering from schizophrenia. The Cayce readings echoed the old osteopathic dictum of "cure by the removal of causes" (Hildreth, 1938). From this perspective, the *possibility* of cure is based upon a thorough understanding of the cause(s) of a particular illness. The purpose of this book is the exploration of this *possibility*. The remaining chapters will document the principles and techniques advocated by Edgar Cayce and provide a therapeutic model which offers a means of applying this approach in a clinical program.

3

Case Studies
◆

CASE STUDIES PROVIDE an effective means of accessing the staggering amount of information in the readings. The case study approach is also consistent with Cayce's preference for dealing with individuals and their problems rather than groups or diagnostic classes. This preference was also apparent in his reluctance to saddle persons with labels (particularly when the labels were derived from poorly understood symptom clusters—i.e., effects rather than causes). Therefore, it is understandable that he refused to use a diagnostic term so vague as schizophrenia. His occasional use of dementia praecox was related to its relative specificity—chronic course with probable brain degeneration. Kraepelin's belief that this syndrome was produced by metabolic dysfunction may also have been relevant because it was consonant with the systemic perspective of Cayce. See Appendix C for a more thorough discussion of dementia praecox and reading selections on the topic.

In formulating an approach to presenting the case studies, it seemed appropriate to preserve as much specificity as possible while seeking to present the cases in a format comprehensible to clinicians and researchers. With this in mind, the numerous readings on psychosis were divided into four categories:

GROUP I: dementia (9 cases) 173, 271, 3315, 3441, 3997, 4097, 5344, 5405, 5690

GROUP II: dementia tendencies (12 cases) 282, 386, 2022, 2200, 2614, 2744, 3662, 4059, 4186, 4333, 5228, 5715

GROUP III: schizophrenic psychosis (33 cases) 300, 1310, 1428, 1513, 1572, 1789, 1969, 2197, 2465, 2712, 2721, 2967, 3075, 3087, 3158, 3163, 3181, 3223, 3421, 3440, 3475, 3589, 3633, 3641, 3996, 4002, 4004, 4100, 4179, 4285, 4342, 5014, 5274

GROUP IV: psychosis not otherwise specified (54 cases) 151, 186, 225, 387, 577, 600, 603, 638, 686, 886, 894, 968, 977, 1168, 1338, 1475, 1488, 1526, 1773, 1873, 1951, 2210, 2248, 2262, 2359, 2544, 2863, 2865, 3365, 3410, 3415, 3481, 3765, 3877, 3905, 3930, 3973, 4147, 4242, 4290, 4519, 4545, 4600, 4624, 4659, 4787, 4800, 4853, 5061, 5167, 5187, 5221, 5533, 5598

Group I consists of cases where the readings specifically noted dementia. This group may be considered as similar to Crow's type II schizophrenia (Crow, 1980), Kraepelian schizophrenia (Keefe, et al., 1988), and process schizophrenia (Langfelt, 1937) while not limited by any of these labels.

Group II consists of cases which the readings stated could lead to dementia praecox if conditions were not changed. Presumably, Groups I and II should have comparable etiologies, with the exception of chronicity effects in Group I (e.g., institutional neglect and abuse, medication effects, etc.). One might also expect to find differences in prognosis and treatment suggestions. Individuals in Group I would have less favorable prognosis with treatment suggestions reflecting the dire condition of these people. For a graphic representation of these dimensions, see Figures 3.1 and 3.2 for etiological factors, Tables 3.1 and 3.2 for prognoses, and Tables 3.3 and 3.4 for examples of treatment plans for these cases.

Group III represents cases where the readings and background information indicate schizophrenia by the following criteria: "positive" symptoms such as hallucinations and delusions, impaired social and vocational functioning, inappropriate affect, cognitive deficits, clinical descriptions and diagnoses, and history of mental illness. In several cases, the readings made remarks indicating physical deterioration in the nervous system and commented on the seriousness of the condition without specifically mentioning dementia praecox. In recognition of the variability associated with schizophrenia (and possibly dementia praecox since there may have been subgroups within this relatively distinct group), these cases were not included in the first two categories. Readers may wish to compare etiological factors associated with Group III (Figure 3.3) to previous subgroups. Group III may represent cases which resemble Crow's type I schizophrenia, though one must be cautious in drawing parallels on such scant data.

Group IV contains cases for which there is insufficient information to include in any of the previous categories. This category consists of "psychoses about which there is inadequate information to make a specific diagnosis" (DSM-III-R, p. 211, American Psychiatric Association, 1987). This group is rather large and only a few examples will be cited. No doubt there are many cases of schizophrenia in this group. Numerous cases might also be designated as organic mental syndrome if one accepts as credible the descriptions of pathology provided in the readings. Group IV provides valuable information for differential diagnosis and readers are encouraged to review these readings.

It must be remembered that this chapter does not represent a random sample of schizophrenic cases. These cases do represent a select sample of individuals suffering from major mental illness during the early decades of this century. Furthermore, these cases are representative of individuals who, very often as a last resort, sought help from a psychic diagnostician. Unfortunately, background data is sketchy in many cases. This may be due, in part, to the limited staff which Cayce employed to maintain correspondence (the Cayce staff often consisted of his wife, personal secretary, and eldest son). Also, keep in mind that toward the end of his life, Cayce was deluged with requests for help, creating additional difficulties in maintaining correspondence with clients.

The format utilized in this section provides an opportunity for commentary on each case. In order to facilitate understanding of the Cayce perspective, this commentary will point out key patterns and serve as a translator of the often convoluted language of the readings. In order to effectively communicate Cayce's perspective, these comments are directed from the position of plausibility of the readings. Of course, readers are encouraged to study the excerpts closely and decide for themselves as to the validity of this material. A brief summary concludes this chapter and will review, in broad terms, some of the most prominent patterns in these cases.

Group I: Dementia

173

Background: Male, 59 years old
Symptoms: Loss of self-confidence, delusions of shame, paranoid delusions, hallucinations
Medical Diagnosis: Unknown
Cayce's Diagnosis and Etiology: "This is the form of hallucination dementia, and is produced, as we see, by a physical condition existent in the physical structure that prevents the normal flow of all blood to the brain in all its parts . . . the supplying nutriment as is necessary to keep normalcy in body is hindered, through the inability of bloodstream to furnish the rebuilding forces to that portion of the brain proper as becomes affected by this subluxation. In times back (some years ago), we find there existed in the body that of a disturbance in the glands of the gestation. In times following this there was an injury to the cerebrospinal system, in the coccyx (3rd from end), also in the last lumbar. With this deflection in the nerve system, with the subluxation of those centers that brought, and do bring in normalcy, those connections with central brain forces (situated here in the normal portion, above the central and to the central portion in the right lobe), we find this brought about, then, to the mental forces of the body, that of first melancholia, of despondency, of fear, through a retraction of the gland running through the body, situated at the base of the medulla oblongata [pineal gland?] and connecting in a threadlike manner through the system to the generatory system, forming, as has been called, to the central portion of the brain . . . This subluxation, bringing this detrimental condition, brings about these depressions, and the gradual softening of this center in brain proper."
Cayce's Prognosis: "With these applied, we would find, in 3 to 6 months, this body, [173], normal."
Treatment Suggested by Cayce:
1. Chiropractic or osteopathic adjustments
2. Soda and gold taken internally

3. Radio-Active Appliance with gold
Treatment Results: [173] was treated at Still-Hildreth Sanatorium—
results not available.
Comments: The adjustments would apparently prevent further
deterioration but would not rebuild the nervous system. For this,
the gold was required. "This [adjustments] will remove strain, yet
would not enliven tissue in itself. We begin, then, giving *internally,*
and through a vibratory force, those forms of soda and gold, internally, that rejuvenate the whole system, as to repropagation of nerve
energy. Stimulating same, see?"
  Also note the presence of significant affective features—a pattern
common in cases diagnosed as dementia. This relates directly to the
issue of "nonspecificity" (Chapter One) and will be addressed in
more detail in subsequent sections. Cayce's diagnosis of "hallucination dementia" is unique and may be a variation of dementia praecox since the softening of brain tissue was specifically noted. The
readings hinted that even the relatively distinct diagnosis of dementia praecox entailed a degree of variability (see Chapter Seven for a
discussion of variability in dementia praecox).

271

Background: Male, 34 years old; he was about 30 years at onset of
symptoms
Symptoms: "Depressed and moody"
Medical Diagnosis: Dementia praecox
Cayce's Diagnosis and Etiology: "In a general manner the condition may be termed dementia praecox (as some have diagnosed it),
but the type and nature of the disturbance—physically *and* mentally, as we find—would indicate that, were there changes made in
the application for the physical reliefs of the body to much that has
been given through these sources as to how certain elements may
be added within the physical forces of a body, not only might the
inroads of this softening of cell cord and brain tissue be stopped but
there might be added sufficient to the system in manners as to bring
about nearer normal reactions for the body. Pressures and incoordinations that are shown from prenatal conditions, and the activities in the physical that have brought about and indicate the
abrasions to the nervous system in such a manner as to make for a
positive condition existent as diagnosed . . . "
Cayce's Prognosis: " . . . we will find that, by the third period of the
recharges from the Battery, there will be a specific change in the

physical and mental conditions of this body [271]." No explicit time frame for recovery was given. "It will be long (as time is counted by individuals) . . . "

Treatment Suggested by Cayce:
1. Change environment (therapeutic milieu)
2. Get plenty of sunshine
3. Companion therapy
4. Wet Cell Battery with gold
5. Radio-Active Appliance
6. Massage
7. Hypnotic suggestions during massage
8. Diet
9. Physical and mental exercise
10. Bibliotherapy and videotherapy
11. Behavioral modeling
12. Establish routine
13. Medicine (lactated pepsin, bromide and iodide of potassium)

Treatment Results: [271] received ten physical readings from 2/13/33 to 7/10/33 and had a companion for most of this period. [271] apparently resisted some of the suggestions such as use of the Wet Cell, eating of fruit, early morning arising, and so forth. Some improvement was noted, especially in the first few weeks. The readings seemed to indicate that the deterioration had stopped but further physical improvement was necessary for recovery. [271]'s mother had him put in an institution in New York. In a letter from her dated 5/1/34, she states, "I am glad to tell you that [271] is doing very well . . . He has certainly improved a lot and is contented . . . " Cayce was deeply disappointed over this case as evidenced from correspondence dated 8/18/33. The tone and content of the readings suggest that the initial choice of companion may not have been judicious and near the end of treatment a new companion was introduced.

Comments: Reading 271-5 has an excellent description of pathological nerve transmission (incoordination) between the CNS and ANS, with implications for sensory input into the ANS. Reading 271-7 also contains information on neurophysiology suggesting deterioration of the "white matter" in the brain, producing incoordination within brain centers, especially those receiving sensory input. Reading 271-9 reiterates the pattern of incoordination of gray matter and white matter in the brain and recommends that "there be applied those vibrations for the correction of the activities in that assimi-

lated by the system for the replenishing of nerve energy cooperation between the cerebrospinal and sympathetic and brain centers
themselves." Note the presence of affective features ("depressed,"
"moody"). The qualifying references to dementia praecox (i.e., "In a
general manner," "may be termed," "as some have diagnosed it,"
"the type and nature of the disturbance") suggest a degree of variability within the relatively distinct diagnostic category of dementia
praecox.

                              3315
Background: Female, 40 years old
Symptoms: Unknown
Medical Diagnosis: Unknown
Cayce's Diagnosis and Etiology: "The conditions here, as we find,
have been so aggravated by animosities, and by hates, that we have
a deterioration in the nerve force along the spinal system; so that
this is dementia—and now possession . . . Q. What was the original
cause, or what brought about this condition? A. Changes in the glandular system, and then aggravated by animosities and hate."
Cayce's Prognosis: " . . . near to hopeless in this experience . . .
Through the application of low electrical forces as . . . may be aid—
if those responsible are active in keeping with divine approbation.
Without these, little may be accomplished . . . Q. What can be done
if the patient is not cooperative? A. Nothing. But do these things."
Treatment Suggested by Cayce:
1. Short-wave electrical treatment ("shocks to the body")
2. Application of love, care, and prayer
Treatment Results: Unknown
Comments: This was a very short reading. The dementia apparently allowed possession to occur (see Appendix E for a discussion
of possession). There appears to have been a strong psychosomatic
element in this case produced by hate and animosity. Cayce stated
that strong negative attitudes could produce lesions in the nervous
system.
    Electrotherapy and spiritual attitudes on the part those giving
treatment were frequently suggested in cases involving possession.
"Q. How often should the electrical treatment be given? A. At least
once a week until there is almost exhaustion to the body, and then
there can be the separation—for, with electricity, dissuasion may be
used on those influences about the body. But there must then be
applied love, care, and prayer."

There was only one reading given. Granted the serious nature of the disorder, one naturally wonders if further suggestions for regeneration of the nervous system would have been given if depossession were accomplished. From a research standpoint, this case should not be viewed as an example of treatment for dementia since the electrical interventions were intended to drive out the discarnate influences and not remedy the dementia. The etiology is significant, however, since it is a common pattern in these cases: glandular dysfunction combined with negative attitudes produced degeneration in the nervous system. The readings also cited a close association between possession and dementia praecox in several cases. According to correspondence from [3315]'s husband the condition was of "some years standing" indicating onset of symptoms in the age range commonly associated with schizophrenia.

3441

Background: Female, 33 years old, located at State Central Hospital in Nashville, Tenn.

Symptoms: Problems with vision, numbness on right side, she was very nervous and couldn't maintain her teaching job

Medical Diagnosis: Dementia praecox

Cayce's Diagnosis and Etiology: " . . . there are disturbances, and there are tendencies towards the destruction of the reflexes to brain centers. These are produced from pressures that are associated and connected with organs of the pelvis . . . subluxations exist in the coccyx, the lumbar, also in the 10th and 11 dorsal areas . . . Sure dementia praecox is indicated, but it is from pressure . . . "

Cayce's Prognosis: " . . . under quite a different environment from that indicated here, we would bring nearer normal conditions for this body . . . It will take time, but be patient, be persistent."

Treatment Suggested by Cayce:
1. Change of environment (Still-Hildreth Sanatorium, i.e., therapeutic milieu)
2. Osteopathic corrections
3. Low electrical forces (similar to Wet Cell but of a "static nature")

Treatment Results: Although the parents couldn't afford to keep their daughter at Still-Hildreth for more than 4 months, some improvement was noted.

Comments: This was apparently a case of lower spine dysfunction affecting the organs of the pelvis and producing dementia praecox. The suggestions for low electrical forces of a static nature were unusual. Cayce stated that such treatment was available at Still-Hildreth.

3997

Background: Male, 19 years old, located at Bryce Hospital in Tuscaloosa, Alabama

Symptoms: "Mental aberrations," sullenness, melancholy, suicidal

Medical Diagnosis: Unknown

Cayce's Diagnosis and Etiology: "There was in the inception, and in presentation at the time of birth, that which produced a pressure on the 1st and 2nd cervicals, that has hindered the normal development of the nerve as especially has to do with the reactions of generation, or gentation in the body—the pineal gland. The pituitary gland has become enlarged from same. The pineal gland being formed, then, in two conditions that produce engorgement in same. Near the indentation or subluxation as produced, brings in the lower portion of same, or in the branches of same that act with the lyden [Leydig] gland, that causing the expansion of same in this region. Hence there has been the continued repression to the body in its development, until—reaching that cycle when the development of the genitory [genitive—generatory] gland and the activity of the lyden [Leydig] gland in the system [puberty?]—has brought about such depression and activity to the action of the imagination, or the activity of the gray matter in nerve reaction, until dementia *is the result."*

Cayce's Prognosis: " . . . the whole of the gland system builded nominally, we would bring—in the third cycle—near normal reaction for this body. Then, unless corrections are made . . . the general breaking down of the gray portion of nerve tissue, nerve cell matter, in the body."

Treatment Suggested by Cayce:
1. Osteopathic corrections
2. Personal care and attention

Treatment Results: Unknown

Comments: This is a good example of a "classic" case of schizophrenia. The young man was 19 years old, exhibiting the symptoms of schizophrenia which resulted from injury at birth (see the discussion of pregnancy and birth complications in Chapter One), and experiencing brain degeneration (he would likely have shown ventricular enlargement if such measurements were available at that time). Cayce's prognosis of improvement in the third cycle (seven-year cycles) suggests that this case would have required at least a couple of years of treatment. The reference to the pineal's role in physical development and its close association with the organs of reproduction and the lower portion of the spinal column is consistent with Cayce's view of that gland. Again, note the presence of affective features.

4097

Background: Male, adult
Symptoms: Unknown
Medical Diagnosis: Unknown
Cayce's Diagnosis and Etiology: " . . . we find the action of the brain itself to be that of dementia praecox—that is, the softening of the tissue used to present the reaction of impressions to the centers as distributed from the action of the sensory system in itself, action of the body itself. That is, impressions as received to this body act refractorily on the centers giving off the impressions received to this body, so that we have only a partial action of the brain to give the proper incentive to the movements of the other forces in the body; or the impossible forces present themselves through the action of other portions of the body. So that the expressions as given off from the body to proceed with its actions become hallucinations, as it were [to other minds] and the expressions from this mind become of a demented force in the actions; yet to the mind itself it is rational. In its impressions to others it expresses the irrational. This, as we find, has been produced by the breaking of cell force itself in the blood supply, as we have given here, to the brain force itself . . . flow of blood through the brain, that can absorb from the system those impurities that have been left and caused the hallucinations of the body at the present time . . . Q. What produced these conditions, Mr. Cayce? A. Extreme nervous tension that overtaxed the system, as received through the sensory forces, until the cells broke here at the 1st cervical. Q. When did that happen . . . ? A. 29½ moons ago. Q. . . . what caused it? A. In the first cervical, where occurred the breaking of the forces, is the entrance of the circulation to the brain receptive forces, as we have given here."
Cayce's Prognosis: "This, you see, would require from six to eight months to effect a perfect balance and flow of blood through the portions of the body." "Do this, as we have given, if we would bring the normal condition to this body."
Treatment Suggested by Cayce:
1. Subject body to extreme heat

2. When under this condition use hypnosis or mesmeristic forces
3. Electric magnetic forces ("laying on of hands" combined with osteopathic manipulation?)
4. Still-Hildreth Sanatorium was suggested
Treatment Results: Unknown
Comments: This is an interesting case of stress-induced somatic dysfunction at the first cervical which produced toxicity within the brain. This case fits the osteopathic model of schizophrenia of that era (which cited spinal lesions, particularly in the cervicals, as leading to pathological circulation of blood to the brain and subsequent toxicity in the brain—see Chapter Five and Appendix C). It is also interesting that the description of the area of the brain affected suggests that the limbic region might be the primary location of degeneration, as is currently posited by many researchers.

5344

Background: Female, 35 years old; she was about 33 years old at the time of the nervous breakdown, the reading was given about 13 months after the breakdown
Symptoms: Unknown
Medical Diagnosis: Unknown
Cayce's Diagnosis and Etiology: "There has already been departure of the soul, which only waits by here . . . The condition has come from pressures which caused dementia praecox."
Cayce's Prognosis: "For already there are those weakenings so of the centers of the cerebrospinal system that no physical help, as we find, may be administered, only the mental or soul help as will be a part of the mental or superconscious self."
Treatment Suggested by Cayce:
1. Show love, care, and attention for the body
Treatment Results: *Unknown*
Comments: This was an unusual case, not only from the standpoint of negative prognosis, but also in regards to the apparently swift degenerative process leading to dissociation of mind and spirit from the physical body. One wonders how many chronic schizophrenics are in a similar condition (catatonic stupor?). Reading 586-1 was given for a woman in Harlem Valley State Hospital who may have been suffering from dementia praecox but was not included in this group due to insufficient etiological and background information. Compare these quotes from 586-1 with [5344]: "For there is much that many would study in such a case departed from the sur-

roundings of this body . . . The coordination has been severed between that which is of the physical-physical [nervous systems] and the mental and spiritual activities as a unit. As we find, little may be added, save for the comfort of this body." It is likely that these two cases epitomize the dissociative potential of dementia praecox in its most extreme degenerative stage.

The reference to [5344] "which only waits by here" is apparently related to Cayce's out-of-body dissociated state during trance. The readings stated that he visited various planes of consciousness during the trance sessions. The "location" of [5344] may have been on the plane of consciousness referred to in the readings as the "borderland." See case [5690] for a further discussion of dissociative phenomena.

5405

Background: Male, 22 years old
Symptoms: "Nervous"
Medical Diagnosis: Dementia praecox
Cayce's Diagnosis and Etiology: " . . . the illness is of the mind, and not so much of body, in the present . . . Q. Do I understand that overstudy and strain was the cause of his condition? A. Overstudy and strain, and, as indicated, an injury in the lower portion of the lumbar axis . . . "
Cayce's Prognosis: " . . . there are measures which might be taken where there may be brought, even under the disturbances, near to normal conditions for this body."
Treatment Suggested by Cayce:
1. Remove from institution
2. Wet Cell Appliance (with gold and silver—alternately)
3. Massage
4. Altruistic nurse or caretaker
5. Apply self in some useful activity
6. "The more out of doors, the better"
7. Prayer by significant others
8. Spiritual attitude and behavior by significant others
Treatment Results: Unknown
Comments: This was probably a case of dementia praecox. "In the present environs, and under the existent shadows, very little may be accomplished, for those individuals in authority take little interest in even possibilities, where there have been, and are evidences of this nature or character of dementia praecox which indicates the

inability of the body to respond to suggestive forces, as indicated, or the reaction of reflexes from brain to the organs of sensory forces in their activity to the physical being . . . There is within the nerve centers that which, in the elements of material, contributes to the white and gray matter of the nervous system, and, as has been indicated, this may be in patient, in gentleness, rebuilded, even when destroyed much more than is indicated here. But with the use of these elements—silver and gold—to the body in such measures and manners as to supply those necessary influences to re-establish in the physical forces of the body those necessary channels along which impulses run, we may replenish, we may supply those forces, for even this body."

The descriptions of brain degeneration suggest softening of the limbic area of the brain (i.e., central portion of the brain involved in emotions and memory). Note that the etiology involves a combination of factors—acquired vulnerability (spinal injury) and mental stress. Also note the location of the insult in the lower portion of the spine (lumbar)—a pattern that will become increasingly familiar in these case studies.

5690

Background: Male, 27 years old; at the time of the reading, he had been in a state hospital for one year

Symptoms: Violent at times, "irrational"

Medical Diagnosis: Unknown

Cayce's Diagnosis and Etiology: "There are physical *defects* in the cerebrospinal nerve system. There are also the lacking of elements in the physical forces, as produced by conditions—some a lacking of elements in the physical forces, as produced by conditions— some a *tendency* in *innate* influences; *not* as wholly hereditary innate, as much as hereditary *tendencies.* Then, with the physical defects, these in their combination bring about that as has been called dementia praecox. This an inability of coordination between sympathetic, cerebrospinal, and the general physical body."

Cayce's Prognosis: "It would require from three to five weeks to eliminate those properties that have been given to produce sedative effect to the nervous reaction and the activities, and from three to five months for the building up where the body would be safe with itself and others, and normal development—as we find—later on."

Treatment Suggested by Cayce:
1. Admit patient to Still-Hildreth Sanatorium

2. Wet Cell Appliance with gold
3. Or, ultraviolet ray with gold taken orally
4. "Mechanical suggestions" (osteopathic treatments)
5. "Mental suggestions" (therapeutic milieu)
Treatment Results: The parents couldn't afford the treatment.
Comments: Note the definition of dementia praecox and the etiology involving a combination of factors. The readings frequently used terms such as incoordination, dissociation, separation, etc., when describing the dementia praecox process. This case provides a dramatic example of the dissociative potential of dementia praecox. "Q. Any advice for the parents? A. We haven't the parents! We have the body! In different places!" Apparently this man was experiencing dissociation (i.e., an "out-of-body experience"). The readings often associated dementia praecox with a weakening of the connections between body, mind, and spirit which would increase the probability of such paranormal happenings.

[5690]'s parents were double first cousins (prenatal condition?). Note that the "innate influences" were stated to be only "hereditary tendencies" and not "hereditary innate." This is congruent with a diathesis/stress model rather than a strictly genetic model of schizophrenia.

The man was healthy, lived a long life, and was physically active but could not care for himself. The process of dementia praecox apparently produced organic personality change as evidenced by correspondence from the family.

Group II: Dementia Tendencies

282

Background: Male, 32 years; he suffered a nervous breakdown
Symptoms: Unknown
Medical Diagnosis: Unknown
Cayce's Diagnosis and Etiology: "We find that from and through the highly sensitive and nervous conditions, owing to material as well as mental reactions, there are incoordinations between the impulses and the physical activities. These produce MENTAL reactions of an UNuniform or of an exaggerated nature with the mental and physical bodies . . . the mental reactions and the nerve strain produce much of the physical condition . . . "
Cayce's Prognosis: "If there would be brought anything near to normalcy, there must be not only a change of environment, a change of

scenes, but a change of thought as well."
Treatment Suggested by Cayce:
1. "Low electrical forces" (Wet Cell or magnetic healing)
2. Change of environment
3. Change thinking
4. Suggestive therapeutics
5. Gold Chloride
Treatment Results: An excellent recovery was noted.
Comments: There was a physical reading given 8 years before the breakdown which indicated a glandular dysfunction: "there are disturbances, and these—unless corrected—must eventually cause distresses that would be much harder to combat with than at present. These have to do with the glands . . . " A life reading (282-2) indicated that there were "innate" tendencies (hereditary) having to do with the "digestive forces becoming clogged—especially in the caecum region." There was a history of insanity in [282]'s family and an aunt apparently suffered from major mental illness. [282]'s sister was concerned about the possibility of inheriting insanity and addressed this issue in readings 457-4 and 457-5.

The correspondence in this file suggests that this man may have become unbalanced by his study of the occult. A letter from Hugh Lynn Cayce to his father states, "The situation with [282] here is peculiar. I am hoping to be of some help to him. He simply has a strange twist which borders on religious fanaticism." The readings state that some forms of dementia are produced in persons "strained by great religious fervor or excitement" (933-1). Reading 282-8 declares that balance will not be restored "unless there is an entire change of environs and outlook, as WELL as the application of those suggestive forces and the low electrical forces, to CLOSE as it were the centers through the system to the influences from without [possession]—which naturally produces a softening of the reaction between the impulses of the nerve forces themselves [dementia praecox]." This appears to be one of several cases where the readings associated the opening of the spiritual centers and possession with dementia praecox.

386

Background: Female, 20 years old
Symptoms: Timid, sensitive, and melancholic; experiencing hallucinations and delusions
Medical Diagnosis: Dementia praecox

Cayce's Diagnosis and Etiology: "This, then, is the difference between an unbalanced condition in a mental reaction [nervous breakdown] and that of dementia—which destroys the reaction in the plasm of the nerve as fixed from the blood supply itself; though, unless there are some material changes, this may become the condition that will ensue." Cayce traced the problem to developments in the eighth to twelfth year; shocks to the nervous system which affected the blood supply: "the effluvia and fluor in the hemoglobin does not make for those activities that carry to the impulses in the nerve forces that which creates a balance in the responsive or reactory forces of a normal body."

Cayce's Prognosis: "And we will find these will respond, in sixty to ninety days, to a near normal condition."

Treatment Suggested by Cayce:
1. Change environment (therapeutic milieu)
2. Near to nature as possible (sun, sea, sand, pines)
3. Wear as few clothes as possible
4. Develop self-dependence
5. Physical activities
6. Companion therapy
7. Massage
8. Wet Cell Battery with gold
9. Suggestive therapeutics
10. Diet (alkaline)
11. Service to others
12. Be joyous ("whistle, sing, holler," etc.)
13. Be sociable

Treatment Results: Three readings were given from 8/9/33 to 10/25/33. Readings indicate compliance with treatment suggestions and gradual improvement in conditions: " . . . the general conditions in the body are improved from that we have had before . . . " [9/28/33] " . . . there are considerable changes in the general physical forces of the body since last we had same here, and these are for the betterment . . . there is still at times coordination in the sympathetics through the activities to the cerebrospinal and the sensory reactions . . . " [10/25/33] Questions asked by [386] during the third reading indicated coherent mental processes.

Comments: This case provides excellent descriptions of nerve transmission dysfunction in reading 386-2. Cayce's explanation of [386]'s hallucinations is interesting: "Q. Does she really hear the things she speaks of, or what causes the hallucinations? A. We have described how that the supersensitiveness of the nerve forces opens the body to such influences; or the body becomes what might be termed a human radio, but in giving expression to what is heard may often deflect what is actually said, felt or thought. For, thoughts are things! And they have their effect upon individuals, especially those that become supersensitive to outside influences! These are just as physical as sticking a pin in the hand!"

This case is indicative of Cayce's tendency to consider serious mental illness as systemic dysfunction rather than simply brain neurotransmitter disorder. This person had numerous physical symptoms such as allergies, complexion problems, constipation, etc. It is interesting that no osteopathic adjustments were suggested (suggestive of primary biochemical dysfunction). Cayce indicated that there was an inflammation of the nerve cell membrane disturbing the nerve impulse. This case also highlights the progressive nature of dementia praecox and the effectiveness of early and consistent treatment. Note the presence of melancholia (affective features were frequently associated with dementia praecox in the readings).

2022

Background: Female, adult
Symptoms: Unknown
Medical Diagnosis: Unknown
Cayce's Diagnosis and Etiology: " . . . these arise from centers in the cerebrospinal system that have become blocked—by subluxations as well as the effect which has gradually been produced by improper glandular activity . . . The subluxations exist in the coccyx end of the spine, the 9th dorsal, and the 1st and second cervical. The glands involved are the thyroids (the inner), the glands in the area above and about the kidneys [adrenal?]—or the effect FROM these to the pineals."
Cayce's Prognosis: " . . . conditions are rather serious. And if there is the continuation of the bromides, this may cause such a softening of the nerve tissue as to produce dementia praecox."
Treatment Suggested by Cayce:
1. Chiropractic or osteopathic adjustments under water
2. Injections of liver extract
3. Wet Cell Appliance carrying gold
4. Blood- and nerve-strengthening diet
5. Open air exercise (especially walking)

6. Constant attendant
7. Diet (semi-liquid, blood and nerve building)
Treatment Results: Unknown
Comments: The suggestions to make the adjustments while the patient was submerged in hot water and give injections of liver extract were rare in these cases. The association of spinal injury with glandular dysfunction (especially pineal) resulting in the process of dementia praecox is a common pattern in the readings. Medications such as bromides were also frequently cited as contributing to brain degeneration.

2200

Background: Male, adult; he was suffering from a nervous breakdown at the time of the reading
Symptoms: Unknown
Medical Diagnosis: Unknown
Cayce's Diagnosis and Etiology: "In the nervous systems themselves do we find the greater disorder or distress. In times back we find there was an accident to the body that produced a lesion in the coccyx . . . lesions have resulted from same in the lower lumbar, in the lower dorsal . . . we find *sympathetic* lesions in the whole of the cervical region. This produces, through these pressures, those spasmodic conditions to the reaction between the sympathetic and the cerebrospinal system—which has been termed a *mental* disorder. The reaction is not mental, but a physical—that acts to, or on, the mental—so that the reflexes that come through the sympathetic system are those that prevent a normal impulse from their reaction, causing that pressure, that condition in the lower end of brain proper that makes for the tendency of the body to move, to react in a wondering manner, to make as for responses of those forces in self of first condemnation in self, then as of that as to *remove* those conditions from self. These come through, then, as repressions in first the sympathetic nerve system, from the lower lumbar plexus to the sacrals and coccyx, then to those activities in the glands themselves that secrete for the functioning through the pineal, and making for an engorgement and an inactivity or an ungoverning of the supply of impulse, as well as blood supply to the brain itself proper. Not dementia praecox, nor even softening of tissue. Unless these conditions are changed in the impulses to the nerve system this deterioration must eventually set in."
Cayce's Prognosis: "Do that, and we will bring—in three to six

months—a near normal body."
Treatment Suggested by Cayce:
1. Osteopathic adjustments
2. Mayblossom Bitters
3. Radio-Active Appliance
4. Diet (nerve-building foods)
5. As much sunshine as possible
6. Uplifting companionship
Treatment Results: Unknown
Comments: This is a good example of lower spinal injury producing psychotic symptoms. Note the presence of "sympathetic lesions" formed in response to the initial trauma. The correspondence from the man's mother is poignant and representative of the logistical problems involved in attempting to treat schizophrenia at home (e.g., oppositional behaviors by patient, lack of professional cooperation, discouragement, etc).

2614
Background: Female, 37 years old
Symptoms: Suicidal ideation, depression, obsessive/compulsive behaviors, hallucinations, social withdrawal, interpersonal problems
Medical Diagnosis: Unknown
Cayce's Diagnosis and Etiology: "These are the result of chemical and glandular reactions in the body; producing a deteriorating reaction in the nerve impulse. Thus the mental aberrations that appear, the hallucination as to lack of desire for associations and activities, faultfinding in self and in environs, as well as those about the body."
Cayce's Prognosis: "If these are allowed to progress they may bring a very detrimental condition—either that of possession or such a deteriorating as to become dementia praecox in its nature."
Treatment Suggested by Cayce:
1. Atomidine
2. Wet Cell with gold
3. Read Bible while lying down using Wet Cell
4. Keep in the open when practical
5. Congenial companionship
6. Practical application of biblical truths
Treatment Results: Unknown
Comments: Note the presence of depression which might lead to a

diagnosis of schizoaffective disorder, manic depressive psychosis, or psychotic depression by current criteria. This is a prime example of "nonspecificity" (see Chapter One) which was frequently the case where glandular dysfunction was the primary etiological factor. The fact that spinal adjustments were not suggested underlines the biochemical nature of the condition. The Atomidine was suggested because the glandular dysfunction was just beginning.

2744

Background: Female, 39 years old, institutionalized
Symptoms: Violent
Medical Diagnosis: Unknown
Cayce's Diagnosis and Etiology: The presenting symptom of skin eruptions was ascribed to prenatal influences (hereditary) which produced poor eliminations due primarily to liver and lymphatic dysfunction. The readings also noted insults resulting from childbirth. The woman's womb was out of position and pressures were noted in the lower spine (coccyx, sacral, and lumbar areas). Sympathetic lesions were then produced in the upper spine (cervicals?). " . . . there were and are pressures that exist from those happenings at the time of childbirth. This pressure upon the centers—the end of the spine and in the lumbar and sacral-ileum axis—has produced those tendencies for deterioration of nerve reflexes . . . It is true that unless there is the ability to relieve this pressure soon, there may be the necessity to give the body the vibratory metals—or the metallic reaction from gold—to aid the system in responding, for the nerves to the plasm in nerve tissue itself, AND to prevent softening or deterioration to brain cells. It is NOT a condition of brain tumors, though some of these MAY arise unless there is an even circulation of nerve impulse and blood supply builded in the body."
Cayce's Prognosis: "This depends entirely upon the response, you see, and as to how soon this [treatment] would begin."
Treatment Suggested by Cayce:
1. Change environment (move to Still-Hildreth)
2. Osteopathic treatments
3. "Leave off the sedatives"
4. Vibratory gold (appliance not stipulated)
5. Therapeutic milieu (positive attitudes of those around her)
Treatment Results: Unknown
Comments: This is a tremendously interesting and important case. Two readings were given for this woman at 25 years of age when she

had no mental symptoms and was functioning quite well. A third reading was given 14 years later when she was in an institution suffering from "insanity."

Note the diathesis/stress etiology in this case. "Prenatal" (hereditary) influences produced a tendency towards poor eliminations. Acquired vulnerability (child birthing difficulties) produced pressures on the spine which, combined with this tendency, resulted in mental symptoms. The process was leading to dementia praecox and possible brain tumors.

Also note the time span of about 14 years between somatic insult and onset of mental symptoms. This is consistent with the etiologies of many other readings on schizophrenia—childhood and adolescent spinal injuries which take a number of years to manifest in a major psychosis.

Cayce apparently foresaw this process in the early readings. In 2744-1, he stated " . . . there are those conditions more of which the body should be warned, and precautions should be taken in time concerning conditions apparent with the body, than that which gives such distress at the present [skin eruptions]. While there are those conditions that bring unpleasantness for the body, these are more of the secondary nature . . . these are not the greater conditions to be warned against . . . The age and the conditions are at that point where corrections need to be made . . . for these other existent conditions will only build that which later would bring detrimental effects to the body."

3662

Background: Female, 28 years old, poor premorbid functioning
Symptoms: Nervous, talkative, irritable, abusive, sexual dysfunction, suicidal, episodic violence
Medical Diagnosis: Manic-depressive psychosis
Cayce's Diagnosis and Etiology: " . . . there are disturbances pathological and psychological . . . there are pressures existing in the coccyx, and in the lower lumbar and sacral areas, that have prevented and that do prevent the normal closing of the lyden (Leydig?) gland in its activity through the body. Thus we have those periods when the body is averse to body-passion and again is as if being possessed by same, causing mental aberrations and imaginations, with the sensory system in its reflexes bringing an illness of whatever nature is indicated in any conversation about the body. These cause fears, dreads and such conditions throughout the body . . . This is posses-

sion, you see. But this comes and goes."

Cayce's Prognosis: "For unless proper corrections are made, there must eventually be caused a full possession or such a deterioration of the gray tissue or cell matter in the spinal cord as to set up deterioration in brain reflexes and reactions [dementia praecox] . . . Do these [the suggestions] and we will bring near to normal conditions for this body."

Treatment Suggested by Cayce:

1. Sympathetic companion (Christian nurse)
2. Therapeutic milieu (more open surroundings)
3. Spinal massage with electrical vibrator
4. Wet Cell Appliance with gold

Treatment Results: Her husband was called into military service and the treatments were not given.

Comments: "Q. Is there danger of suicide, as before? A. Not if we do these things. Without—well, the body is not responsible, as indicated. This is possession, you see. But this comes and goes." The possession was apparently episodic and not a total possession.

This may have been a case of "kundalini crisis" (see Appendix B) in which possession occurred when the Leydig gland was functioning. The pattern of lower spinal pressures affecting the glandular system (particularly the Leydig gland) was present.

Note the diagnosis of manic-depressive psychosis. This was probably due to the cyclical nature of the psychotic episodes ("waxing and waning") and may have been related to glandular cycles. The tendency for violence was common in such cases.

This case may represent a significant subgroup which is congruent with the diagnosis of schizoaffective by current psychiatric criteria. Note the similarities with cases [1513] and [1789] which responded well to treatment and had similar etiologies. The parallel with [1789] is particularly significant since the diagnosis in that case was manic depressive insanity and Cayce noted tendencies for possession. See Chapter Seven for a discussion of nonspecificity (regarding bipolar disorder).

The correspondence from her husband provides important information about premorbid functioning: "My mother-in-law told me that when my wife was 5 years old, she fell from a bridge on a bed of rocks, cutting the back of her head in such a way as to require several stitches. Subsequently she became very nervous and high strung. By the time she attended high school, she preferred studying to school activities, was unfriendly and had developed an antisocial attitude. During our courtship, she was an attractive, considerate young woman, yet withdrawn and moody at times. At the age of 27, she suffered a nervous breakdown, and became so violent that it was necessary to commit her to a sanitarium." She improved and was discharged 4/11/43. On 2/2/44 she relapsed and was in a sanitarium at the time of the reading.

4059

Background: Female, 57 years old, institutionalized at the time of the reading
Symptoms: Depression, weight loss, nervousness, skin blemishes
Medical Diagnosis: Manic depressive, chronic
Cayce's Diagnosis and Etiology: " . . . tendencies for inactivity of impulses from the central nervous system . . . it is the beginning of deterioration. These general conditions deal with the whole entity—body, mind and soul . . . the deterioration coming in the reflex reactions through the central nervous system. For these, in the present, are smoothing cells or indentations of the circulation in the reflexes of the brain." [dementia praecox]
Cayce's Prognosis: "We find that these may respond but much will depend upon the love, the care, the consistency and persistency with which the attendant or nurse would care for the body."
Treatment Suggested by Cayce:
1. Sympathetic nurse (companion)
2. Massage
3. Wet Cell with gold
4. Diet (normal with plenty of seafoods)
5. General activities in the open when possible
6. Keep good eliminations
Treatment Results: Treatments not given
Comments: The medical diagnosis of "manic depressive, chronic" relates directly to the comments regarding the previous case. Unfortunately, the reading for [4059] does not provide an etiology. The statement that "These general conditions deal with the whole entity—body, mind and soul" suggests that there may have been karmic involvement (i.e., genetic tendencies) in this case. The lack of suggestions for osteopathic or chiropractic treatments and the prescription for the Wet Cell with gold points to a biochemical dysfunction (probably glandular) as the prime etiological factor.

4186

Background: Male, adult

Symptoms: Nervousness, hallucinations, loss of appetite, incoherence

Medical Diagnosis: Unknown

Cayce's Diagnosis and Etiology: " . . . the abnormal conditions as we find them in this body have to do principally with the nervous system . . . There has been within this body an accident to the physical body itself, that with the fear of the condition that will bring this body to the end of justice, if done to the body that which would be justice to the body, until the weight of this on the mind has affected the whole nervous system." These combined factors led to abnormal kidney function and uremic poisoning. "The body is near to becoming in a state of dementia, which if allowed to go on will mean the destruction of the physical brain action of the mental and moral forces of this body. Not so much of physical action, but of the mental and moral forces."

Cayce's Prognosis: " . . . with consistent use of the medicinal properties taken into the system, restore to this body within 2 moons its normal condition and station in life."

Treatment Suggested by Cayce:

1. Medicine (tincture of valerian, bromide of potash, and elixir of calisaya)
2. Osteopathic adjustments
3. Hypnotic suggestions during osteopathic treatments

Treatment Results: Unknown

Comments: The presence of uremic poisoning is important in this case since kidney dialysis has proven effective in treating schizophrenia in certain cases (see Chapter One). Note that the etiology involves a combination of factors: acquired vulnerability (spinal injury) and mental stress (worry).

4333

Background: Female, adult, she was in a state hospital at the time of the reading; "she was a college graduate making a good salary when she got sick"

Symptoms: Unknown

Medical Diagnosis: Unknown

Cayce's Diagnosis and Etiology: " . . . overtaxation in the mental, with the physical in the state of taxation, the weakened condition then forms that pressure wherein incoordination occurs in the body

. . . cell force broken, came when there was discharged from the system that of the genitive system that is of the reproductive nature, and that in this taxation, then, we find these glands of reproduction that of the first cause . . . These glands are about the genitory system, and especially are these in that activity when the ovarine form . . . cast off their effulgence in its discharge from the system [menstruation]. The pressure, then, on account of the fall the body had in the sixth (6th) year that injured the spinal center near the lower lumbar and the sacral, produces a pressure in the overtaxed condition that produces reflexes in the pineal gland. Then we have these occurrences of the hallucinations, or the inability for the body to function normal."

Cayce's Prognosis: "Do not allow this to go so far as to produce the softening or the reaction in the center in brain from which coordinating radiation is made [dementia praecox] . . . [with treatment] within three to four moons, there will be found the *returning* of the full equilibrium in this body."

Treatment Suggested by Cayce:
1. Osteopathic treatments during periods of menstruation
2. Hydrotherapy during menstrual cycle (each day the body was to sit over earthen or crock container which contained 1 gallon of boiling water with 20 drops of tincture of myrrh, 40 drops of fluid extract of tolu, and 1 aloe; allow fumes to enter vagina)
3. Remove from present surroundings
4. "Keep the body where it will not harm self or others"
5. "Do not allow the body to remain alone too often or for too long" (companion)
6. "Keep the mind directed towards spiritual application of better things"

Treatment Results: Unknown

Comments: This case has many important etiological factors which are associated with dementia praecox. There was a spinal injury to the sacral and lumbar regions at age six which predisposed the body to problems in the reproductive system (i.e., acquired vulnerability). "Overtaxation in the mental" (i.e., psychological stress) combined with this condition to activate the pineal and produce psychotic symptoms (i.e., "hallucinations, or the inability for the body to function normal"). Violent tendencies were noted and the suggestion given to "Keep the body where it will not harm self or others"). The progressive nature of this syndrome was noted and caution given regarding softening of the brain.

The pattern of lower spinal injury affecting the reproductive glands resulting in chronic psychosis was common in the readings and was often associated with affective features similar to (and perhaps identical to) the symptoms of schizoaffective disorder. Manic psychosis was often present with violent or self-destructive tendencies. There was often a "waxing and waning" of symptoms which may have been related to glandular involvement. Pineal involvement in pathological cases such as this resembled a condition currently referred to as "kundalini crisis," or an opening of the person to universal forces and the possibility of florid psychosis (see Appendix B).

5228

Background: Male, 31 years old; he had a nervous breakdown in high school
Symptoms: Doesn't speak, abnormal behavior
Medical Diagnosis: Hebephrenic dementia praecox, mute form
Cayce's Diagnosis and Etiology: "Such violent reactions have existed until they brought that dissociation or short circuit in the areas between the cerebrospinal and sympathetic nervous systems, both in those areas in lumbar axis and in the brachial centers, here, or a violent nervous breakdown by overtaxing and more from worry about those things which were 'not too good to think about.' "
Cayce's Prognosis: None given
Treatment Suggested by Cayce:
1. Wet Cell with gold
2. Neuropathic massage to base of brain and spine
Treatment Results: Treatment not provided
Comments: This may have been a case of stress-induced somatic dysfunction which was moving toward dementia praecox. "Here are those conditions which if neglected will lead to such poor reflexes from brain to activities of the inferior muscles of the locomotories as to bring about dementia praecox, or such softening of reflexes as for there to be little effect of the gray matter impulse indicated in thought, or activity, either voluntary or involuntary."

5715

Background: Male, "in his 20s"
Symptoms: Unknown
Medical Diagnosis: Unknown
Cayce's Diagnosis and Etiology: " . . . there are distresses caused in

the coordination of the sympathetic and cerebrospinal nerve system, produced by *pressure* in the lumbar and sacral region, which prevents that proper reaction as should come with the activities of the pineal gland and the lyden [Leydig] gland, through the medulla oblongata to the brain . . . will these be taken in time, before the pressure produces the softening of the brain tissue itself; until there is dementia in its reaction."

Cayce's Prognosis: "Will the body respond, it should be brought to normal, should this be taken in time."

Treatment Suggested by Cayce:
1. Osteopathic manipulations
2. Wet Cell with gold
3. Additional gold taken orally
4. Diet (blood and nerve building with balance between potashes and iodines)
5. Put him in state institution
6. Medicine (bromides to quiet body)
7. Cleansing of throat

Treatment Results: Not known

Comments: Here again is the typical pattern of pressures on lower spine affecting the glands (Leydig and pineal) leading to dementia praecox. This man must have been violent and uncontrollable since the readings suggested bromides to quiet him. This suggestion points out the flexibility of the readings when dealing with an acute case.

Group III: Schizophrenic Psychosis

300

Background: Male, 35 years old; he had been ten years in a state hospital at the time of the reading, his mother died early, alcoholic father, "concentrated" early religious training, he had suffered a head injury resulting from an elevator accident (date unknown)

Symptoms: Delusions (religious and grandiose), lack of motivation, cognitive deficits, interpersonal conflicts

Medical Diagnosis: Unknown

Cayce's Diagnosis and Etiology: " . . . from a metaphysical as well as some particular conditions the case might be better understood; and in particular offer an opportunity or channel for the study of deeper or reincarnated influences, that go for the hereditary and environmental influence . . . Then, having been an entity, a body (in

the present) with those surroundings or environs that brought about the warping of the instinct and intelligency of the active forces that coordinate with the imaginative and the material influences, we find an incoordination between the mental images as builded by the body and those that are able to be raised from the invisible to the visible as manifesting in a material plane . . . the abilities to co-ordinate the mental from the activities visible to material conditions or aids are almost nil . . . Or, there is little of the first impulse that are towards normalcy; that is, of self-preservation. To go into the patho-logical conditions for the moment, then, that they may be better understood, these are lacking in those centers along the sympa-thetic and cerebrospinal where there are the coordinations between the impulse and the stamen that cares for the abilities to carry on in a given line or direction."
Cayce's Prognosis: Not provided
Treatment Suggested by Cayce:
1. Suggestive therapeutics
2. "Suggestive magnetic treatments"
Treatment Results: Good results were obtained, this man was re-leased from the hospital and was living in Cleveland, Ohio, at last report (1960).
Comments: This is an important case, not only because of the good results, but because of the etiology. One must remember that the readings stated that entities have a choice of parents in the incarna-tion process. The fact that this entity chose such a dismal environ-ment suggests a "karmic" aspect to this case ("metaphysical" or "reincarnated influences"). The magnetic treatments were appar-ently recommended to remedy a deficiency in the sympathetic gan-glia. Treatment would result in better coordination between ANS and CNS (i.e., mind and body). The suggestive therapeutics (i.e., hypnotic suggestions) may have stimulated the "inner self" to insti-gate and maintain the healing process.

1310
Background: Female, 59 years old; she was located in an "insane asylum" at the time of the reading
Symptoms: Melancholic, almost comatose at times, loss of moti-vation
Medical Diagnosis: Unknown
Cayce's Diagnosis and Etiology: " . . . there is a weakening of the reflex actions from the central nerve system to the brain forces, and

the reflexes along the sympathetic or vegetative nerve system . . . These have been, as we find, brought about by nerve strain, anxiety, and a weakened constitution; especially in affectations through the glandular system and that which produces through same the replenishing of tissue for activity in the nerve force which carries the impulses to and from brain's reaction."

Cayce's Prognosis: "But if there is the change seen, then the more hopefulness being held, the greater the change may be."

Treatment Suggested by Cayce:
1. Wet Cell with gold
2. Oral administration of chloride of gold and bromide of soda
3. Massage
4. Suggestive therapeutics
5. Take her home

Treatment Results: The treatments not given—she was taken home and some improvement was noted in her general attitude.

Comments: This appears to have been a case of chronic schizophrenia with an etiology of mental stress producing glandular dysfunction leading to weakened nervous system and improper neurotransmission in the brain. The affective features point to schizoaffective by current diagnostic criteria.

1428

Background: Male, 30 years old
Symptoms: Delusions
Medical Diagnosis: Dementia praecox
Cayce's Diagnosis and Etiology: "In the bodily functions there have been those effects of activities to allay an infection that acted upon the organs of the body as related to the higher or the more emotional nervous systems and forces of the body through the genitive system. These with pressures, while the conditions have allayed or eliminated, pressures left in the coccyx, the lumbar and lower dorsal area, continue to make for the effect of these highly active forces upon the system. These are rather from the serums and the medicines taken, rather than the dis-ease or disturbance itself. This, then, is not a true dementia praecox condition. While there is incoordination between the cerebrospinal and the sympathetic nervous system, this arises rather from the conditions that have been indicated."

Cayce's Prognosis: "This would be done for at least thirty days. Then a rest period of two to three weeks, then AGAIN these applied.

And we will find, in this manner, we may bring the better conditions for this body."
Treatment Suggested by Cayce:
1. Chiropractic adjustments
2. Wet Cell Appliance
3. Massage, especially over abdominal area
4. Constructive, prayerful attitude by significant others
Treatment Results: Unknown
Comments: This would appear to be a case of medicinally induced somatic dysfunction resulting in psychosis. The possibility of viral involvement is interesting since some researchers believe a seasonal virus may be an etiological factor in schizophrenia.

1513

Background: Male, 47 years old; he was in Rockland State Hospital, New York, at the time of the reading
Symptoms: Unknown
Medical Diagnosis: "Insanity"
Cayce's Diagnosis and Etiology: "For through pressures upon nerve energies in the coccyx area and the ileum plexus, as well as that pressure upon the lumbar axis, there has been a deflection of coordination between the sympathetic and the cerebrospinal nervous system . . . Q. What was the original cause, or what produced this condition? A. A fall on the ice, injuring the coccyx end of the spine. Q. What caused the original pains in the head? A. Reflexes from those injuries to the pressures made upon the pineal centers."
Cayce's Prognosis: "It will require at least sixty to ninety days."
Treatment Suggested by Cayce:
1. Osteopathic adjustments
2. Wet Cell Appliance with gold
3. Exercise, "in the open . . . but NEVER alone."
4. Service to others
5. Suggestive therapeutics during treatments
6. Keep the body-mind active in constructive thinking
Treatment Results: An excellent recovery was noted.
Comments: Correspondence in this case states, "Mr. [1513] had a nervous breakdown while in the Postal Service from overwork, or so the doctors stated." The reading cites an injury to the lower spine as the cause of the condition. [1513] confirmed that he had fallen on ice some years ago. The initial reading in this case stated that [1513] would relapse when he realized that there was an improbability of

his being restored to active service.

The etiology of lower spinal injury affecting the pineal was often associated with a waxing and waning of symptoms, with the probability of florid psychosis during the acute episodes (see reading 294-141 in Appendix B for a discussion of pressures upon the pineal). The osteopathic manipulations were supposed to stimulate "the ganglia especially in all areas of the brush end of the cerebrospinal system; to prevent same forming or producing clogging again in the system."

No diagnosis was provided in this file and it is difficult to guess how it might be diagnosed by current criteria (perhaps schizophreniform, atypical psychosis, or brief reactive psychosis). Since the readings indicate a high probability of relapse and chronic course (without treatment), this case is included as late-onset schizophrenia (see Harris & Jeste, 1988). Case [3641] provides an interesting parallel to [1513] since that case also involved lower spinal injury which was produced by a fall on ice—the injury occurred much earlier in life and produced a chronic course that matched the "schizophrenic pattern" more closely.

1572

Background: Female, 50 years old
Symptoms: Insomnia, hallucinations
Medical Diagnosis: Unknown
Cayce's Diagnosis and Etiology: "As has been indicated, much of the disturbance is the incoordination between the cerebrospinal nervous system and the sympathetic nervous system, or vegetative nerve system. Hence pressures are indicated in the lumbar and the lower dorsal area. These are the areas, then, with the brush end of the cerebrospinal system and the plexus of the lower portion of the abdomen, to produce the convulsions in the activities when the body attempts to rest, or often when the body begins to lose consciousness in sleep. Such disturbances are produced as to excite the activities of the glandular forces as related to the plexus at the pubic bone itself. Thus a great disturbance is caused through the activity of the organs of the pelvis . . . this is the incoordination between the cerebrospinal and the sympathetic nervous system. And as the glandular system is affected as related to the genitive system, and especially affecting directly the center above the puba, there is produced—with the toxic forces in the system—this burning, and the EFFECT of POSSESSION!"

Cayce's Prognosis: "Do these things and we will bring the better conditions for this body."

Treatment Suggested by Cayce:

1. Russian white oil and enemas
2. Spinal massage with electric vibrator
3. Violet Ray treatment
4. Diet suggestions

Treatment Results: Unknown

Comments: Remarks by [1572] before the reading states: "Been troubled this way a long time, gradually getting worse—and unbearable; come here as last resort." She felt a "power" take possession of her, and was bothered with tiny images like tiny dwarfs crawling all over her; she couldn't rest. At night when she should be sleeping, or resting from sleep, she had terrible experiences while asleep—felt that she was a man and wandering in search of someone with whom to gratify sex desires. "My trouble is witchcraft . . . When they put this power on one, he can do what he wants to. This is why I came to you. I thought you could help me to get rid of it—this thing on the inside of the abdomen and it is same as a man."

The pattern of lower spinal pressures affecting the genital glands was present in this case. The disorder was apparently triggered by menopause. The chronic course of the condition with bizarre hallucinations and delusions would likely be diagnosed as schizophrenia by current criteria.

1789

Background: Female, 32 years old; she was an artist and was apparently attacked while showing her artwork, she was in a state hospital at the time of the reading

Symptoms: Hallucinations, irrationality, amnesia, hysteria, "She tore a mattress half in two once she got her finger nails into the cloths. She was absolutely a wild maniac."

Medical Diagnosis: Manic depressive insanity

Cayce's Diagnosis and Etiology: This woman was attacked and "in the attempt to escape, and finding self trapped, as it were, the physical exercise and activity in the attempt shattered the connection between the cerebrospinal and sympathetic system; especially in the coccyx and lumbar areas. Losing consciousness the entity became a prey to those suggestive forces as were acted upon, and by the injection of outside forces to keep that hidden as attempted upon the body [hypnosis?]. Then, in its present environs, there have been only moments of rationality; and then NO one to respond brought greater and still greater depression to the better self."

Cayce's Prognosis: "[following the suggestions] The body then should be able, physically and mentally, to return to regular activities."

Treatment Suggested by Cayce:

1. Constant companion
2. Osteopathic adjustments
3. Diet: nerve-building foods
4. Wet Cell Appliance with gold
5. Change in environment (from state institution)
6. Prayer for patient
7. Activity in open air (not in city, but in country)
8. Artistic activities as condition improves
9. Become more socially active
10. Study Bible
11. Massage
12. Attitude toward others (helpfulness and hopefulness)
13. Diet (normal)
14. Eliminations (keep normal)

Treatment Results: An excellent recovery was produced after many months of treatment.

Comments: This is a good case for study for anyone interested in applying this approach since it contains many readings, wide range of therapeutic modalities, persistent application of the suggestions, and excellent results.

It is difficult to guess how this person would be diagnosed by current criteria. She would no doubt be heavily medicated. There was apparently a waxing and waning of symptoms with periods of near normal functioning. This episodic course no doubt produced the diagnosis of manic depressive insanity. The presence of violent mania is also noteworthy in this regard. The prevalence of psychosis might lead to a diagnosis of schizoaffective by current criteria.

The reference to possession in reading 1789-1 suggests that she was near to having a dissociation of the mental, spiritual, and physical bodies. "The beauty of this soul, its abilities as a creative influence in the lives of those who may bring it back as it were from the very borderland, is worth all the effort ... Such is so near possession that there needs to be great care taken." The pattern of lower spinal injury producing insanity and possession was often cited in the readings as leading to dementia praecox.

1969

Background: Male, 38 years old; he was in a state hospital at the time of the reading

Symptoms: Unknown

Medical Diagnosis: Unknown

Cayce's Diagnosis and Etiology: "For here we have a condition that is as much POSSESSION as a weakening of the nerve forces in the system; and the general nerve breakdown will NOT be eliminated by the administering of drugs nor by the mere activity of suppression... For it is as a split personality in the present, with the reflexes forming that which has been indicated—that causes the incoordination in the mental and spiritual and physical forces of this body."

Cayce's Prognosis: "Yet this may be materially aided, if it is taken in time to use suggestive therapeutics combined with a very low form of electrical vibration."

Treatment Suggested by Cayce:

1. Violet Ray
2. Suggestive therapeutics (hypnosis)
3. Injections of liver extracts
4. Therapeutic milieu

Treatment Results: Unknown

Comments: This man had a life reading (1969-2) after the physical reading (1969-1) which suggested a karmic basis for his problems. "Then the entity was in the name of Randall Campbell, bringing in that experience the disturbing forces which in the present are finding expression in the madness within self—as an activity upon the forces in the brain's activity upon the emotions of the body-force. Thus there may be applied the suggestive forces in putting the consciousness into that position where the awareness of the subconscious force may become a part of the consciousness, and thus maintain a better equilibrium of the flow of activity of the impulses to the supersensitive forces of the body-force itself; bringing then, through such subjugation, the awareness of itself, its condition, its needs and its desires. Then, keep the entity as far as possible from that which mitigates or subjugates the body-forces with the spiritual influences—or from sedatives or bromides. For these will only add to the confusion of the reactions as were indicated in Randall's life."

This excerpt seems to suggest that sedatives and bromides can lead to possession in such cases. It is not entirely clear whether possession in this case involves discarnate entities or past-life personalities which are bleeding into the present experience. The reading does mention a "weakening of the nerve forces in the system," a process associated with the process of dementia praecox and discarnate possession. Although the recommendation of formal hypnosis in cases of discarnate possession was common, the suggestion in this case appears to refer to past-life regression—a highly unusual therapeutic technique in the readings. Cayce actually used one of [1969]'s past-life names (Randall) to refer to him in the reading. [1969]'s past life as Randall apparently was a strong influence on his current experience.

2197

Background: Female, adult; she was in an "insane hospital" at the time of the reading

Symptoms: Depression, hallucinations, suicidal

Medical Diagnosis: Unknown

Cayce's Diagnosis and Etiology: " . . . with this body the physical is very good throughout. There is in the physical those obstructions to the indentations of the action of the nerve system that produces aberrations and hallucinations in the manifestations of the mental, and the physical becomes abased with these conditions . . . The nerve systems in the physical we find that depression first caused in the lyden [Leydig] gland that pressed, or indentations made on the perineurial and the pineal nerve center connecting with the lyden [Leydig] gland. This then gives the hallucinations in the vibration to the brain center or through the cerebellum oblongata [medulla oblongata?], you see. In the impression as this receives, there comes those conditions of melancholia, of self-destructive forces, of aberrations of depression as received and hallucinations to all the functioning of the sensory organism, through which these nerve connections find manifestations with the pineal nerve in its course through the system."

Cayce's Prognosis: "[With the treatments], the physical may be brought to the normal functioning."

Treatment Suggested by Cayce:

1. Surgery to remove "glands in the pelvic organs of gentation [genitation]"

Treatment Results: Unknown

Comments: This case may have involved "kundalini crisis" (see Appendix B) since the injury to the pelvic organs had activated the Leydig and pineal centers producing florid psychosis with strong affective components. This case might be diagnosed as psychotic depression or schizoaffective by current criteria. See case [886] for similar etiology and treatment suggestions.

2465

Background: Female, 28years old; she was institutionalized at the time of the reading
Symptoms: Unknown
Medical Diagnosis: Unknown
Cayce's Diagnosis and Etiology: "There has been a lesion in the lacteal duct and that as coordinating with the organs of the pelvis . . . Hence at times such a state is produced as to almost become an obsession, but possession in same. The reaction to the pineal becomes so severe as to short-circuit the nerve impulse; carrying or producing a fluttering or an engorgement in static waves to the base of the brain. Thus periods are caused when there is lack of self-control."
Cayce's Prognosis: "Q. May she be brought to normal in mind and body? A. As we find, near to normal; and entirely so if PERSISTENCY is kept up."
Treatment Suggested by Cayce:
1. Bring home from institution
2. Provide constant companion
3. Castor oil packs over lacteal duct and the caecum area
4. Massage
5. Chiropractic or osteopathic adjustment
6. Dry cell battery and chloride of gold
Treatment Results: There apparently was improvement due to application of the suggestions. See the records of Dr. Phillips in this file.
Comments: The etiology in this case sounds similar to some of the readings given by Cayce on epilepsy (i.e., lesion in lacteal ducts, loss of self-control, and tendency for possession). The involvement of the pelvic organs producing an engorgement of the pineal is a common pattern in the readings on schizophrenia. See the discussion of "schizophrenic epilepsy" in Chapter Seven (i.e., nonspecificity).

2712

Background: Female, 22 years old; she was in a "mental hospital" at the time of the reading, onset of symptoms at about age 18
Symptoms: Unknown
Medical Diagnosis: Unknown
Cayce's Diagnosis and Etiology: " . . . this is a condition—under the nerve strain, and with those great expectations in the body-mind

development, and then receiving a shock—there was caused disassociation in the mental forces of the body. Thus there was produced inharmony between the cerebrospinal and the sympathetic impulses of the body. Hence a condition of a pathological nature was produced in which there was nerve deterioration, or in which the brain cell activity was disturbed in its associations—or the harmony was disturbed . . . most of the centers along the cerebrospinal system—where there is the closer association of the ganglia of the sympathetic AND cerebrospinal connections—show knots or lesions of a form . . . those indicated in the 2nd, 3rd and 4th cervicals, in the 2nd, 3rd, 4th and 5th dorsals, 9th dorsal and throughout the sacral area . . . Q. What caused this shock, or what was the nature of it? A. An unexpected disappointment, and a fear of individuals."
Cayce's Prognosis: " . . . normalcy mentally and physically, may be brought to this body, if these influences will be consistently kept about this body."
Treatment Suggested by Cayce:
1. Change environment (therapeutic milieu)
2. Companion
3. Osteopathic treatments
4. Wet Cell with gold
5. Prayer and meditation
6. Color therapy
7. Music therapy
Treatment Results: Unknown
Comments: This case fits the "schizophrenic pattern" in many respects: the age of onset at about 18 years old, a high level of psychosocial stress (i.e., *expressed emotion*), a stressful life event ("shock caused by disappointment and fear of individuals), an episodic pattern of breakdowns, etc.
    The seriousness of this case is apparent in the suggestion for a constant companion, the use of the Wet Cell with gold (nerve cell deterioration was noted), the large number of lesions cited, and the dissociation of the mental and physical forces of the body. It is likely that the lesions had a psychosomatic etiology since the readings frequently stated that mental stress could cause lesions in the nervous system and, in this case, the numerous lesions were described as "tensions along the spinal system." There are two important implications for a psychosomatic etiology: (1) the lesions may not show up on an X-ray or chiropractic examination oriented towards subluxations and (2) the treatment would have to address the

psychological nature of the pathology.

2721

Background: Female, 18 years old, good premorbid functioning until age 16 when she had a breakdown; she was in a mental institution at the time of the reading

Symptoms: Her mother's letter states: "she is listless, restless, won't or can't talk. The doctors can find no defect in her body . . . " A subsequent assessment was provided at the Still-Hildreth Sanatorium and is included verbatim since such detailed clinical observations are rare in these cases: "The patient presents a morbid detachment and inaccessibility. The attention is occupied with a practically impenetrable reverie of random phantasy. No satisfactory discussion of her experiences is obtainable and there is mainly absence of response to questions. Alert and understanding cooperation is lacking and the execution of simple requests often ignored. There is mute indifference or an occasional mumbled and indistinct remark which has no apparent connection with immediate realities. The level of consciousness is insufficient to maintain adequate awareness and all sensibilities are in a measure clouded. Emotional reactions are impoverished. Personal needs are neglected and soiling of clothing at times occurs. There are dully delusional interpretations. The problem represents a well-established dissociation of schizophrenic type."

Medical Diagnosis: Schizophrenia

Cayce's Diagnosis and Etiology: "We find that in the beginning, a pressure in the coccyx end of the spine, combined with a delayed activity in the glandular system as related to the menstrual flow, caused these nerve pressures—in the lumbar axis, in the 9th dorsal, and the pressures upon the adrenals that hinder the glands which control the emotional forces of the body as to the secondary or sensory system . . . There has not been the destruction entirely of the normal reflexes between the sensory and the sympathetic or imaginative system AND the central or cerebrospinal system [dementia praecox] . . . Q. What was the original cause of her condition? A. An injury to the coccyx from a fall when only about three-and-a-half to four years old." Drugs (sedatives) had aggravated the condition by hindering the assimilative and eliminative systems.

Cayce's Prognosis: "We find that we may bring help if there will be the changing of the body to those environs such as in Macon, Missouri [Still-Hildreth] . . . "

Treatment Suggested by Cayce:
1. Refer to Still-Hildreth Sanatorium (therapeutic milieu)
2. Osteopathic treatments
3. Wet Cell Appliance with gold
4. Massage

Treatment Results: Improvement was noted in reading 2721-2 and subsequent correspondence with Still-Hildreth Sanatorium.

Comments: Since there was a preponderance of "negative symptoms" (withdrawal, emotional flatness, etc.), she would probably not respond well to drug therapy and would be regarded as chronic schizophrenic by current standards. Note the early spinal injury and the resultant problems in glandular development. This might be a typical pattern in many schizophrenic cases—childhood spinal injury affecting the glandular system during puberty resulting in psychosis during the late teenage years. The detailed clinical assessment is significant in this case since the etiology is clearly stated in the readings. This apparent correlation between etiology (i.e., childhood spinal injury with later glandular dysfunction) and well-defined schizophrenic process is important since many of the readings given for persons suffering from schizophrenia had similar etiologies.

2967

Background: Male, 27 years old, mental problems started at about 23 years of age; he was in a state hospital at the time of the reading

Symptoms: Social withdrawal

Medical Diagnosis: Schizophrenia

Cayce's Diagnosis and Etiology: Original cause of the illness was "lack of those elements in the system that cause the coordination between the areas about the lacteals." A long-standing condition produced depletion of fibrin in the nerve impulses resulting in incoordination among cerebrospinal, sensory, and autonomic nerve systems.

Treatment Suggested by Cayce:
1. Wet Cell Appliance with gold
2. Massage
3. Companion

Treatment Results: Some improvement noted before the patient became oppositional and noncompliant—he ran away from the companion, hid in someone's house, and had to be taken home.

Comments: There were no spinal injuries noted and no suggestions for osteopathic adjustments. The problem may have been primarily biochemical, resulting from inadequate assimilations and affecting neurotransmission. Lacteal dysfunction was often cited by Cayce in cases of epilepsy, although there was no mention of epileptic symptoms in this case (see Chapter Seven for a discussion of the overlap between schizophrenia and epilepsy).

3075

Background: Male, 24 years old; he suffered a breakdown at age 13, "He couldn't sleep and went completely to pieces, mentally. He seemed to have hallucinations, couldn't stop singing." He was placed in a sanitarium and his illness was marked by episodic relapses during the years. He had a twin brother who was normal.

Symptoms: Hallucinations, paranoid delusions, "obsessed with girls (although he has not had close contact with any)," depression

Medical Diagnosis: Unknown

Cayce's Diagnosis and Etiology: "As we find, the conditions that disturb this body are as much of a psychological nature as of a pathological nature. Pathologically, these would have to do with conditions which existed during the period of gestation. Psychologically, these have to do with the karma of this body, and those responsible for the physical body. Hence we have here conditions that at times approach near to that of possession of the mind by external influences, or that very close to the spiritual possession by discarnate forces. To be sure, these interpretations would not be accepted by some as an explanation. And yet there will come those days when many will understand and interpret properly . . . Owing to those conditions which existed in the manner in which coordination is established in the physical reactions between impressions received through sensory system and the reaction upon the reflexes of brain, we find these at times become very much disassociated. And those impressions received sympathetically, or through vision, through hearing, through sensing by impressions, become the motivative force in the reaction. At such times possession near takes place. With the capsule of the inner brain itself, these cause distortions, the associations with not the normal reflexes but with the impressions received in the suggestive forces."

Cayce's Prognosis: "Hence, as we find, with patience these may be materially aided."

Treatment Suggested by Cayce:
1. Hypnosis

2. Hand-held machine (Violet Ray)
3. Spinal massage
4. Association with nature (but not animals, "close to the soil, and that necessarily would be away from cities")
Treatment Results: Unknown
Comments: "The character of the [reflexes] will depend much upon the type of suggestion that will be made while under the influence of another mind. We find that the body WILL respond, and it may be directed into any of those channels that may aid the body in becoming a useful, dependable citizen, and a helpful influence with others." Hypnosis and the Violet Ray were often suggested in cases which Cayce diagnosed as possession. The electrical vibrations of the Violet Ray were said to drive out the discarnate entities (see Appendix E).

The etiology in this case is unusual: karmic factors influencing the gestation process manifesting as incoordination in the nervous systems, particularly in the brain. In light of the research indicating a high concordance rate for schizophrenia between twins, it is interesting that a twin brother was normal.

3087

Background: Female, 25 years old
Symptoms: Unknown
Medical Diagnosis: Unknown
Cayce's Diagnosis and Etiology: "In the nerve forces of the body— this inability of coordination with the mental and physical self arises from those subluxations which exist in the sacral and lumbar area, causing a lesion in the lower dorsal and the 3rd cervical. This suppression of energies has caused the functionings of the pelvic organs to act in those manners in which there is a suppression of the glandular forces, as related to those conditions which disturb, through the inability of proper coordination the tubes and the ovaries themselves. Thus we have a suppression that arises from the supplying of energies to the activity of these organs. Thus we get those reflex reactions to the sympathetic and cerebrospinal system, as to produce the lack of coordination between the mental—or the reasoning self—and the physical self in the body."
Cayce's Prognosis: "This done, we will find bettered conditions coming for this body, and the mental and physical reactions attaining more to normal conditions."
Treatment Suggested by Cayce:

1. Osteopathic adjustments
2. Dry cell appliance with gold
Treatment Results: The mother could not afford the battery and the treatments were not given.
Comments: This young woman was apparently in the early stages of schizophrenia at the time of the reading and was subsequently sent to a state hospital. The last correspondence in this case (1948) was five years after the reading and she was still in the state hospital; doctors there described her condition as a case of "split-mind," a term congruent with Bleuler's definition of schizophrenia. The pattern of spinal injury (particularly in the lower areas) affecting the glandular system (pelvic organs) resulting in incoordination of the nervous systems was present in this case.

3158

Background: Male, 37 years old; he had a history of nervous break-downs, onset of symptoms began at age 13
Symptoms: Delusions, religious obsessions, anxiety, self-condemnation, obsessive/compulsive tendencies
Medical Diagnosis: Unknown
Cayce's Diagnosis and Etiology: " . . . here we have a lesion in the brain centers. This causes not only these spells of lapse of control of the body but the inability for the body to control itself in an emotional manner. This is a karmic condition . . . These as we find are between sympathetic and cerebrospinal nervous centers. Hence oft the things the body would do seem apparently unable to reach the consciousness. Things the body in itself promises not to do, it does. The voluntary and involuntary reaction or impulse, as carried in the white and gray matter of the nervous systems, tends in certain centers to run together and become confusing to the body."
Cayce's Prognosis: "This is a karmic condition. While the body might be benefited, it would require long, persistent and consistent effort on the part of some very loving, very careful individual."
Treatment Suggested by Cayce:
1. Osteopathic corrections
2. Wet Cell Appliance carrying gold
3. Violet Ray
4. Massage
Treatment Results: Treatment was provided and improvement noted: " . . . he is much improved. His mental attitude is much better and he is working harder to help himself, so we are encouraged to

expect that he will soon be strong in mind & body . . . [3158] is much improved now, and I am very thankful to all who may have helped him in any way."
Comments: In a check reading these questions were asked: "Q. Any improvement in the brain condition? A. It's the reflexes from the brain that need improvement, for it is not the brain itself deteriorating, but the medulla oblongata reflexes in the brain forces, in the central portion of the brain cells [limbic region?] . . . Q. Why does his mind seem to run down when he's reclining? A. The inability of the flow. For when he is up—It's to be considered as to the difference between animal magnetism and man. He is supposed to stand upright as a man. When he's down, there's possession. Q. In what way is his condition karmic? From this life or another? A. From what he has brought from other experiences that he meted to others." The recommendation for the Violet Ray was common in cases of possession.

3163

Background: Female, 42 years old
Symptoms: Cognitive deficits, "mental aberrations"
Medical Diagnosis: Unknown
Cayce's Diagnosis and Etiology: " . . . these are more mental aberrations, or lack of coordination between the cerebrospinal and the sympathetic nervous systems. These come from a condition existent when very young . . . For, as we find, the disturbances are in the nerve ends of the coccyx area; and the reactions are confusion, with the inability of the body to coordinate the impulses received from instructions by others or to apply that obtained by impressions received through the sensory activities. Not an imbecile, not lesions in the brain; though there is a very smooth reaction [dementia praecox?] in the reflexes in brain centers . . . But these nerves [at the coccyx] will necessarily have to be straightened; that is, as it were, will have to be straightened where the pressures have been produced from an injury to the end of the spine. Don't remove it [surgery], but DO make those changes so that there is not a short circuiting in the impulses from the brush end of the spine to the nerves of the lower portion of the sympathetic system."
Cayce's Prognosis: "As to whether this may be entirely corrected at this late date, will depend upon the persistency with which administrations may be made for the body."
Treatment Suggested by Cayce:

1. Wet Cell with gold
2. Osteopathic corrections
3. Patience

Treatment Results: Unknown

Comments: This appears to be a case of chronic schizophrenia resulting from a spinal injury during childhood. The injury was to the coccyx and produced an incoordination between the CNS and ANS. Since this was a long-standing condition, the readings note the difficulty in achieving recovery and insist upon patience and persistence in applying the suggestions. This may have been a case of dementia praecox since the reading describes a very smooth reaction in the brain centers—a description often used in dementia cases.

3181

Background: Male, 40 years old; he was in a state hospital at the time of the reading and had a long history of mental illness

Symptoms: Hallucinations, anxiety

Medical Diagnosis: Unknown

Cayce's Diagnosis and Etiology: "Suppressions—as we find are the sources, bases of the conditions. These are of such a nature as to cause an undulating condition in the normalcy, and in the opposites in the reflexes in the mind. We find that these are from pressures that have existed in times back, and then the aggravations produced in the mental environ of the body [state hospital] . . . Q. Is his condition the result of frustration with respect to the solution of personal problems? A. This only accentuated it. As indicated, these conditions arise from pressures upon the connecting chords between cerebrospinal and sympathetic system; especially in the coccyx area. The conditions affecting sympathetics [personal problems] caused frustration. The tendency towards the less of the use of return impulses in the nerve system, or a short circuit between impulses and personal activity. Hence hallucinations."

Cayce's Prognosis: "Do these things and we will make better conditions for this body."

Treatment Suggested by Cayce:
1. Osteopathic corrections
2. Wet Cell with gold

Treatment Results: The treatments were given and a slight improvement was noted.

Comments: This appears to be another case of lower spinal injury producing chronic schizophrenia. The effects of psychosocial stressors are noted in the reading and represent a significant etiological factor in this case. This man apparently had many horrible experiences in the various mental institutions in which he was confined; "the worst one being an experience with Metrozol which left him with a badly mangled arm so he is always frightened and upset over the idea of more treatments" (sister's correspondence).

3223

Background: Male, 31 years old; onset of illness at about age 21
Symptoms: Unknown
Medical Diagnosis: Unknown
Cayce's Diagnosis and Etiology: "Now, as we find, there are disturbances which prevent the normal reactions between the sympathetic and cerebrospinal nervous systems. The injury to the spine, in the coccyx area that happened some time ago has destroyed those connections and coordinating centers in two particular areas . . . Q. Was this injury referred to a result of the bicycle accident years ago? A. On the end of the spine and the lumbar center. This naturally caused the segment in the third cervical also to be destroyed."
Cayce's Prognosis: "We find that these conditions may be materially aided. For, in most other respects, the body is very good . . . These as we find should bring better conditions for this body . . . Beginning with the second series of these treatments we should find helpful forces for the body."
Treatment Suggested by Cayce:
1. Cease treatment with sedatives
2. Osteopathic corrections
3. Use Bromidia after osteopathic adjustments
4. Wet Cell with gold solution
5. Massage
6. Keep in the open quite often
7. Keep the body active at some definite activity
8. Diet (few meats—use seafoods, especially oysters)
Treatment Results: Unknown
Comments: This appears to be another case of spinal injury producing an incoordination between the CNS and ANS resulting in psychosis in early adulthood. The correspondence from his sister is interesting since it provides information on prodromal functioning and onset of symptoms. "He became mentally troubled about 10 years ago [age 21], shortly after he had an accident on his bicycle. He did bruise his head and body rather badly then, but doctors have

not been able to find anything physically wrong with him—he sometimes complains of headaches. You can imagine what a great sorrow this has been to my poor mother and father, who have watched this happen and have been unable to help him. The doctors have pronounced him harmless and as far as they know helpless. It is such a terrible pity that he has to be so afflicted, for as I remember him before he changed he was a lovely, kind, talented young man. He attended . . . Institute of Art and planned to teach art and planned to teach fine arts here—we have even now many beautiful drawings that he made before he changed."

The reference to him being harmless is interesting since the reading notes that if he responds to treatment, some violent behavior may manifest and precautions should be taken. This pattern is mentioned in several cases where the patient exhibits a preponderance of negative symptoms (i.e., social withdrawal, cognitive deficits, flat affect, etc.) before treatment but may become more animated with treatment. The readings usually regarded this as a positive sign and a transitory stage in the recovery process.

Also note the reference to destruction of white matter in the cerebrospinal system which was exacerbated by the use of medications.

3421

Background: Female, 39 years old, theosophist; "she's had this problem for 23 years" (onset at about age 16)

Symptoms: Insomnia (only 1-3 hours of sleep each night), she was awakened by a "creature" that "tears my body to pieces unless I keep moving and exercising, the reaction of my nerves is maddening," she had been to many doctors who were unable to help

Medical Diagnosis: Unknown

Cayce's Diagnosis and Etiology: " . . . the pathological [subluxations in hip and coccyx] as well as psychological conditions must be considered with the mental conditions of the body. We find there has been the opening of the lyden (Leydig?) gland, so that the kundaline forces move along the spine to the various centers that open with this attitude, or with these activities of the mental and spiritual forces of the body—much in the same manner as might be illustrated in the foetus that forms from conception. These naturally take form. Here these take form, for they have not in their inception been put to a definite use. The psychological reaction is much like that as may be illustrated in one gaining much knowledge without making practical application of it. It then forms its own concepts. Now we

combine these two and we have that indicated here as possession of the body; gnawing, as it were, on all of the seven centers of the body, causing the inability for rest or even a concerted activity . . . Pathologically, we may find this center in the reproductive gland or activity of the body—the ovarian activity."
Cayce's Prognosis: "Do these. Be consistent, be persistent . . . For there is hope."
Treatment Suggested by Cayce:
1. Hot pack applied to ovarian area (pack consists of mutton tallow, spirits of turpentine, and spirits of camphor put on flannel cloth)
2. Osteopathic corrections
3. Radio-Active Appliance
4. Meditation during electrotherapy
Treatment Results: Her letters state that she followed the suggestions faithfully and received no relief. She also acknowledged, "that we didn't quite understand the explanations and directions, and so couldn't follow them more carefully or accurately. The osteopath couldn't understand, but did the very best he could."
Comments: She had received some relief previously using an electrical appliance. The doctor who did the corrections noted the trouble as indicated by Cayce.

Cayce's description of the "creature" that "gnaws" on the woman was, "that which is as a positive possession—but a creation of the own mental and physical self." In metaphysical terms, this may have been a "thought form" of the woman's own mind.

The woman said the Radio-Active Appliance irritated the "creature" and made for violent flare-ups of the condition. On a follow-up questionnaire in 1952, she maintains that the condition had spread to other family members (i.e., her husband, mother, and two brothers).

This case might be described as a case of "kundaline crisis" (see Appendix B). The bizarre nature of this woman's "hallucinations" and "delusions," along with onset of symptoms at age 16, would likely lead to a diagnosis of schizophrenia by current psychiatric criteria. The reading also noted the presence of subluxations in the hip and coccyx—somatic dysfunctions of the lower spine affecting the reproductive glands—were often cited in cases of kundalini awakening which became pathological.

3440
Background: Female, 29 years old; her sister reported: "All of her

life she has suffered from an emotional disorder diagnosed as schizophrenia," she had a history of head injuries during childhood
Symptoms: "Emotional disturbance or frustration coupled with lack of self-confidence, oversensitiveness, lack of vitality," lack of motivation, insomnia
Medical Diagnosis: Schizophrenia
Cayce's Diagnosis and Etiology: "As we find, there are segments in the cerebrospinal system where the jar and the injuries to the body have caused the connections between sympathetic and cerebrospinal systems to become disturbed. These produce those conditions of nervousness that have long been existent through the body. Also they produce the insomnia, and the upset of the imaginative forces—so that the body becomes easily aggravated, easily tired out, or becomes supersensitive to slights, slurs and the like . . . These repressions and impoverishments produced by pressures at times cause the exaggerated disturbances through various functioning of reflexes. And as there are those areas where coordination between sympathetic and cerebrospinal is disturbed, at times the body apparently is slow in grasping the reflex or the LAW or WHY pertaining to subjects, conditions, things and activities through the associations of the body."
Cayce's Prognosis: "While these have not necessarily caused permanent injuries, the longer the body has gone without the correction of the impingements existent through the system the greater has become, and greater will become, the disturbances—and the harder it will be to adjust or control them."
Treatments Recommended by Cayce:
1. Osteopathic adjustments
2. Hydrotherapy
3. Radio-Active Appliance
4. Meditation
5. Learn music
6. Outdoor activities: tennis, golf, horseback riding
7. Diet: well balanced, not too many sugars and starches
Treatment Results: Apparently the suggestions were followed to some extent since a letter from her sister (dated 10/9/73; 29 years after the reading) stated: "In recent years [3440]'s condition has deteriorated, and I am now her legal guardian. She told me the reading prescribed osteopathy treatments which did her some good, and she wants to resume the treatments."
Comments: This is a classical case of schizophrenia (early onset,

positive and negative symptoms, chronic course of development) which Cayce attributed to spinal injuries during childhood. The full spectrum treatment regimen is representative of the holistic approach advocated by the readings.

A life reading (3440-2) noted a karmic basis for much that the woman was experiencing—the expression "the entity is meeting self" is mentioned a couple of times. One particularly dramatic incarnation involved slaughter in a Roman arena where the entity condoned killing. Attitudinal problems (e.g., condemning others) are cited as originating in a variety of lifetimes. Service to others was recommended and vocational abilities noted in the arts, especially songwriting.

3475

Background: Female, 22 years old; mother's letter stated: "She suffered a nervous breakdown, diagnosed as dementia praecox 3 years ago. She was confined to sanitariums and under various forms of treatment for 2 years, then recovered sufficiently to be at home for a year, only to crack up again last January when we were compelled to return her to a sanitarium. Her condition is pitiful. She shows no sign of improvement yet."

Symptoms: Unknown

Medical Diagnosis: Dementia praecox/schizophrenia

Cayce's Diagnosis and Etiology: The reading stated that the nervous collapse was due to "adhesions related to the organs of the pelvis."

Cayce's Prognosis: " . . . if this condition continues we may expect deterioration in the nerve plasm itself [dementia praecox?]."

Treatment Suggested by Cayce:
1. Refer to Still-Hildreth Sanatorium
2. Give mild sedative before treatments
3. Corrections by osteopathic gynecologist

Treatment Results: The physical condition improved but no change in the mental condition was noted.

Comments: Only one brief reading was given and there was no follow-up—Cayce passed away. There are detailed assessment documents from Still-Hildreth in this file which indicate "The condition is a well-established case of schizophrenia." This was an important case since the connection between somatic dysfunction (adhesions in the pelvis) and the schizophrenic process was well established. The pelvic problems would likely have produced glandular dysfunctions. The readings make a cryptic reference to the probability of "deterioration in the nerve plasm" if the condition is not corrected. This expression was associated with dementia praecox in the readings. A brother [3589] also suffered a nervous breakdown—see following case.

3589

Background: Male, 21 years old; he was in a state hospital at the time of the reading, his sister [3475] was diagnosed as having schizophrenia

Symptoms: Unknown

Medical Diagnosis: "Insanity"

Cayce's Diagnosis and Etiology: " . . . there are great distresses between the physical and the mental body. There are those disintegrations of the sources or channels through which impulses are carried to the centers in the body for control of a balanced mental activity of physical being . . . The administration of bromides only tends to heighten this incoordination . . . To be sure, there are individuals who are possessed with influences or entities that would be torments to others, but this is more such. Thus the use of violence at times only tends to heighten this incoordination in the impulses along brain forces [he was in Manhattan State Hospital]." Cayce noted "tendencies for inflammation to the organs of the genital system" and pressures in the 1st, 2nd, 3rd cervicals, and the coccyx.

Cayce's Prognosis: "The controlling of these impulses by stimulating activities to the gonads and the brain centers in the 9th dorsal might give the body those opportunities for responding."

Treatment Suggested by Cayce:

1. Move to Still-Hildreth
2. Osteopathic corrections
3. May require operative measures
4. Quietness, patience, and gentleness instead of severity (therapeutic milieu)

Treatment Results: Unknown

Comments: This patient's sister had a similar condition. In both cases, abnormality of the genital system and spinal pressures were noted. This was a brief reading given near the end of Edgar Cayce's life and the etiology is, therefore, limited. Possession and dementia praecox appear to have been involved in this case.

3633

3633-1 was a life reading for an eleven-year-old boy who would later be diagnosed as schizophrenic. At an early age, the parents recognized that the child was special and were concerned for him. The reading portrayed great potential which could be manifested in extreme forms: "For here is the opportunity for an entity (while comparisons are odious, these would be good comparisons) to be either a Beethoven or a Whittier or a Jesse James or some such entity! For the entity is inclined to think more highly of himself than he ought to think, as would be indicated. That's what these three individuals did, in themselves. As to the application made of it, depends upon the self . . . the body will go to excess in many ways, unless there is the real training in the periods of unfoldment. And the entity is beginning to reach that period when, while the spirit must not be broken, everyone should be very firm and positive with the entity, inducing the entity through reason to analyze self and to form the proper concepts of ideals and purposes and in doing this, we will not only give to the world a real individual with genius, but make for individual soul development. Otherwise, we will give to the world one of genius in making trouble for somebody."

About four years after the reading (age 15), [3633] became mentally ill. At age 18 he shot his father and grandmother. He was confined in mental hospitals for years and was diagnosed as suffering from schizophrenia and dementia praecox. Unfortunately, Edgar Cayce died shortly after the reading and therefore was unable to provide check readings on this boy. This reading does provide some insight into Cayce's perspective on karma, and its relevance to major mental illnesses such as schizophrenia. Astrological influences and four previous lives are cited in the reading.

3641

Background: Female, 38 years old; she suffered an initial breakdown at age 26 and yearly breakdowns since age 32, she was in a sanitarium at the time of the reading
Symptoms: "Mental derangements," violent at times, waxing and waning of symptoms
Medical Diagnosis: Unknown
Cayce's Diagnosis and Etiology: "While there are physical disturbances, there is also a mental derangement—and this means just what it implies. In the physical force, there has existed from long ago, those disorders that have caused a disturbance in the body

dealing with the activity of the cerebrospinal and sympathetic nerve system, as related to the activities of the body in its glandular functioning. There was, or still is, a disturbance in the second and third coccyx segments that is the seat or source or beginning of the disorder. Then, without this being corrected, there has been caused a severance of nerve centers in the abdominal area, where nerves of the sympathetic and cerebrospinal system, in the brush end of the spine, parallel in such manners as to have reflexes that cause periods when the sympathetic system is the more active. At times there are lapses or losses of control of the emotional system, because of the overactivity of the emotional system without the control of the physical activity . . . Q. What caused these pressures in the coccyx? A. When about fourteen years old, the body set down too hard on the ice."

Cayce's Prognosis: "Do that [the treatments] and we will bring near to normal conditions for this body."

Treatment Suggested by Cayce:
1. Osteopathic corrections
2. Wet Cell Appliance used in the same manner as the Radio-Active Appliance (i.e., without gold, alternate connections)

Treatment Results: Unknown

Comments: This is a fascinating case for many reasons. Note the similarity with [1513] who also injured the coccyx by falling on ice. The waxing and waning of symptoms, with periods of relatively normal functioning in the early stages of the syndrome, was also a commonly cited pattern in cases with this etiology. The age of onset and chronic course fit the schizophrenic pattern but also resemble schizoaffective disorder due to its affective features and tendency for episodic cycles (which may resemble manic psychosis). The woman had been given a total of 58 shock treatments and the husband wanted to know if these should be continued since they did have a calming (and depressing effect) on his wife. Cayce replied, "For goodness sake don't, unless you want her to stay in a worse condition." The reading stated that there was no brain deterioration but that the pressures needed to be removed.

Although the original injury was to the coccyx, sympathetic pressures were also noted in the 4th lumbar; 9th and 3rd dorsal; 3rd, 2nd, and 1st cervical with the 3rd cervical of particular importance. Cayce recommended "osteopathic coordination of each segment along the spine." Very often in the readings, lower spinal injury would produce pressures in other centers along the spine ("sympathetic" or "reflex" lesions—see the discussion of manual medicine in Chapter Seven) and would require treatment which coordinated the whole spine—an intervention which was congruent with osteopathic philosophy and technique of that era.

3996

Background: Female, adult; she was in a state hospital at the time of the reading
Symptoms: Paranoia, hallucinations, self-condemnation
Medical Diagnosis: Unknown
Cayce's Diagnosis and Etiology: "IN THE NERVE SYSTEM: This, too, we find under distress, both from pressure in portions of body by physical condition, also the reaction as received through blood forces not eliminating properties brings pressure on centers that deviates the sensory system in such a manner that the expression as found in the body gives those hallucinations that become so detrimental to self and self's satisfactions. In the pelvic organs we find the physical condition causing distress on the body. This produced in times back, at the time when there was the condition of pregnancy, and the pressures as produced brought the pressure in the form of a lesion to the pituitary or pineal glands, and reacting through pituitary glands in brain centers."
Cayce's Prognosis: "Do that and we will bring this body [3996] to its normal conditions."
Treatment Suggested by Cayce:
1. Medicine (yellow dock root, burdock root, stillingia, poke root, iodide of potassium, and simple syrup)
2. Deep manipulations to the pelvis (with moist heat)
3. Choride of gold and bicarbonate of soda
Treatment Results: Unknown
Comments: This may have been a case of paranoid schizophrenia resulting from somatic dysfunction. Pregnancy produced lesions in the pelvis which affected blood flow to the brain (poor eliminations/toxemia) resulting in lesions in the pineal and pituitary glands. See case [2744] for a similar etiology.

4002

Background: Female, 28 years old; she suffered a breakdown at 23 years of age and had been hospitalized for about 5 years at the time of the reading
Symptoms: Sporadic violent behavior, wouldn't talk

Medical Diagnosis: Unknown
Cayce's Diagnosis and Etiology: " . . . there are very definite causes that produce the abnormal reactions between the mental and the imaginative or the sympathetic and imaginative reactions to the brain. These have been existent for some time. We find that there are adhesions in the organs of the pelvis causing definite reactions to the pineal gland. These as they react to and through the reflexes of brain cause those periods when there are the exaggerated repressions, and there enters all of those experiences through which the entity in transition has passed [reincarnational material?] . . . Q. What brought on the mental breakdown? A. As just indicated the adhesions in the pelvic organs, as directly connected or associated with the lyden (Leydig) and the pineal glands."
Cayce's Prognosis: " . . . if there would be the application of the short-wave electrical shocks for the body, along with the osteopathic adjustments that might be made in Macon, Missouri [Still-Hildreth], there might be brought back near to normal conditions for this body . . . "
Treatment Suggested by Cayce:
1. Referral to Still-Hildreth Sanatorium
2. Short-wave electrical shocks
3. Osteopathic adjustments
4. Rest
5. Treat with gentleness and kindness (therapeutic milieu)
Treatment Results: Unknown
Comments.   Adhesions in the pelvis affected the Leydig gland and activated the pineal system—this may have been a "kundalini crisis" (see Appendix B). Note the tendencies for violent behavior associated with this case—this was a fairly common pattern in cases of pineal activation. Also note the reference to past-life memories, which would be interpreted as delusions and hallucinations by most clinicians.

4004

Background: Male, 39 years old
Symptoms: Unknown
Medical Diagnosis: Dementia praecox
Cayce's Diagnosis and Etiology: "In times back there was an injury to the area between the last of the dorsals and the lumbar. A pressure exists from a subluxation . . . From these pressures there are these causes for a mental breakdown, so that great imaginations are

produced [delusions?] at times and at others there is a sullenness [social withdrawal?] that becomes aggravating to others and equally as depressing to the body-forces of the entity itself."

Cayce's Prognosis: "With care this may still be reduced, but in times back could have been easily corrected if precautions had been taken—or at least it could have been much more easily eliminated . . . Do give the body the opportunity of these adjustments and we may bring the opportunity for a normal, complete expression of the entity's self, which has been denied—either by negligence or lack of expression."

Treatment Suggested by Cayce:
1. Osteopathic corrections
2. Special attendant (companion)
3. Short-wave electrical therapy

Treatment Results: The suggestions were not followed.

Comments: This reading points out the importance of early intervention. The medical diagnosis of dementia praecox was apparently not indicative of actual brain degeneration since some improvement was noted without treatment. Note the lower spinal injury which was a long-standing condition. The recommendation for short-wave therapy was unusual since the Wet Cell was often suggested in such cases.

4100

Background: Female, 20 years old; she was in a "mental hospital" at the time of the reading

Symptoms: Behavioral perseverations, catatonic withdrawal

Medical Diagnosis: Unknown

Cayce's Diagnosis and Etiology: "In the physical and mental conditions with this body, [4100], we find there is the lack of coordination between the expressive forces in the imaginative or sympathetic and cerebrospinal; so that the reactions which occur from the activities of the body-mental, the body-physical, are out of accord with that ordinarily seen in the activities of one endowed with the physical abilities and the reactions to same. This condition, as we find, has been brought on by those external influences that affect the coordinating between the sympathetic and cerebrospinal, in the cervical region . . . These effects are seen more in the activities of the sensory system; as in sight, speech, hearing, feeling, all find a response, but not in a coordinative way and manner; and since these do not find their concordant activity, the responses are as one blank, or unmindful of those activities that are brought to the body in an ordinary way or manner. There are responses, though, as there may be pointed out to the body those activities of any nature pertaining to purely the physical revibrations, or the physical activities, and these will be carried on in the manner designated without change [perseveration]."

Cayce's Prognosis: "Q. To what extent can she be rehabilitated? A. About 99 and 44/100 percent. Q. Will she ever recover sufficiently for her to live away from a hospital? A. It can be done now, if put under the proper precautions or conditions." (18 months to 2 years was given as a time frame)

Treatment Suggested by Cayce:
1. Therapeutic milieu
2. Wet Cell with gold
3. Companion

Treatment Results: Unknown

Comments: This may have been catatonic schizophrenia or the adult stage of a pervasive developmental disorder (i.e., autism). Since psychiatry has little understanding of either of these disorders, the diagnostic label is not so important as a sense of the person's experience and the treatment suggestions.

There is no correspondence with this file, so the developmental course in this case cannot be ascertained. Questions asked during the reading do provide some insight into the condition, however. "Q. Are my visits helping or retarding my daughter? A. Helping, whenever there is helpfulness held; for the body responds very much to a great deal it is not accredited with! What to do with it, is what it doesn't know! Q. Does it make her sad or glad, and is she desirous though unable to make her thoughts and emotions known to me? A. It makes her glad when good comes; sad when misunderstood or misinterpreted, for it is no different! Q. What are the thoughts most prevalent in my daughter's mind generally? A. Attempting to correlate . . . the ability to give expression to that which passes on is broken. The activities of that given to create those feelers in a material body, or to bring about—as it were—the correlating of a short circuit in the conditions between a well-balanced mental and a well-balanced physical mind. Q. Is my daughter conscious of the fact that it is her mother who visits her when I come there? A. Often it is days before she becomes conscious as to just who it is, but the consciousness is there! It is being builded! All the good that may be done for this body will not be lost; for even at this hour it would be well to consider and to take note of the change in demeanor of the body, during this next twenty minutes."

This last answer is worth noting, since [4100]'s mother was present with [4100] at the time of the reading and later commented, "Around 4 o'clock or a little after, a change did take place in [4100]'s demeanor, so much so that she [the mother] couldn't keep from noticing it. She [4100] suddenly became completely calm and smiled—which was very unusual, a rare thing for her to do." The reading was given between 3:45 and 4:24 P. M. Eastern Standard Time and coincided with the change noted by the mother.

The reading states that treatment should not be given unless the suggestions are followed persistently and consistently since a worsened condition may be produced by a failure to follow through with the suggestions persistently.

4179

Background: Female, adult; she was in a state sanitarium at the time of the reading
Symptoms: Unknown
Medical Diagnosis: Dementia praecox
Cayce's Diagnosis and Etiology: "In the action of the cerebrospinal forces we have a condition which has been called dementia praecox . . . the action of the forces is not of this exact nature . . . We have the action through the nerve centers over portions of the body as we have here through the thyroid as in the throat and neck, the nonactive force of the cellular forces in the body with the circulation to carry all forces to the brain producing the condition that has been expressed by the suppression through the organs of gestation or through the generatory organs. Through this has been brought the reaction which is acting on the nerve forces through the solar plexus center through organs affecting the predisposition as given by generation by spiritual forces as brought from one world to another when it became an individual and [made] its own individuality. The functioning of the organs, that is the brain forces, are hindered by the action of the incentive that is carried to the action of the brain forces, so that proper action as carried to the forces, yet to carry out the impression as received, the body does not act [catatonic?]."
Cayce's Prognosis: "[The treatment] must be of long and very persistent force."
Treatment Suggested by Cayce:
1. Hypnosis

2. Surgery to remove "clotting of certain cellular forces along the spine, notably along the lower dorsals . . . from the frontal side."
Treatment Results: Unknown
Comments: This is an extraordinary case in many respects. Here we have a woman suffering from a major mental illness resembling dementia praecox (which very likely fits the current diagnostic criteria for schizophrenia). Her condition appears chronic and she may be in a catatonic stupor. The reading states that her condition resulted from an inherited tendency which manifested through a deficiency in the glandular system. This inadequacy is described as the "nonactive force of the cellular forces in the body." The readings often indicate that karmic (i.e., hereditary) patterns are manifested in the glandular system and that this system is responsible for providing "incentive" to the brain forces (secretions necessary for proper neurotransmission?).

As in most cases with karmic involvement, recovery entails "long and very persistent force." The use of hypnosis in such cases is not unusual—the recommendation for surgery points up the intractability of the condition.

4285

Background: Female, adult
Symptoms: Unknown
Medical Diagnosis: Unknown
Cayce's Diagnosis and Etiology: " . . . the abnormal conditions as we find them in this body has more to do with the mental condition in the body than it has to do with the physical . . . the impressions that reach the brain reach there in such a condition that the reaction for the body to act under those impressions become hallucinations to the action of the physical forces within the body itself. They have produced within the body from times back, and it is not the fault of this body itself, but rather that of the individual before, which has to do with the hereditary forces as we have expressed or shown in this body here . . . the impressions to the brain forces that bring the hallucinations to the body. The nerve force, and the influence as is carried by the nerve matter and forces in the body itself has to do with the white matter as carried in the body . . . We find at the 9th dorsal an impingement of the nerve forces there. We find at the upper end of the sacrum, or the beginning of the dorsal region, the impingement that causes all of the forces as expressed in the brain matter and forces the impressions to the body of self-destruc-

tive forces, for their actions are received from the glands where re-production is originated in the body."
Cayce's Prognosis: "To gain assistance for the body and ease and rest, and to rid it of the hallucinations, do as we have said."
Treatment Suggested by Cayce:
1. Hypnosis
2. Deep manipulations while hypnotized
3. Or, surgery to remove fallopian tubes and "genital glands"
Treatment Results: Unknown
Comments: The reading stated that the spinal manipulations would not "make the body perfectly normal in the functioning of the brain forces themselves, again." Perhaps this is why the hypnotic suggestions were to be given, "through that force known as hypnotic influence control may be gained that will assist the body to balance the mental forces not yet in perfect condition." The reading did emphasize that the condition was more mental than physical, "for the action of the mental in its expressions or manifestations through the physical has to do with the abnormal that is within the body . . ." The axiom "mind is the builder" may be appropriate here since this appears to be a case of mentally induced somatic dysfunctions (i.e., lesions along the spine and in the reproductive tract).

4342

Background: Female, adult; she was in a state hospital at the time of the reading suffering from a chronic condition which manifested as "yearly breakdowns"
Symptoms: Unknown
Medical Diagnosis: Unknown
Cayce's Diagnosis and Etiology: "IN THE NERVE SYSTEM: In this we find the seat of the trouble. In times past, in the beginning, as it were, of this earth's existence, we find the seat of the trouble—not a prenatal or congenital condition, yet one produced at the birth of the individual . . . this has produced . . . distortion to impressions . . . the brain, with improper distortion—these elements, the gray, the white tissue itself—sets in motion, and when these become un-balanced, or distorted, the reaction in the brain, and then the ac-tivities to those incentives of the physical forces in body become distorted also, and to another mind becomes unbalanced. In this body, the pressure as produced at birth was in the presenting of the body itself, in that known as breech birth, and the pressure was pro-duced in the last lumbar, and the 2nd portion or structure of the

sacral, and the sacral then producing a pressure to those of the generatory system brought about that enlargement in those centers about these organs in pelvis, that direct connect with the base of the brain in this gland situated there [pineal]. The thread of same, which traverses the system from brain to the end of the cerebrospinal cord proper. With the pressure created in this position in this body, with the gradual development of the body, we have then this condition becoming aggravated. In the passing years, we find, as the body developed to the womanhood, this incentive has remained, making or producing in its reaction that of the eccentric, high strung, overactivity in every exercise of a mental prodigy, as might be termed. In later years, there came an accident to the end of the spine (four years ago—sixteenth of September, four years ago) which was to the end of the coccyx, that which excited, as it were, these centers in the sacral and the lower lumbar. These reactions, then, are produced through this reaction to the base of the brain—a fullness, or an enlargement, that produces first headaches, then nervous indigestion, then a racking, as it were, to the whole sympathetic system, and an unbalanced mental reaction . . . "

Cayce's Prognosis: "In six weeks the body should be perfectly normal."

Treatment Suggested by Cayce:
1. Remove from current environment (state hospital)
2. Osteopathic corrections after wet heat to relax body
3. Mayapple bitters
4. Alpine rays

Treatment Results: Treatments not given

Comments: Here is a case of double insult to the spine occurring years apart (at birth and as a young woman) with the second incident aggravating the existing condition: "In the main, these are of two different conditions of the same material, yet different structure in their action in the system." For a discussion of pregnancy and birth complications, see Chapter One.

This woman may have been prone to violent behavior since the reading states that she had been given bromides and was in restraints at the time of the reading. There are several important etiological factors here: lower spinal injury affecting pelvic organs resulting in pineal involvement. Note the cyclic pattern of breakdowns and violent tendencies which were often associated with this etiology. The prodromal symptoms ("eccentric, high strung, overactivity in every exercise of a mental prodigy") suggest mania during late adolescence and early adulthood but is also congruent with gender differences noted in schizophrenia (see discussion of gender in Chapter One). Involvement of the pineal suggests "kundalini crisis" in this case.

5014

Background: Male, 11 years old; "the child was greatly neglected and underfed for the 5½ years he lived under his grandmother's supervision . . . very retarded physically and also in all mental endeavors and in mental and social adjustments . . . please suggest treatment for child's extreme lack of effort and utterly irresponsible attitude toward school work"

Symptoms: See background

Medical Diagnosis: Unknown

Cayce's Diagnosis and Etiology: " . . . there are disturbances preventing the better normal development of the body. These suppressions are in the areas where reflexes to the various activities or impulses through the body find their reactions; that is, the incoordination between impulses received by suggestions activative along the sympathetic nervous system and the responses through the central nervous system . . . For this was a breech or foot, breech and foot presentation. This brought about pressures in the coccyx and sacral areas that have prevented the normal reactions through the pineal. Not that portion having to do with growth but the exterior portions or the left side, where there are connections in the lumbar axis, 9th dorsal, the brachial center and the upper cervical center."

Cayce's Prognosis: "Thus we will find a change in the activities of the body, bringing the reflexes to the brain centers with the nervous system in the ganglia where there are the closer associations with the sympathetic and suggestive nerve forces of the body."

Treatment Suggested by Cayce:
1. Wet Cell Battery used in same manner as Radio-Active appliance
2. Massage
3. Suggestive therapeutics during treatments
4. Atomidine
5. Diet (keep away from too much sweets and starches)
6. Keep good eliminations (massage colon to aid in emptying it)

Treatment Results: The suggestions were followed closely for seven years and consistent improvement was noted. At that time he ceased to respond to treatment and had a nervous breakdown at age 20. Subsequent relapses resulted in confinement in a state hospital, diagnosis of schizophrenia, and treatment with Thorazine. His condition stabilized and he was able to maintain a fairly high level of functioning in the hospital.

Comments: This is a very significant case since it provides insight into the developmental course of schizophrenia. The reading indicated that spinal injury at birth resulted in glandular dysfunction (pineal) and incoordination between the autonomic and central nervous systems. This case fits the model developed by Mednick and associates (see the discussion of ANS dysfunction and PBCs in Chapter One). The PBC was a breech birth which produced pressures along the spine. The ANS abnormality was described as "the incoordination between impulses received by suggestions activative along the sympathetic nervous system and the responses through the central nervous system." This incoordination between the ANS and CNS led to cognitive deficits and social withdrawal: "We find that these are the sources of the retardments, the inability of concentration, the inability to coordinate the body's reaction with others; for the body becomes confused with groups or crowds. Thus those reactions in which the body attempts to shield itself, to get away from or to be closer to those who have respect for or interest in the body itself (as he sees it)." Note that the ANS was not viewed as simply a peripheral system in which abnormal functioning resulted from a primary brain dysfunction. On the contrary, it was ANS pathology which produced the brain dysfunction. The dynamic partnership of these major systems was often cited in the systems approach advocated in the readings.

The presence of a major PBC and the high probability of abnormal ANS reactivity would likely place this case in the "high risk" category according to Mednick's research. It is difficult to assess the level of retardation in this case, but it is possible that this case would carry a dual diagnosis. The poor premorbid adjustment would be associated with a poor prognosis by current criteria.

See Appendix B for a discussion of the pineal's role in growth and development, an important consideration in this case. Cayce died a few months after this reading, so check readings were not given. One wonders if osteopathic adjustments would have been recommended if such readings had been given; this was the pattern in similar cases and may have reversed the schizophrenic process (i.e., "cure by removal of cause").

5274

Background: Female, 39 years old; she was in a mental hospital at the time of the reading
Symptoms: Hallucinations, delusions
Medical Diagnosis: Unknown
Cayce's Diagnosis and Etiology: "There are pressures in the coccyx end of the spine from an injury received thirty-seven years ago. This has become static . . . Q. What causes the hallucinations and the persisting in wearing a cardboard or metal pad over her right eye? A. These are the reactions from former appearances of the same entity in the earth. Q. Why does she imagine she is being abandoned and tortured by people who dislike her? A. This, again, is the impression from other appearances in the earth."
Cayce's Prognosis: "As we find, there are disturbances, but whether these will respond to the applications that may be suggested will depend a great deal upon the faith and hope and persistency of the parents, for this has gone on for so long . . . It will require long periods and patience."
Treatment Suggested by Cayce:
1. Remove from institution (therapeutic milieu)
2. Osteopathic corrections
3. Wet Cell used as the Radio-Active Appliance
4. Suggestive therapeutics (presleep suggestions)
5. Prayer by those about body
Treatment Results: Unknown
Comments: The spinal injury would have occurred at age two. One wonders how often past-life memories and experiences are interpreted as hallucinations and delusions in such cases.

Group IV: Psychosis Not Otherwise Specified

577

Background: Female, adult; she suffered for years with a physical ailment which doctors were unable to find the cause or cure
Symptoms: Dizziness, "acute pains," insomnia, melancholia, social withdrawal, waxing and waning of symptoms
Medical Diagnosis: Unknown
Cayce's Diagnosis and Etiology: " . . . in the NERVE SYSTEM subluxations existent in the lower end of the spine, in the coccyx area . . . This has occurred from a condition that existed some times back in the body, and these reactions to the body bring gland

troubles . . . [these gland secretions] affect the glands in the organs from which impulses are received from the ganglia along the whole of the cerebrospinal system . . . Q. Was this condition in the coccyx produced by an injury? A. By an injury—fell on a dance floor—years ago."

Cayce's Prognosis: Not given

Treatment Suggested by Cayce:
1. Osteopathic manipulations
2. Massage
3. Plain Violet Ray
4. Radio-Active Appliance
5. Diet (normal diet with alkaline tendency)

Treatment Results: Not available

Comments: This case would appear to represent the prodromal stages of schizophrenia (based upon the level of functioning and the etiology given in the reading). Note the lower spinal injury, which over a period of years produced glandular dysfunction. This pattern might be diagnosed as schizoaffective by current criteria due to the presence of affective symptoms and cyclic episodes.

A quote about the significance of injury to the coccyx is worth noting: " . . . most any condition may arise from injury or swelling or plethora (as more of this is here) [to the coccyx] than from most any portion of the body, unless in the head or brain itself."

Kundalini involvement might also have been a factor in this case since the reading notes the activity of the pineal "making to the activities of the imaginative forces the greater reaction . . . not hallucinations, not wholly neurotic conditions (as may be sometimes called); for the gland itself is affected, you see."

600

Background: Male, adult; he had been troubled for 7-8 months

Symptoms: Anxiety, "dreams or visions even in the waking state"

Medical Diagnosis: Not provided

Cayce's Diagnosis and Etiology: "Two years two months and eight days ago, in moving a heavy box a wrench was made. With the condition in the genital system becoming exaggerated, this produced in the area from the 9th to the 12th dorsal a subluxation." This pressure produced toxemia through clogging of kidneys and liver which affected the adrenals and lacteals. "Q. Why are my conscious and subconscious minds continuously working? A. As has been indicated, from the pressures that are seen in the system—that have produced, and do produce, the effect. The pressure is on the sympathetic or the sensory systems, which are the activities of the subconscious forces; and the conscious forces are through the cerebrospinal system. So this makes for a continual combativeness one with another, and dreams or visions even in the waking state."

Cayce's Prognosis: "Do these, and—as we find—we will bring the normal condition to this body in three to four weeks."

Treatment Suggested by Cayce:
1. Osteopathic manipulations
2. Massage
3. Sinusoidal treatment
4. Medication (simple syrup, tincture of stillingia, essence of Buchu leaves, podophyllin, plus essence of lactated pepsin)
5. Avoid heavy labor
6. Diet (alkaline)
7. Be out of doors when possible
8. Refrain from sex during treatment
9. Wet Cell could be used in lieu of sinusoidal

Treatment Results: Unknown

Comments: This man was apparently depressed and obsessing about his condition. Hypochondriacal tendencies were noted. The comment in the reading pertaining to waking dreams and visions is interesting since there has been some speculation that hallucinations in schizophrenia may result from wakeful dreaming (i.e., REM intrusion into the waking state; see Wyatt, 1971, for a review of this literature). This man may have been headed for a psychotic breakdown—there was no follow-up correspondence in the file to determine the course of the condition.

886

Background: Female, adult, suffering from "nervous breakdown"

Symptoms: Hallucinations

Medical Diagnosis: Unknown

Cayce's Diagnosis and Etiology: " . . . the body has been under a great strain not only from repression but from the denial of conditions, circumstances and surroundings with the body. And there has come a separating of the coordination between the sympathetic—or the sensory reaction and the normal physical reaction. Hence we have hallucinations, we have periods when there are those reactions of little or no coordination in the responses to the sensory forces of the body; or there is a mental, or it may be better described as a psychopathic condition and also a pathological reaction from a nonsupply of the glandular secretions for keeping a normal balance. Hence, going under this strain, we have had this nervous breakdown."

Cayce's Prognosis: "In two to three weeks, should there be the response, we may give that which will be the more helpful."

Treatment Suggested by Cayce:
1. Referral to gynecologist
2. Rest
3. Medication (hypnotics)

Treatment Results: Excellent results were noted

Comments: Correspondence states that the "girl had a nervous breakdown and was in a terrible state. On receiving the reading the family took her to Dr. C. J. Andrews who treated her with immediate results. The girl soon returned to her job." She maintained her job as clerk-typist and died in 1969.

This appears to be a case of stress-induced somatic dysfunction of the pelvic organs. The exact nature of the "great strain" was not cited in the reading. Note the similarities to case [2197] (Group III). "Nonsupply of the glandular secretions" was a common etiological factor in the development of the psychosis and was often cited in the readings as leading to brain degeneration (dementia). This case was included in Group IV since there was insufficient background information to determine the developmental course—the psychosis might have been in the initial acute stages at the time of the reading and therefore be appropriately diagnosed as schizophreniform.

1168

Background: Male, 27 years old; "has had several nervous breakdowns since he was about ten to eleven years old . . . these spells seem to come about every three to four years and last about two to three months."

Symptoms: "Unusual manner in which the body walks," tenderness over right side of body

Medical Diagnosis: Acute mania

Cayce's Diagnosis and Etiology: " . . . the causes [are from] conditions that surrounded the body during the period of gestation and at the time of birth. For there were periods when there was a despairing of proper delivery, and yet the body itself as well as that it depended upon apparently outgrew those conditions produced by an improper presentation and the manner of taking same . . . The indica-

tions through the blood supply show how that the body is constantly under a nerve strain, but that the reactions which come about that produce the incoordination in the reflexes between the muscular forces or the body-physical and the body-mental occur rather at those periods of cycle readjustment between the lower portions of that cord called the pineal with its coordination with the adrenal and the lacteal plexus or larger portion of the assimilating system."
Cayce's Prognosis: " . . . if there is the response, if there is the patience, if there is the persistence, this should before the body is thirty-two be near to normal" (i.e., within 5 years).
Treatment Suggested by Cayce:
1. Use medications judiciously (sedatives and hypnotics)
2. Castor oil packs
3. Osteopathic manipulations
4. Massage
5. Radio-Active Appliance
6. Diet (alkaline tendency, body building)
7. Keep up the eliminations
Treatment Results: Improvement was noted.
Comments: This is an interesting case of birth trauma producing lower spinal injury which affected the glandular system producing episodes of manic psychosis. These episodes were cyclical and were produced by the pineal (this gland is responsible for certain developmental cycles) which was considered by Cayce to be a system rather than a discreet glandular entity (see Appendix B). This pattern of lower spinal injury and pineal involvement producing episodes (at times violent) of manic psychosis was common in the readings and was said to be prodromal for dementia praecox and possession (this pattern was also nonspecific and overlapped to some degree with bipolar, see Chapter Seven).

The long period of recovery predicted in the reading is consistent with cases involving birth trauma. The relatively high level of functioning between breakdowns is not consistent with current criteria for schizophrenia and would probably be diagnosed as manic psychosis. The etiology and systemic pathology in this case is similar to several cases where there is a clear indication of schizophrenia and therefore is interesting from a nosological perspective.

1475
Background: Female, 30 years old; she was hospitalized at the time of the reading

Symptoms: Unknown
Medical Diagnosis: Unknown
Cayce's Diagnosis and Etiology: " . . . the combination of disturbances is both pathological and psychopathic—in their reactions,
with this body . . . First, in the blood supply we find a deficiency;
caused or produced by great strains that have been produced in the
body through the attempts of the body in supplying, as it were, the
necessary forces for the rebuilding of other bodies [pregnancy]. This
strain has produced in the sources of red blood supply a deficiency
in the hormones of the blood forces, in the hemoglobin, in that
which makes for the proper coordination in the replenishing
through glandular forces of the system . . . Hence the strain that is
produced upon the nerve system of the body; an incoordination
between the deeper circulation or the cerebrospinal and the sympathetic or vegetative, or the superficial circulation . . . Hence as we
have indicated, the first consideration is to save the SANITY of the
body, or keep that coordination between the assimilating system
and that in which the cerebrospinal AND the sympathetic may KEEP
coordination. That there are, then, distinct disturbances in specific
centers of the body becomes evident—from those causes that have
been indicated; as in the lumbar, the 9th dorsal, the upper cervicals
. . . Q. What specifically has caused this condition? A. As we find, the
great strain upon the body in childbearing WITHOUT the proper
consideration of even keeping an equal balance in the salts and elements of the body; thus depleting the circulation, taking from the
system the influences necessary for proper glandular rebuilding;
thus drawing upon the system to an extent as to cause deterioration
rather than the ability to rejuvenate itself . . . For that is the process
or the activity of the glands, to secrete that which enables the body,
physically throughout, to REPRODUCE itself."
Cayce's Prognosis: Not provided
Treatment Suggested by Cayce:
1. Osteopathic massage
2. Wet Cell with gold and Atomidine (alternated)
3. Medicine (cinnamon water, lime water, iodide of potassium, and
bromide of potassium)
4. Keep body quiet
5. Pleasant surroundings
6. Ventriculin
7. Move to osteopathic hospital in Philadelphia or Macon, Mo.
Treatment Results: Unknown

Comments: Immediately after the reading her husband commented: "I feel the reading fits her case exactly. She had 3 children within 3 years and was very 'faddish' about her diet throughout the period—not careful at all about building herself up."

2863

Background: Female, 44 years old
Symptoms: Insomnia, nervous exhaustion, visual and auditory "hallucinations," anxiety
Medical Diagnosis: Unknown
Cayce's Diagnosis and Etiology: ". . . there are some pathological or physical disturbances that must be considered. There are also psychological conditions that have much to do with the physical forces of the body. Those anxieties brought about by some conditions about the body produce such discouraging. And while there are those attitudes of the body, these become conflicting forces and contribute to that general 'all over' condition experienced at times." Subluxations were noted in the dorsals and cervicals which produced a toxic condition via liver and kidney dysfunction. The glands became involved (adrenals and thyroids) resulting in systemic dysfunctions.
Cayce's Prognosis: "Do these [treatments] and we will make for better conditions with this body."
Treatment Suggested by Cayce:
1. Hydrotherapy
2. Massage
3. Colonic
4. Short-wave electric treatments
5. Vitamin supplements (A, D, B, B-complex, and Niacin—One-A-Day brand was suggested)
6. Constructive attitudes
7. Constructive behavior
8. Diet (general)
9. Glyco-Thymoline vaginal douche
10. Ultra-violet light (mercury light with green glass)
11. Petrolagar (for constipation)
12. Hand-held Violet Ray (for insomnia)
Treatment Results: Excellent results were noted.
Comments: Correspondence dated 7/12/43 states: "At times I [2863] can sense or see people that have passed on—minute details of hair, eyes, teeth, skin, clothing—so that they are recognized by

other people. Have seen numbers and trees or views—never know when these things will appear. Have heard distinct voice in last 12 years, never get a message—Sometimes I am alone or talking on phone or with someone. Have no control over it."

Reading 2863-2 confirms the transpersonal nature of the "hallucinations": "As the centers are opened, that is, why we are giving the electrical treatments in the two forms—one external to act upon the structural portion, the other to the centers that will prevent any form of possession or impression from the psychic forces outside the body." This case could be classified as a "spiritual emergency" (i.e., "kundalini crisis") resulting from the awakening of psychic forces complicated by somatic dysfunctions (see Appendix B). This case also has many of the etiological factors which the readings associated with dementia praecox: psychological stress (attitudinal problems), spinal subluxations, toxicity resulting from poor eliminations, glandular dysfunctions, kundalini involvement, and a predilection for possession.

3415

Background: Female, 22 years old; "she has had mental aberrations for which we cannot account, the most persistent being the notion that she is being used as the subject of experimentation for the advancement of science. She resents this 'experimentation' and has had a reproachful attitude towards us for not discussing it with her." She was placed in a rest home and "interrogated by psychiatrists, and also was given about 6 shock treatments to her head." She was taken to a chiropractor who treated her for "severe displacement of vertebrae at the base of the skull." She refused to have any more treatments but her delusions seemed to be less frequent as a result of this application.

Symptoms: Paranoid delusions, "nervousness and hysteria"

Medical Diagnosis: "psychoneurosis"

Cayce's Diagnosis and Etiology: " . . . there are definite disturbances in the physical organs of the body that are causing the hallucinations as well as those reflexes to the mental body . . . This was caused by an injury to the end of the spine . . . Q. Then this is not a hereditary condition? A. It is purely a physical condition, from a pressure existent in the coccyx end of the spine, affecting directly the organs of the pelvis. Here we find, under a sympathetic gynecologist, there would be found such adhesions in the organs of the pelvis and the activity of the genital organs as to produce these disturbances."

Cayce's Prognosis: "If this condition is taken in time, we find that this body can be saved from a life of confinement. For the cycle of life here will run long, unless there is self-effacement [suicide?]."

Treatment Suggested by Cayce:
1. Have examination at Still-Hildreth
2. Osteopathic corrections

Treatment Results: The suggestions were not followed.

Comments: The pattern of lower spinal injury affecting the genital organs is present here. Still-Hildreth was often recommended in such cases. This case might be viewed as delusional disorder or prodromal schizophrenia since the readings often cite this etiological pattern as leading to a chronic condition. In such cases, "nervousness and hysteria" would amplify to a manic psychosis with violent tendencies ("she dislikes being thwarted or crossed") and brain degeneration (dementia praecox) would often result.

3877

Background: Female, adult
Symptoms: Hallucinations
Medical Diagnosis: Unknown
Cayce's Diagnosis and Etiology: "In the nervous system we find taxed forces as produced to the cerebrospinal nerve, yet itself reaching from the ileum plexus to the first cervical plexus. This is shown to have been produced by injury to this plexus at some time back . . . This gives then an overcharge of blood flow to the brain force itself. It then produces a reaction in the brain forces and produces hallucinations . . . When we have an overtaxed, or an oversupply of the nutriment that causes the condition that is produced in the system, the connection is broken between the sympathetic and cerebrospinal forces where they join here in the sacrum."
Cayce's Prognosis: "Do this as we have given, if we would bring this body to its better self."
Treatment Suggested by Cayce:
1. Osteopathic manipulations
2. Salt taken orally
3. Salt packs to vagina
Treatment Results: Unknown
Comments: There are several important etiological factors present here which are associated with the schizophrenic process as described in the readings: injury in the pelvic region, affecting the sacrum and pelvic organs, interfering with proper nutrition to the

brain, resulting in psychotic symptoms. There is no correspondence with this reading and the severity of the process cannot be ascertained; it is therefore included in Group IV as a case of prodromal schizophrenia.

3905

Background: Female, 21 years old, in a mental hospital at the time of the reading

Symptoms: Her mother reports: "[3905] is emotionally very unstable. Sometimes when in a highly nervous state she trembles all over and momentarily loses the power of locomotion. At times she has temper tantrums or violent rages during which she is apt to become destructive and break objects, strike and kick and tear up her clothes, and to give way to loud and prolonged screaming. She has at various times threatened self-destruction."

Medical Diagnosis: "Not insanity, [3905] needs psychotherapy"

Cayce's Diagnosis and Etiology: "At the time of birth there was a pressure brought about in the areas of the coccyx and the lower end of the spine that makes, even yet, a dissociation in that area of the coccyx and the end of the cerebrospinal nerve segments . . . Q. Has the environment been a factor in bringing about this condition? A. Every phase might be a factor but this is the pathological [i.e., physical] condition. The others are the result of the attempt of the association of physical and mental reactions in body forces."

Cayce's Prognosis: "Thus [with treatment] we will bring near to normal reactions for this body."

Treatment Suggested by Cayce:
1. Insulin shocks
2. Osteopathic corrections
3. Diet (well balanced)

Treatment Results: Unknown

Comments: Apparently the psychiatrists considered this a case of personality disorder. The reading emphasized the importance of a holistic approach while insisting that the etiology was primarily somatic. "Thus we find a body well endowed with faculties and yet in the present on the verge of a disintegration of the unity of purpose . . . For remember, as indicated, the physical, the mental and the spiritual body should be considered in making the applications. Consider it as an entity, not merely as a physical body. For the body has a mind, a soul and a physical body; they war one with another oft because of this dissociation, or this open end of the spine which came at birth ... Even an x-ray will show this dissociation indicated." The references to "disintegration" and "dissociation" were expressions which the readings often associated with dementia praecox and the etiological factors also point in that direction. Note the presence of birth trauma and the relationship between somatic dysfunction and environmental influences. The suggestion for insulin shock treatment was highly unusual in the readings and points up the seriousness of the condition.

4600

Background: Female, 25 years old; she had a goiter operation the previous year

Symptoms: Bulging eyes and headaches

Medical Diagnosis: Unknown

Cayce's Diagnosis and Etiology: "The beginning, or the cause of these troubles, as we find, is that the system became unbalanced through the metabolism of the blood and the reaction in the nerve system caused the clogging of the glands in the system. The effect of same was to produce in some of the glands that of the plethora condition that brought about the enlargement of same. With the removal of these conditions [surgery] there was produced the still further clogging in the internal system. Hence, the body is thrown out of equilibrium almost to the point where there is not coordination between the cerebrospinal and the reaction of the organs of the body. Dementia and melancholia are bordered close to the balance of forces from within the system by this unbalanced, unequalized, condition throughout the organs of the body ... "

Cayce's Prognosis: "Follow these directions consistently and persistently, for through same we will bring about the normal forces for this body ... "

Treatment Suggested by Cayce:

1. Radium appliance
2. Osteopathic adjustments
3. Diet (general with iodized salt)

Treatment Results: The suggestions were not followed.

Comments: This was a case of glandular imbalances which affected the other major body systems, including the central nervous system. Note the linkage of dementia and melancholia in this case which again indicates nonspecificity.

4624

Background: Female, 45 years old; she would have been in her mid-thirties at the onset of symptoms and was in a state asylum at the time of the reading

Symptoms: "Hallucinations," hyperactivity

Medical Diagnosis: Unknown

Cayce's Diagnosis and Etiology: "We find that in times back there were lacerations to the womb, and adhesions—that affect the nerve system, especially when the ovum from the system is discharged [menstruation]—that bring on conditions that, in the inability of the system to coordinate through the normal nerve centers affected by these lesions, bring on first hallucinations and repressions to the reaction in brain centers."

Cayce's Prognosis: ". . . yet the condition has not reached that stage whereby, were these pressures removed, and the system builded back in nerve energy to that responding in the system, but what the condition could be removed, and the body mentally and normally restored."

Treatment Suggested by Cayce:
1. Operation to straighten the womb and break up lesions
2. Radio-Active Appliance with gold chloride and sodium (internally and vibratorily)

Treatment Results: Unknown

Comments: The Cayce readings often associated lesions in the reproductive system with glandular dysfunction and psychosis. [4624]'s husband thought that stress may also have been a factor in this case: "She became insane during the time of the World War. She read newspapers telling about the war. She is now in the insane hospital at Tuscaloosa, Ala. She is never satisfied being at one place a long time, she likes to roam about very much."

Dennerstein, Judd, and Davies (1983) provide a brief review of cyclical psychosis (also referred to as periodic psychosis, recurrent menstrual psychosis, and atypical endogenous psychosis). Features include delusions, hallucinations, insomnia, hyperactivity, emotional lability, and ANS symptoms such as flushing, anorexia, or nausea. The authors also describe a case study which is relevant to the present discussion since the woman involved presented with numerous pathological symptoms and had a strong family history of schizophrenia. Danazol, a synthetic steroid derived from ethisterone, was effective in preventing the cyclical psychosis—her symptoms had previously resolved with chlorpromazine and electroconvulsive therapy, but recurred each month just before the onset of menses.

4659

Background: Male, adult; he was institutionalized at the time of the reading
Symptoms: Unknown
Medical Diagnosis: Unknown
Cayce's Diagnosis and Etiology: " . . . the causes of the conditions as are produced in the functioning of the nerve system, and the coordinating of the mentality, and its actions toward the physical forces of the body are deep-seated, caused by a pressure and the lack of coordination in certain of the glands as produce, with the functioning of other organs, that pressure in the system necessary for the sympathetic and cerebrospinal and the dissemination of the reasoning forces with the normal sensory organism of the body. This produced by this pressure and by the taking into the system of properties [mercury] that caused a lack of the body furnishing sufficient of the elements to produce the proper metabolism in the body. With the destroying of this metabolism and of the katabolism, the nerve reaction in sensory and in the sympathetic produced an overenlarged sympathetic reaction, without dissemination in sensory. Hence the conditions as have brought about that of nerve reaction to the point of wherein the differentiation is below the normal, while the physical functioning of many organs remain near normal . . . [there is a lacking of] coordination between the brain forces in the body, the sympathetic system, and the sensory organism—for all are involved in the condition . . . [this condition has] been coming on since that condition as existed in the indigestion in the body, and since the body really reached that age of puberty . . . Q. What produced this pressure and caused this trouble? A. First was produced by a pressure in the region of the brush end of the cerebrospinal system. Then, taking mercury in the system brought about this retraction in the whole nervous system, with a nerve breakdown, see? inability of coordination."
Cayce's Prognosis: "Should be normal within one year, would these [suggestions] be followed out closely."
Treatment Suggested by Cayce:
1. Change environment (rest and quiet/therapeutic milieu)
2. Companion therapy
3. Chloride of gold and bicarbonate of soda (taken orally)

4. Radio-Active Appliance with nitrate of silver
Treatment Results: Unknown
Comments: This man must have been in a very serious condition. The reading states that manipulations and other medicinal properties would be required later as changes came about. A question in the reading points up the gravity of the situation: "Q. Does the body realize his condition? A. Only partially, for there is not the full coordination between the sympathetic and the sensory system . . . At times he wakes to the realization, especially following those hallucinations to the entity as regarding other people's attitude toward the body, see?"

4787

Background: Female, adult; she was in a hospital at the time of the reading
Symptoms: "Unsightly" skin condition
Medical Diagnosis: Unknown
Cayce's Diagnosis and Etiology: "In times back we find there has been a lesion formed in and about the pelvic organs that allowed lacerations to the organs and this has gradually brought about the condition existing in the body at present, so to give the better condition to this body, we would first have the removal of that producing the hallucinations to the mental forces . . . Q. What do you mean by this body having hallucinations . . . A. We mean the body has hallucinations. Things appear that are not . . . " There were systemic dysfunctions noted including liver and kidney disturbance resulting in toxemia. Improper assimilation and drosses in the system resulted in "brain force impoverished and the hallucinations . . . " Drug effects (bromides) aggravated the condition and contributed to the skin problems by clogging the circulation, especially in the capillaries and lymphatics. Unspecified pressures on certain nerve centers affected the cerebrospinal system resulting in incoordination in the sensory system.
Cayce's Prognosis: "Do as we have given, we will remove these conditions."
Treatment Suggested by Cayce:
1. Manipulative therapy
2. Medicine (rain water, wild cherry bark, yellow dock root, dogwood bark, calisaya bark, alcohol, chloride of gold, bromide of soda, and balsam of myrrh)
3. Massage

4. "Strong" Violet Ray
Treatment Results: Unknown
Comments: In the Cayce readings, pelvic organ lesions resulting in systemic dysfunctions were a common etiological factor in psychosis. Lack of nutrients to the brain and toxicity in the body were also frequently cited factors consistent with the osteopathic model of schizophrenia during that era.

4853

Background: Female, adult
Symptoms: Suicidal tendencies, paranoid delusions, withdrawal, nervousness, melancholia, nausea, comatose spells, night terrors
Medical Diagnosis: Unknown
Cayce's Diagnosis and Etiology: "There existed a prenatal condition from the condition of the sire, or father, that brought into the system those effects in the nervous system as related to the genitive organs and genitive relations those forces as made for a weakening of the associations or connections in the nervous system; so that, as the body reached that age wherein nature was to discharge in the system those forces as made for creative energies in the system [puberty], these failed to respond in their proper way and manner." Cayce stated that there was a "muco-effect" in the plasms of the nervous forces to the organs of genitation affecting the brain centers and associated glands: the pineal, pituitary, the adrenal, and the lacteals.
Cayce's Prognosis: "Be persistent, be consistent, and we will—within the next twelve to eighteen months—bring about a near normalcy for this body."
Treatment Suggested by Cayce:
1. Wet Cell Appliance carrying gold and silver
2. Osteopathic treatments
3. Diet (general)
4. Colonic irrigations
5. Determination and expectancy by those giving treatments
6. Neuropathic massage
Treatment Results: Treatments were initiated in the Cayce Hospital and continued by a sister at home. Improvement was noted in weight gain and a decrease in nervousness, but depression remained with "black spells" of unreality.
Comments: The hereditary factor in this case is significant and may be related to the relatively lengthy period of treatment recom-

mended in the reading. The involvement of the glandular system during puberty was also cited as an important etiological consideration. This was apparently related to the periods of depression which she experienced. A pressure in the lower spine was also noted as contributing to her problems. This might be diagnosed as psychotic depression using current criteria. "Q. What causes the feeling of blackness that comes over her two or three times a day, when everything seems unreal and strange to her? A. The pressure as has been described in the coccyx region, acting reflexly on the hypogastric and pneumogastric plexus to the brain centers themselves, producing that flow *of* blood, or flow of blood *from* the brain—to or from the brain. These come in different reactions."

5221

Background: Female, 53 years old
Symptoms: Insomnia, headaches, feelings of persecution
Medical Diagnosis: Unknown
Cayce's Diagnosis and Etiology: "It is indicated that the body is a supersensitive individual entity who has allowed itself through study, through opening the centers of the body, to become possessed with reflexes and activities outside of itself. As we find, these are the sources of the anxieties. These are the sources of the feelings of possession. These are the sources of the oppressions . . . Q. How did I happen to pick this up? A. As has been indicated, the body in its study opened the centers and allowed self to become sensitive to outside influences. Q. What is it exactly that assails me? A. Outside influences. Disincarnated entities . . . Those pathological conditions as indicated are a part of the disturbances. These are through the areas of the assimilating system, and thus the adjustments osteopathically or neuropathically should be given at least once or twice a week."
Cayce's Prognosis: "If the body will do these [treatments] and set itself in mind to be rid of these conditions and to live a normal-reacting life, these will bring conditions which will be satisfactory for the body . . . Do as given and we will gain help."
Treatment Suggested by Cayce:
1. Ultra-violet Ray treatment in the mornings
2. Violet Ray treatments in the evenings
3. Hypnotic suggestions given during Violet Ray treatments
4. Massage following Violet Ray treatments
5. Osteopathic or neuropathic treatments

6. Live a normal reacting life
Treatment Results: She was noncompliant to the suggestions.
Comments: The correspondence of this woman is fascinating and deserves study. She noted poltergeist activities and feelings of persecution which she mistakenly attributed to a living man. The persecutions were sexually oriented. There is extreme malice inherent in this correspondence. The reference to the "opening of centers in the body" suggests the possibility of kundalini involvement (i.e., "kundalini crisis") leading to possession.

Summary

There are several important themes which run through these case study summaries. A brief discussion of the major dimensions can serve to elucidate these patterns.

Etiology

There was considerable etiological variability in these cases. Etiological factors implicated in this disorder included: karma, heredity ("innate" and "hereditary tendencies"), gestation and birth trauma, childhood injuries (particularly to the spine), psychosocial stressors (both "EE" and life events), mental stressors (e.g., worry, fear, self-condemnation), glandular dysfunctions of various natures (especially in response to lower spinal injuries, puberty, and menopause), poor eliminations (toxemia), discarnate possession, transpersonal experiences resulting from activation of the "kundalini" energy (pineal system), institutional effects (including neglect, abuse, and medication effects), and a host of systemic dysfunctions.

The common effect produced by all of these etiological factors was an incoordination, dissociation, or separation of the nervous systems of the body. The brain was ultimately affected resulting in chronic psychosis. In its most extreme form, this process led to brain degeneration and a dissociation of the physical, mental, and spiritual bodies (dementia praecox). Obviously, not all the etiological factors were involved in each case. However, there were certain predominate factors such as spinal injury and glandular dysfunction. Very often, it was a combination of factors which produced the psychopathology. In many respects, this perspective anticipated the diathesis/stress models and systems approaches currently in vogue. Figure 3.4 summarizes the frequency of etiological factors in these cases by combining data from the first three groups. Based upon the Cayce readings, somatic dysfunctions (primarily spinal injuries) and glandular dysfunctions appear to be highly significant etiological factors in the development of schizophrenia.

Diagnosis

There was also considerable nonspecificity in the symptomology in these case studies. This was most evident in the frequency of affective features such as mania and depression (including melancholia). One can either view this as a conceptual quandary or a nosological opportunity. If one wishes to adhere to existing nosology which relies almost entirely on diagnosis of symptom clusters, the nonspecificity in these case studies could be worrisome. On the other hand, if one seeks a deeper understanding of the underlying biological, psychological, and spiritual dimensions of major mental illnesses (such as schizophrenia), nonspecificity provides the opportunity to explore the dynamic interactions of the systems involved in psychopathology. By understanding the relationships between major diagnostic categories, marginal subgroups such as schizoaffective disorder can become more meaningful. Chapter Seven contains a discussion of variability and nonspecificity in schizophrenia and provides recommendations for resolving this diagnostic dilemma.

Prognosis

The readings were generally favorable in regards to outcome in these cases—if the treatment suggestions were followed accurately and persistently. Logically, the most difficult cases involved longstanding conditions (e.g., produced by heredity, birth trauma, childhood injuries, etc.). The message here is obvious—treat as soon as possible, keeping in mind that prevention is the most effective intervention. There were a couple of cases in which the degenerative process had gone too far. There had already been a dissociation of mind, body, and spirit with no hope for physical recovery. Even in those cases, however, the caregivers were encouraged to treat the body lovingly and prayerfully, for spiritual growth was still possible for all involved.

Treatment

In contrast to the diversity of etiological factors leading to schizophrenia, the suggested treatments were often simple, repetitive, and nonspecific. A basic treatment plan can be summarized as:

1) provide a therapeutic milieu (emphasizing spiritual qualities such as service and altruism; a companion was often suggested in cases where the individual was incapable of following the suggestions consistently or if suicide was a factor)
2) apply physical therapy (osteopathy, chiropractic, massage, etc.)
3) use electrotherapy (usually the Wet Cell with gold) to regenerate the nervous system
4) utilize suggestive therapeutics to access the inner resources of each client
5) provide opportunities for growth and development (e.g., recreational, social, vocational, and artistic activities commonly associated with rehabilitation)

Treatment Results

Positive therapeutic outcome was dependent upon two factors:
1) Persistent and consistent application of the suggestions provided in the readings
2) A response of the body to the treatments
In most cases, the suggestions were not followed to any appreciable degree since many of the afflicted persons were institutionalized in state hospitals. Such an environment was not disposed to following obscure suggestions from a psychic diagnostician. In the few cases where the suggestions were faithfully followed, positive results were forthcoming.

Institutions which utilized principles and techniques consonant with the Cayce readings (such as the Still-Hildreth Sanatorium) provide valuable data on treatment outcome which will be addressed in Chapters Five and Six. However, first it is necessary to consider the therapeutic principles which form the foundation of Cayce's approach.

4

Therapeutic Principles

◆

THE CAYCE READINGS indicate several key principles which form
the basis for a holistic approach to treating schizophrenia. Principles are guidelines which provide direction for the therapeutic
process and facilitate the application of the various treatment techniques.

Edgar Cayce considered the universe to be a lawful expression of
a creative energy or force commonly referred to as God. Principles
are generalities based upon this lawful structure and must be applied if successful therapeutic results are expected. Specific therapeutic techniques will vary from person to person and illness to
illness, but the principles involved do not vary—they are unwaver-
ing. To attempt to apply techniques without a concern for principles
can lead to confusion such as abounds in the contemporary mental
health system. The prevailing approach generally does not take into
consideration the meaning of illness (which represents the spiritual
dimension of experience) and therefore is limited in its ability to
provide care for the whole person. The Cayce readings insist that

purpose and meaning are an integral part of the therapeutic process.

The format of this and subsequent chapters will be to present a summary of a specific topic, with relevant citations and comments, which is followed by excerpts from the Cayce readings. Keep in mind that even though topics are dealt with separately to make the material easier to assimilate intellectually, they all interface and work together in practice. The considerable overlap in content of each topic points to the underlying unity inherent in these principles.

"One Activity Becomes Then Dependent upon Another"

This principle exemplifies the interconnectedness which is the essence of holism. Some individuals receiving readings applied only those portions of the readings which were easy or convenient. During subsequent check readings, Cayce would usually give a stern admonition to follow all of the suggestions if success was desired. This is especially important in the treatment of serious disorders such as schizophrenia where multiple systems are involved and interventions aimed at producing normal functioning in all systems are essential.

Reading 271-3 is an excellent example of this principle. The person administering the somatic treatment was advised to give hypnotic suggestions during the electrotherapy treatments. In this case, failure to follow the readings thoroughly not only prevented healing, but exposed the person to the possibility of worsening the condition. Cayce often recommended hypnotic suggestions (Chapter Five) for cases of schizophrenia (i.e., dementia praecox). Such persons were sometimes incapable of coherent mental processes and were noncompliant to treatment due to lack of motivation. Hypnotic suggestions provided "programming" at two levels: (1) at the interpersonal level they increased patient compliance to the therapeutic program, and (2) at the subconscious ("sympathetic") level, they provided precise directions to the nervous system so that the regenerative processes could proceed safely. Without the positive suggestions, the electrotherapy could do more harm than good.

Excerpts from the Cayce Readings
271-3   M. 34   3/3/33
In the administering of those suggestions that have been outlined, as indicated, it is presumed that all will be adhered to in the

manner given; and one activity becomes then dependent upon another.

With the revivifying of urges from physical to mental, through those reactions in the activity of the forces from the appliance to the brain's activity, unless the suggestions are carried with same it may be made more harmful than beneficial.

If these are carried together in their activity, then they will produce those reactions—as given—for the betterments of the body.

These, as we find, should be adhered to more in the manner that has been outlined for the body, and there may be expected to be the better reactions from same.

For, without this there comes that of not knowing what to do with the impulses; and the body then becomes at times irresponsible for the activities of the mental reactions.

Then, we would carry out more closely those suggestions that have been given will bring for this body the better physical and mental reactions ...

Q. Are we doing everything possible for him in his present state of mind?

A. If the whole of the suggestions given had been adhered to, there would not be the recurrent conditions that are apparent in the present! The suggestions must be made; else leave off, or change, or do without the whole thing!

Q. Why did he seem to lose the cheerfulness of the past ten days?

A. As we have just given, when there is that application for the body that will make for reactions in nerve impulse to a tempered condition in brain's reaction—and the suggestions not adhered to for those activities as outlined, there may be expected these results! Either DO it, or don't try to do it!

"Patience and Persistence"

Patience and persistence were spiritual qualities frequently mentioned in the readings and were regarded as essential for treatment success. These qualities provided the basis for therapeutic milieu (Chapter Five) and offered an opportunity for personal growth to those providing treatment.

Excerpts from the Cayce Readings
271-5   M. 34   5/1/33
Yet, as we have given, there may be brought about conditions

wherein the body may be set to—and will—return to its mental balance, and mental equilibrium.

It will be long (as time is counted by individuals), it will mean persistence, it will mean patience, it will mean keeping the mental balance in spiritual creative forces that are the builders for the body.

271-7   M. 34   5/29/33

As to how the associates are to accomplish same, it requires patience and persistence, and prayer, and understanding; and if these are not being accomplished they are untrue first to selves and to the duty and obligation that is about those who would direct the changes that are being made in the applications of those things that have started in the bringing about of the reactions in the body.

Then, in making the applications for the conditions in the system, where the electrical forces are adding to the motivative forces of the body, these should be kept as near intact with that which has been given as possible. To be sure, fear of what will be the result is the basic principle that prevents the body from being docile; but, if the body were docile—then you'd know he was already an ass and would never be much else!

But the conditions to be met are in that of patience, persistence, and reasoning with the body for the better improvement of its own abilities to meet the needs of the varied conditions that arise in the activities of the body itself. Not because "Your mammy wants it," not because "You've got to do it," but because "This will make for the better reactions in yourself!" For there are periods when the reactions are near normal.

The periods then of what may be termed rationality, in reasoning, are longer; they may not be but a moment longer, but to this experience that may mean many years of sane rationalism, if those moments are taken advantage of. Ready for questions.

Q. What approach should Lu make to get [271] to take the battery . . . ?

A. This has just been given, as to how the approach is to be made; with patience, with persistence. Rather than losing patience and saying harsh words, walk away! Then, when self has gained control of self, just reason—and reason—and reason.

Q. When he absolutely refuses to have the battery, is it best to wait until the next night?

A. Best to wait if it's a hundred years; wait until you have succeeded in conquering self, and you will then be able to conquer the body and the mind! If it's a day, or a night, or a week, a month, a year, conquer self!

Q. Is there any way this fear in the body can be removed?

A. By the patience, persistence of suggestion to the body. Is there any way that to the mind of a child that has been burned, it can be taught there is a way to handle fire? This is gradually builded by the overcoming of fear, through the suggestions—patiently, persistently; patiently, persistently; prayerfully.

2465-1   F. 28   3/17/41

Q. May she be brought to normal in mind and body?

A. As we find, near to normal; and entirely so if PERSISTENCY is kept up.

2721-2   F. 19   9/23/42

Keep up the coordinations of the massage and the suggestive forces. Doing these—with patience, care, persistence—we will bring the abilities of this body to care even for itself. Be persistent. Do be prayerful.

"Consistency"

Consistency is a close relative of patience and persistence and refers to the actual physical manifestation of those spiritual qualities. Consistency entails alertness and precision (in some cases, the readings noted that the suggestions were being persistently followed, but with insufficient attention to detail). In disorders such as schizophrenia, where the nervous systems require rebuilding and reprogramming, consistent application of the treatments is important.

Excerpts from the Cayce Readings
271-2   M. 34   3/27/33

The centers to which these attachments are applied; these are very well. Be careful that these are applied, however, in the same place each time ...

2248-1   F. 24   5/27/40

Do these, consistently; and we will bring—and in a little while, six to nine months—a near to normal mental and physical body.

"In the Application Comes the Awareness"

This principle echoes through the readings and is especially important in the treatment of complex disorders where variability is the rule. In other words, one must continually be open to information about how to best help each client. Cayce stated that the ability to intuitively obtain information is a birthright of each person and that one could not ask a question which could not be answered from within. Since Cayce is no longer around to provide check readings on persons wishing to follow the suggestions found in the readings, it is very important that other sources of intuitive information become available. Open-minded application represents a safe and effective avenue to such information. In other words, don't anticipate problems by worrying. Apply the suggestions with an open mind and sincere desire to be of service and the necessary information will be provided.

1789-3 F. 32 4/21/39
Q. Is there danger of her going back into the hysterical state in which we found her at first, and how can we prevent such a recurrence?
A. This depends upon whether or not there is the application of those suggested influences about the body.
DO as has been indicated! and not ask questions until something is done!

"Moderation in All Things"

This principle is synonymous with the word balance and is one of the most important principles contained in the readings. It refers to coordination among the numerous aspects of spiritual, mental, and physical being. Immoderate diet can adversely affect the acid/alkaline balance in the body and produce an internal environment favorable to disease. Immoderation is often thought of as synonymous with indulgence of physical appetites without due consideration of mental and spiritual balance. The opposite can also happen as was the case for [3481]—an example of overzealous pursuit of spiritual and mental growth without due consideration of the physical body. Her involvement in Theosophy and adherence to a vegetarian diet were so extreme that she deprived her body of nutriments and unbalanced the spiritual/mental/physical unity. The condition described in case [3481] may not be all that uncommon due the current interest in "new age" lifestyles.

The importance of balance is so crucial to the understanding of mental illness that one could build a pretty good case that Cayce's theory of psychopathology could be defined as *imbalance.* Likewise, his therapeutic model was based on the restoration of balance. It is important to realize that the establishment of balance in the life of a person suffering from schizophrenia also requires balance in the life of those providing treatment. The maintenance of a consistent and persistent treatment program without becoming overzealous and immoderate is just as challenging as avoiding a treatment program that is lax and deficit in its application. Reading 1916-3 emphasizes the importance of mental and physical balance by affirming the importance of both—constructive thinking *and* purposeful application.

Excerpts from the Cayce Readings
294-130   M. 54   1/14/32

Better to be moderate in all things, whether eating or drinking, or smoking, or what! MODERATION is the key to success or longevity!

1398-2   M. 38   8/12/37

. . . the reactions have not been so well. These as we find arise from too strenuous an application of those things suggested.

In taking of the Atomidine (and this should be a part of the applications), take as indicated; not just at any time and not being particular as to quantity. Take as GIVEN, if there would be the proper reactions!

As for the baths, the rubs—take as indicated! While the applications have been well, the manner of taking has not been regarded in the way and manner as it should—with the conditions to be met. The manner outlined is the manner that will be the more helpful for the body.

Do not be too strenuous in the exercises, but take sufficient to make for the proper reactions from adjustments and massages that have been indicated; as well as in the diet, we would follow closely that which has been indicated as the better for the body—if the body would receive the better results.

These, to be sure, are the manners as we have found. If the body chooses otherwise, then take the consequences . . .

Overstrenuousness is not well for the body, any more than over-eating, undereating or overdosing or improper dosing at any time.

1916-3   F. 19   7/5/29
We can only do things by doing them! Thinking them will not accomplish, unless put in action! Activity brings strength. Overactivity may weaken the very thing attempted to be strengthened. Moderation in all things—let that be for self and for others. Keep the mind in that atmosphere and channel as holds ever before same the image of that desired. That is Truth!

3481-1   F. 46   12/23/43 [Theosophist, vegetarian]
Individuals can become too zealous or too active without consideration of the physical, mental and spiritual. True, all influences are first spiritual; but the mind is the builder and the body is the result. Spiritualizing the body without the mind being wholly spiritualized may bring such results as we find indicated here, so as to raise even the kundaline forces in the body without their giving full expression.
The lack of elements is causing such disturbances in this body
. . . These, then, are the sources of disturbances here: etherealizing mentally and the lack of materializing physically in body-forces; from excesses of diets that do not supply the full or complete needs of a body physically active in the vibrations that surround this body . . .
Q. Are the pituitary, pineal, thyroid and adrenal glands working?
A. Overworking!

"Mind Is the Builder"

Much interest is currently being focused on the role of mind in the processes of health and illness. The "mind/body" connection is being explored in the laboratory under the guise of psychoneuro-immunology and in the clinic as psychosomatic medicine. Although the precise mechanisms of this interaction are still being debated, one can feel comfortable with the assertion that mental processes are important in the etiology and treatment of a wide range of disorders.
The Cayce readings are full of examples of this connection and give explicit instructions for utilizing mental processes in the healing process (Chapter Five). To be sure, when there was significant

physiological impairment, as in advanced cases of schizophrenia, healing of the body was often the first priority. As soon as the body was healed enough to permit even a slight amount of coherent thought, the attendants were instructed to provide positive, constructive information for the mind to use.

Excerpts from the Cayce Readings
3440-2   F. 29   1/4/44
While the entity is supersensitive and at times little disappointments, fears, doubts, and even an upset liver, may cause moods— even the shedding of tears, we find that these, too, may be met in the spiritual aspirations and desires of the body.

Know that with what measure you mete it is measured to you.

If you would have friends, be friendly. If you would even have fun, make fun for someone else.

Read the comic papers; not as to become sarcastic, no—but remember, ever, even thy Master, Jesus, could laugh in the face of the cross. Can ye find a better example?

Then see the joy, even in sorrow. See the pleasure that may even come with pain.

These are mostly matters of the mind. For mind is ever the builder. As you think in your heart, so are you.

4083-1   M. 55   4/12/44
In analyzing body, mind, soul, all phases of an entity's experience must be taken into consideration. In analyzing the mind and its reactions, oft individuals who would psychoanalyze or who would interpret the reactions that individual entities take, leave out those premises of soul, mind, body . . . Mind as a stream, not mind as purely physical or wholly spiritual, but it is that which shapes, which forms, which controls, which directs, which builds, which acts upon . . . A thought enters the mind. You either entertain it or you discard it. If you discard it, it has little or no effect . . .

5380-1   M. 54   7/20/44
In giving an interpretation of the disturbance as we find here, the mental attitude has as much to do with the physical reactions as illnesses in the body. For as we find, in the physical or purely pathological little disturbs the body, save sympathetically, but in the mental attitude there is so much of the making for the degrading of self that self-destruction becomes a part of the reaction, but it is wholly

mental. And thus the nerve forces for the body, this body as any body, any individual, who makes destructive thought in the body, condemning self for this or that, will bring, unless there are proper reactions, dissociation or lack of coordination between sympathetic and cerebrospinal system, and it may develop any condition which may be purely physical by deterioration of mental processes and their effect upon organs of the body.

"Provide the Treatments in Cycles"

The readings suggest that treatments be given in cycles that allow the body to rest and recover. Rest is required because some of the treatments (particularly the somatic therapies) can be stressful to the body. Recovery involves the ability of the body to maintain its own equilibrium without continued outside support. Continual treatment can rob the body of the ability to maintain itself and form a dependence on the specific treatments. The cycles of treatment recommended by Cayce varied considerably for individuals and for the type of treatments they were receiving. This is due in part to the variation in cycles between individuals and within an individual at different stages of healing.

The utilization of treatments in cycles was prominent in the philosophy of A. T. Still: "Find it, fix it, and leave it alone" (in Brantingham, 1986), a frequent admonition of the founder of osteopathy. The latter portion of this phrase refers to the necessity of allowing the body to heal itself. A. G. Hildreth, a close associate of Still and co-founder of the Still-Hildreth Sanatorium, summed it up by noting that a major problem facing clinicians is "knowing when to leave the tissues alone, that is, timing and spacing the treatments so they will be consonant with the time periods required by the healing processes of the body." (1930, p. 7) Hildreth goes on to comment that, "It is important to know when you have treated the patient enough, when you have done the right thing to correct the physical interference and to have the brains enough to know how much time nature needs to recuperate before a repetition of your treatment is given. Scientific facts are made useful only through complete knowledge and understanding of their applications." (p. 11)

The Cayce readings provide many examples of the utilization of cycles of treatment, not only from the standpoint of a single type of intervention (i.e. osteopathic treatments), but from a multidisciplinary perspective incorporating the various somatic, mental and spiritual modalities which comprise a holistic approach. For example, a series of osteopathic treatments might be given, and during the rest period between series, electrotherapy would be recommended. The sequence and duration of these cycles were important. The readings would often chide individuals for not adhering to the suggested cycles.

Excerpts from the Cayce Readings

271-1   M. 34   2/13/33

As to the matter of treatments, we would make application each day in periods of three to five weeks—and then a rest period of a week to ten days when a different vibration would be given the body—and then begin again with the original treatment, and so on.

271-6   M. 34   5/15/33

The periods in the treatments for rest, as we find, should have begun in this present week; not before; the rest period for five days, then begin again with the battery that carries the electronic influences through the medicated applications . . .

1439-1   M. 38   9/6/37

These osteopathic manipulations would be given for periods of six to ten such adjustments, left off for a period of a month, and then given again.

After the second of such adjustments or treatments are begun, we would THEN begin with the application of the low electrical vibrations of the Wet Cell Appliance that would carry Gold into the system . . .

These vibrations would not be given for more than twenty minutes in the beginning, and given only every other day; preferably as the body is ready to rest of an evening—taking the time to do same.

Give these vibrations in periods also; that is, give for thirty days—or fifteen treatments; leave of for thirty days; and then give again.

3440-1   F. 29   1/4/44

After these treatments [osteopathic adjustments] have been taken twice each week for six to eight treatments; then leave them off a period of three to four weeks.

During the rest period from osteopathy, take at least two hydrotherapy treatments—letting the body be thoroughly relaxed in a Pine Oil Bath; that is, with Pine Oil in the Bath in which the body would lie for twenty to thirty minutes every day. The two hydrotherapy treatments (colonic irrigations) should be about ten days to two weeks apart.

Each day following the Pine Oil Bath, attach the Radio-Active Appliance for one hour—and go to sleep. This will put the body to sleep. This will regain a great deal of that rest which the body in the last ten years has lost. This will make better coordination between the extremities of the body, through the circulation—the lymph and deeper circulation.

After the three weeks leave off the baths and the Radio-Active Appliance, and begin again with the osteopathic adjustments—this time making the adjustments, gradually, slowly, in the upper cervicals, upper dorsals, and then gradually in the 9th and 6th dorsals, and in the lumbar and sacral areas.

Then, after at least six of the adjustments have been made (not before), begin to add body-building energies and vitamins. Don't add these through the early periods, else they will contribute to more anxiety in the body . . .

After the second series of osteopathic adjustments, begin the Appliance again—and also the baths occasionally.

"All Healing Comes from Within"

The medical model of healing, which underlies most contemporary therapeutic modalities, suggests that treatment produces healing. The Cayce readings prefer to emphasize that it is attunement within the body that produces healing—not the treatments. In other words, in certain cases the correct treatment can be given and the body may not respond. In a serious illness such as schizophrenia, one must not only provide treatment in a mechanical fashion (as if the treatment is all there is to it), but seek to produce attunement within the inflicted individual.

The most obvious ramification of this principle is the problem of reaction within individuals suffering from the most serious form of schizophrenia (which Cayce diagnosed as dementia praecox, see Appendix C). When there is actual brain degeneration, the reaction of the body to treatment may be difficult to maintain. In several cases, Cayce cautioned that a "wait and see" attitude would be necessary because deterioration was so advanced that a positive prognosis was problematic. Persons were cautioned to follow the principles listed in this section and see if the body would respond.

The spiritual dimension of the applications was stressed in these cases. One can sense Cayce's transpersonal perspective in these instances—the unconscious (or "soul forces") would have to be stimulated to regenerate the physical body. Without such a response from the "Divine from within," recovery was impossible.

In reading 2153-6, note the reference to cycles of rest which allow the body to respond. This reading focuses on the role of cycles in allowing attunement to take place.

1310-1 F. 59 12/23/36

Q. May the body expect a complete cure? If so, how long will it be?

A. This depends, naturally, upon the reactions and the manner in which the applications may be made—as to the responses to and by the body. These, of course, are always questions—where body-building has to be accomplished. But if there is the change, see, then the more hopefulness being held, the greater the change may be.

2153-6 F. 13 11/12/40

Q. Would it be satisfactory to continue—

A. [Interrupting] You see, it is not that there are just so many treatments to be given and they can all be gotten through with and that's all there is to it! NO application of ANY medicinal property or any mechanical adjustment, or any other influence, is healing of itself! These applications merely help to attune, adjust, correlate the activities of the bodily functions to nature and natural sources!

All healing, thence, is from life! Life is God! It is the adjusting of the forces that are manifested in the individual body.

These directions as we have indicated take these conditions into consideration. Then, there must be periods of reaction of the bodily forces, the bodily functionings, the bodily response to influences without and within; and then the necessary attuning again and again.

The BODY is a pattern, it is an ensample of all the forces of the universe itself.

If all the rain that is helpful for the production of any element came at once, would it be better? If all the sunshine came at once, would it be better? If all the joy, all the sadness in the life experience of an individual were poured out at once, would it be better?

It is the cooperation, the reaction, the response made BY the individual that is sought. Know that the soul-entity must find in the applications that response which attunes its abilities, its hopes, its desires, its purposes to that universal consciousness. THAT is the healing—of any nature!

2359-1   M. Adult   9/9/30

Q. Will his mental condition improve or be cured entirely?

A. This, as we find, will materially improve. As to cure entirely, that will depend upon the responses in the system. The pressures as exist in the present prevent the normal reaction between sympathetic and cerebrospinal impulses. Not dementia; not a softening, not even a distribution of disorders as of a malignant nature, or of a conservatory nature—yet these are as distortions of the sympathetics, attempting to coordinate in or under pressures.

Q. If this treatment is followed, how long will it be before he will be cured?

A. The responses should show their beginning in three to five weeks. As to be cured, that will depend upon the response of the system.

2642-1   M. 45   12/30/41

KNOW—KNOW—there CAN be NO healing save from the awakening of the Divine within self. This is not only true for this body but every individual entity. It is a fact that these influences or centers may be aroused by varied means, through which body, mind and soul function in the physical being. Thus the needs of these considerations for this body, particularly, in making administrations for beneficial results for this body!

5598-1   M. 23   8/8/30

Q. Can he be taught to dress, feed, and care for himself in other respects?

A. If there is any response, much may be accomplished through this. If there is no response, little—or none—can be accomplished. It will require patience and persistence. See? . . . This, as is seen, must be builded within the mental being of the body.

5

Therapeutic Techniques

$\blacklozenge$

ALTHOUGH THE CAYCE readings propose a holistic framework from which to view the human condition, the readings also discuss the three aspects (body, mind, spirit) as if they can be examined separately.

267-2   F. 38   4/6/34
 . . . we have a soul body, a mental body, a physical body—each working and functioning in its own realm; all dependent one upon another, to be sure—but separate.

307-10   F. 57   1/15/36
 . . . so seldom is it considered by all, that spirituality, mentality, and the physical being are all one; yet may indeed separate and function one without the other—and one at the expense of the other. Make them cooperative, make them one in their purpose.

This chapter will examine therapies which address each of these aspects of the SELF (or as the readings seemed to prefer, the *ENTITY*). Keep in mind that humans are whole beings. The apparent division into body, mind, and spirit is a distortion necessitated by a three-dimensional perspective (which parallels the Western tradition of making distinctions between levels of experience).

It becomes increasingly obvious as one studies the readings that there is an inherent overlap in the treatment modalities. In practice, this overlap is exemplified by the principle "one activity becomes then dependent upon another" (Chapter Four). Holism involves treating the whole self—from different angles. Healing involves making these different aspects "cooperative," making them "one in their purpose."

An introduction precedes each of the sections of this chapter and serves to orient the reader to the excerpts from the readings which follow. Relevant clinical and research sources are cited when available to provide a context for the discussion.

SOMATIC THERAPIES

Therapies which primarily address the physical dimension of the self are called somatic therapies ("pertaining to or characteristic of the body [soma]," Miller & Keane, 1972, p. 890). The most common form of somatic therapy currently used to treat schizophrenia is medication. In the contemporary mental health field, the pervasive use of psychotropic medication is often equated with therapeutic efficacy. Other somatic therapies which are (or have been) employed with varying degrees of success include: manual medicine (e.g., osteopathy and chiropractic), physical therapy (e.g., exercise, massage, hydrotherapy, etc.), nutrition therapy (including vitamins), electrotherapy (primarily ECT), insulin shock therapy, and psychosurgery. Since the Cayce readings emphasized manual medicine as a primary treatment for major mental illnesses such as schizophrenia, this form of somatic therapy will be discussed first.

Manual Medicine

Manual medicine has been defined as "the use of mechanical forces applied through the hands to diagnose and treat functional disorders of the mechanical and soft tissue system" (Glossary of Osteopathic Terminology, 1990). Manual medicine encompasses a

Therapeutic Techniques ◆

variety of somatic therapies based upon a structural consideration
of physical dysfunction. Osteopathy and chiropractic represent the
most prominent examples of manual medicine today, and although
these professions represent divergent applications, their origins and
basic philosophy have much in common.

> Andrew Taylor Still (1845-1917) [osteopathy] and Daniel
> David Palmer (1845-1913) [chiropractic] were contemporaries,
> founders of dissenting schools of healing, school heads, phi-
> losophers, father figures to marginal professions, editors and
> authors. Both were spiritualists, doctrinaire eccentrics . . . and
> both taught that man and his healing was the product of a su-
> preme being. (Brantingham, 1986, pp. 18-19)

Osteopathy is the system of treatment developed by A. T. Still late
in the nineteenth century. Still believed that most diseases of the
human body result from improper or inadequate flow of the "nutrient arterial flow" (Sutherland, 1976). Disturbance of arterial flow
was often associated with structural defects of the musculoskeletal
system, impaired neurotransmission, and numerous other dysfunctions.

> As an electrician controls electric currents, so an Osteopath
> controls life currents and revives suspended forces . . . Study to
> understand bones, muscles, ligaments, nerves, blood supply,
> and everything pertaining to the human engine, and if your
> work be well done, you will have it under perfect control. (Still,
> 1897, pp. 275-276)

Although Still was referring to disease in general, subsequent
generations of osteopaths recognized the role of structural defects
in mental illness—particularly spinal injury and its relationship to
ANS dysfunction. F. M. Still, a grandson of A. T. Still and an osteopathic psychiatrist at Still-Hildreth Sanatorium, provides insight
into the relationship between schizophrenia (dementia praecox)
and autonomic dysfunction as cited in Chapter One:

> My theory of dementia praecox is necessarily based upon
> an osteopathic concept of this disorder . . . the autonomic ner-
> vous system is fundamentally involved and the distorted men-
> tality and accompanying physical phenomena are symptoms

of this difficulty. The basic regulatory functions of the nervous system, designated as autonomic, with their intimately associated circulatory and endocrine control, when in disorder gradually have their unfavorable effect upon the higher centers and account for the profound biological changes in the absence of constant and definite cerebral pathology. Early in this illness there should always be a hopeful prognosis. Deterioration is usually a slow and irregular process and certain to advance only to the degree in which the autonomic stress is unrelieved. The very theory of osteopathy is based upon physical causes which have their influence largely through autonomic action. The same fundamental principle which applies to the treatment of other organic disorders applies also to disorders of the intellect. In my opinion no field more truly demonstrates the value of osteopathic care than dementia praecox. (1933, p. 4)

This quote is a concise statement of the traditional osteopathic perspective on schizophrenia. It should be kept in mind when examining extract 1158-24 later in this section, where Cayce defines osteopathy as "the keeping of a BALANCE—by the touch—between the sympathetic [ANS] and cerebrospinal system!" The philosophy underlying osteopathy, as developed by Still, parallels that of the Cayce readings. Cayce's enthusiasm for the osteopathic approach will be abundantly clear in the excerpts which follow. J. Gail Cayce's *Osteopathy: Comparative Concepts—A. T. Still and Edgar Cayce* (1973) is a useful introduction to the subject and is highly recommended for persons interested in this aspect of Cayce's perspective.

It is important to keep in mind that osteopathy has changed considerably from the early decades of this century when Cayce was giving the readings. Today, osteopathy has assumed a professional stature which is legally recognized as equal to allopathic medicine. D.O.s (doctors of osteopathy) are provided the same privileges and responsibilities granted M.D.s, including the prescription of medication and performance of surgery. The evolution of osteopathy has produced practitioners that are generally considered to be sympathetic to "holistic medicine" while placing increasing emphasis on interventions utilized by traditional M.D.s. There is, undoubtedly, much less emphasis on manipulative techniques today than during Cayce's era. The formation of the North American Academy of Musculoskeletal Medicine, an organization composed of D.O.s (doctors of osteopathy), registered physical therapists, and M.D.s, attests to the integration of osteopathy into contemporary medicine and the greater acceptance of manipulative therapy by mainstream professionals.

Another change since Cayce's era is the evolvement of chiropractic as a major treatment option. Chiropractic has expanded to include a more holistic perspective. Its practitioners often provide a wide range of services including dietary counseling, acupuncture, massage, and electrotherapy.

The readings' recommendations for osteopathic treatment over chiropractic, in most cases, may have been due to the stature of chiropractic during that era. Gladys Davis Turner, Cayce's secretary for many years, provides insight on the role of chiropractic in the Cayce readings (Turner, 1957). She reports that a chiropractic member of the A.R.E. (Dr. J.E.F.) was disturbed by Cayce's apparent disregard for chiropractic:

> Being a chiropractor, naturally I wondered why osteopathy was preferred and why such a statement was made as was in case 304-1, where it says: "Chiropractic treatment is adjustment, not relaxation of the muscular forces." We chiropractors have been taught that chiropractic treatments do relax muscles, and I know it does. But if we go into the past a little on chiropractic and osteopathic history, we can see why the statement was made—at the time of the reading . . .
>
> I have no way of comparing the standards between osteopathy and chiropractic as they existed at that time, but osteopathic schools had at least a six-year head start over chiropractic schools and therefore very likely were of better quality than chiropractic ones. Then, too, B. J. Palmer [son of founder D. D. Palmer] was more interested in turning out chiropractors and it made no difference to him as to what type of a person took his course. He was interested in quantity and not in quality and length of time at the school was short. Finally after a number of years (about 1926), some of the faculty from the Davenport School broke away from school and started their own because they were "fed up" with some of B. J.'s ideas . . . In the meantime other schools were springing up all over the country because this or that individual developed, in his private practice, a special type of adjustment or technique, and he became so enthused with it, he thought the word "chiropractic" meant his

own method of treatment so he started a school to teach "Chiropractic" centered around his techniques.

So the reading 5211-1 where it says: "But there are chiropractors and there are chiropractors" could well mean this period when so many schools of different chiropractic thought were in existence. Also reading 5229-1 saying, " . . . but there are few chiropractors who make them properly," could mean this period when there so many chiropractors being "milled" out of the Davenport school, and only a few being "good adjusters" . . .

As I said for a while I was irked, but now I'm not, for again considering the time (1924) when the reading was taken, the advice given, and the status of chiropractic at that time, no doubt the reading was right.

With 3,300 graduates from the Palmer school in 1921, which was the largest class to graduate of all the healing arts of that period, it is quite possible that the most noted chiropractic adjustment (at that time) was what is known as the Palmer recoil, a type of adjusttment developed by B. J. Palmer and taught to all his students. Without going into detail to describe a recoil adjustment, it is sufficient to say that it is a harsh type of adjustment, and if one were witnessing a recoil adjustment being given in the cervical region, one might think the neck would break by such a thrust. They definitely were not the kind of adjustments to bring about relaxation . . .

However, thank goodness, other methods of adjusting were being developed in the chiropractic profession which were not so severe, which accomplished the same result and were relaxing to the patient. So now I'm quite confident that very likely if readings were taken today and the question asked as was in reading 304-1, the answer would not be so much against chiropractic.

Pagano echoes this sentiment by noting that in certain respects, chiropractors have assumed the role formally served by osteopaths.

Today the role of chiropractor, as I see it, encompasses the full role formerly practiced by the osteopath relative to the Cayce readings, and the osteopath has, for the most part, followed the path of medical practice. By these standards one would have to reevaluate the profession of choice as they pertain to the Cayce readings. The answer may be simply to find the right individual practitioner, whether chiropractor or osteopath, who will exercise the therapy called for in the readings. (Pagano, 1987, p. 14)

Pagano is a well-established chiropractic practitioner utilizing the Cayce approach to manual medicine. His informative discussion of manipulative therapy in the Cayce readings is highly recommended.

The role of manual medicine in the treatment of schizophrenia cannot be underestimated. A careful reading of the case studies in Chapter Three will highlight the involvement of lesions, adhesions, subluxations, and "pressures" in the production of psychotic symptoms.

Although the term lesion was used by early osteopaths, the current osteopathic term for lesion is *somatic dysfunction*. It is defined as "impaired or altered function of related components of the somatic (body framework) system; skeletal, arthrodial, and myofascial structures, and related vascular, lymphatic, and neurol elements" (Educational Council on Osteopathic Principles, 1990).

Subluxation was the term of preference by the early chiropractors and has continued to the present day although the expression "subluxation complex" has been adopted by some practitioners. Current terminology in both professions represents a recognition of "systems theory" and the concept of holism. Cayce frequently used the term "pressure" to designate the nature of the pathology in these cases although a wide variety of designations are scattered throughout the readings. Irvin Korr, the outstanding physiologist who invested many years researching osteopathic concepts, discussed the role of *pressure* in the formation and maintenance of the osteopathic lesion.

Now lest you anticipate that I am going to talk about the old-fashioned "pinched nerves" and such, I am not. I am going to talk about much more subtle influences that exert profound effects on cord function and its communications. These foramina contain not only the nerves and roots and their sheaths, but also quantities of fat, connective tissue, periosteum, blood vessels and so forth. We now know that it takes very slight, localized pressure or mechanical deformation to disturb the excitability and conductivity of the neurons that happen to be passing through a foramen at the focus of the pressure or deformation . . . In this environment the neurons are subject to quite considerable mechanical and chemical influences of various kinds, compression and torsion and many others. (Korr, 1970, pp. 57-58)

This excerpt from the osteopathic literature provides insight into what Cayce meant by the word "pressure" when used in the context of somatic dysfunction (see Tables 5.2, 5.3, and especially 5.4). The writings of Irvin Korr are a valuable resource for persons seeking insight into the role of the sympathetic nervous system, the effects of spinal lesions, and systemic incoordination resulting from somatic dysfunction.

And what is the source of these *pressures?* A. G. Hildreth, co-founder of the Still-Hildreth Sanatorium, used the word "strain" to designate the root of many mental problems.

To what are nervous and mental breakdowns due? This cannot be answered in a single word. The one word which comes nearest is "strain"—physical strain, mental strain. Mental overwork, grief, worry, religious excitement, etc., physical overwork, injury to head or spine, exhaustion from hemorrhage, operations, childbirth, etc., acute and chronic infections, and diseases of metabolism are causes.

Physiological crises, such as puberty and menopause, inheritance of nervous instability, toxins or poisons, whether taken as drugs, formed by bacteria, absorbed from sluggish bowels, or formed in the tissues and retained in the blood through failure of elimination—all these are possible factors in the production of mental disorders. Of these, heredity is just a predisposing cause. Nervous instability is all that is inherited. Probably every case is the cumulative result of a number of causes acting in concert.

Break into the circle of causes. Remove all that are removable. Leave the rest to nature. Thus assisted, she is usually able to "come back." Such is the philosophy of treatment at Still-Hildreth. (1929, p. 518)

One could not hope for a more succinct description of the causes and treatment of schizophrenia as portrayed in the readings. It encompasses variability of etiology, the role of heredity (i.e., diathesis/stress), cure by removal of causes, and healing by natural processes. It is understandable that the Cayce readings so frequently referred difficult cases to the Still-Hildreth Sanatorium (Cayce apparently had a cordial relationship with Still-Hildreth, see Documents 5.1 and 5.2).

As noted, the pathology produced by strain was referred to as a lesion in the osteopathic tradition. Cayce often used this term in his psychic diagnoses. Practitioners of manual therapy will appreciate the language of the readings in this regard since the diagnostic terms were often associated with the kind of referrals made by Cayce. As an example, reading 2022-1 diagnosed subluxations at the coccyx, 9th dorsal, and 1st and 2nd cervicals. As in many cases where the term subluxation was used, Cayce's use of the term was consonant with chiropractic usage and the reading recommended "adjustments—either chiropractically or osteopathically." In reading 3997-1, where the dysfunction was less specific and more systemic, Cayce suggested: "Osteopathically should the corrections, or only may the corrections be made properly—though correction might be made nominally under that called chiropractic; yet the reactions to the glands from the pressure would intensify . . . " (readers should keep in mind the previous discussion about the type of chiropractic that was prevalent during Cayce's era).

The recoveries resulting from adherence to the suggestions provided in the Cayce readings (e.g., [386], [1513], [1789], etc.) closely resemble cases in the osteopathic and chiropractic literature. Hildreth, in his excellent book *The Lengthening Shadow of Dr. Andrew Taylor Still* (1938), cites numerous cases where manipulative therapy provided seemingly miraculous cures. Quigley (1973), a staff member of the Clear View Sanitarium for 21 years and director for ten years, shares his experience by stating:

> When I first joined the staff of Clear View Sanitarium in 1940, I held strongly to the view that mental disorders were primarily of emotional origin. I frequently saw agitated schizophrenics, dangerous to themselves and others, arrive at Clear View in straitjackets, completely out of contact with the world of reality. They were not responsive to words, care, or any type of ministration. However, after chiropractic adjustments a dramatic change occurred, in which the patient began to orient himself by asking questions as to who we were, where he was, what happened to him. Soon he was released

from restraints, had freedom of the ward and was eventually released from the Sanitarium. At first I felt this represented those persons who will make spontaneous recovery with or without care. When this type of experience was observed in patients who had been under psychiatric hospitalization for years, the change was difficult to reconcile with a psychological rationale alone . . . These recoveries were not limited to schizophrenic types but also to psychotic depressions. (pp. 115-116)

In 1933, a study was conducted at the Still-Hildreth Sanatorium to measure the prevalence of osteopathic lesions in 1,000 cases of schizophrenia (Still, 1933). Table 5.1 presents the results of this study and suggests a high level of dysfunction in the upper cervical and upper dorsal areas of the spine. Dunn (1950) believes the relatively sparse incidence of lower spinal dysfunction found in this study supports a physiological etiology of schizophrenia.

It may seem remarkable that the lumbar region was infrequently lesioned in schizophrenics, considering the relative frequency of low lumbar problems in general practice. But the fact of low lesion frequency here only lends additional support to the theories of physical etiology in psychiatric disorders. The lumbar segments are of little importance in connection with the autonomic nervous system. (p. 356)

It is impossible to make a direct comparison of this study with the frequency of somatic dysfunction diagnosed in the Cayce readings because the information in the readings was not provided in a form amenable to the format used at Still-Hildreth. One can study Tables 5.2, 5.3, and 5.4 and review Figure 3.4 to get a sense of the frequency and location of somatic dysfunction in cases of schizophrenia in the Cayce readings (Chapter Three, Groups I, II & III). These tables and figure show a divergence from the earlier osteopathic study. There is a relatively high level of lower spine pathology in the Cayce readings. Injury to the coccyx, lumbar, and sacral areas appeared to be associated with dysfunction in the pelvic organs (e. g., reproductive glands). This model of psychosis marks one of the distinctions between the bulk of the osteopathic literature which viewed schizophrenia as resulting from dorsal and cervical lesions (which then affected the brain via the cardiovascular system—i. e., dysfunctional arterial flow to the brain resulting in lack of nutrients or autointoxication) and the Cayce readings which recognized the prevalence of endocrine involvement in this process. Reading 3609-1 illustrates this pattern: "pressures upon the brush end of the cerebrospinal system as to affect glandular forces, such pressures in the sympathetic and the vegetative nerve system as to cause disassociations between impulses and the cerebrospinal reflexes."

Glandular involvement resulting from lower spine dysfunction has important assessment implications because these cases tend to overlap with affective pathology (i.e., schizoaffective disorder and psychotic depression). Anxiety, depression, and even cases of violent psychotic mania were cited in the readings when this process was noted.

In summary, the Cayce readings are in agreement with the traditional osteopathic analysis of schizophrenia which viewed brain degeneration as resulting from dysfunctional blood supply to the brain producing a lack of adequate nutrition and/or improper elimination of metabolic waste. This process was often associated with cervical and dorsal lesions affecting the ANS. The readings went on to suggest another major process which could also result in psychotic symptoms and brain degeneration. This process focused on lower spinal insult and affected the glandular system (usually via the pelvic organs). These two major patterns of pathology were not mutually exclusive and did not preclude other etiologies in the development of schizophrenia.

In other words, the variability associated with schizophrenia has a somatic basis which involves all the major body systems. From the perspective of the Cayce readings, the philosophy and techniques of manual medicine provide a crucial avenue of intervention in the treatment of schizophrenia.

Excerpts from the Cayce Readings
902-1 2/17/41

As a system of treating human ills, osteopathy—WE would give—is more beneficial than most measures that may be given. Why? In any preventative or curative measure, that condition to be produced is to assist the system to gain its normal equilibrium. It is known that each organ receives impulses from other portions of the system by the suggestive forces (sympathetic nervous system) and by circulatory forces (the cerebrospinal system and the blood supply itself). These course through the system in very close parallel activity in EVERY single portion of the body. Hence stimulating ganglia from which impulses arise—either sympathetically or functionally—must be helpful in the body gaining an equilibrium.

1158-24   F. 50   4/20/40
Q. Should other glands be stimulated which have not been?
A. As just indicated, these should be stimulated—but from the centers from which the IMPULSE for their activity emanates!

Let's describe this for a second, that the entity or body here may understand, as well as the one making the stimulation:

Along the cerebrospinal system we find segments. These are cushioned. Not that the segment itself is awry, but through each segment there arises an impulse or a nerve connection between it and the sympathetic system—or the nerves running parallel with same. Through the sympathetic system (as it is called, or those centers not encased in cerebrospinal system) are the connections with the cerebrospinal system.

Then, in each center—that is, of the segment where these connect—there are tiny bursa, or a plasm of nerve reaction. This becomes congested, or slow in its activity to each portion of the system. For, each organ, each gland of the system, receives impulses through this manner for its activity.

Hence we find there are reactions to every portion of the system by suggestion, mentally, and by the environment and surroundings.

Also we find that a reaction may be stimulated INTERNALLY to the organs of the body, by injection of properties or foods, or by activities of same.

We also find the reflex from these internally to the brain centers.

Then, the SCIENCE of osteopathy is not merely the punching in a certain segment or the cracking of the bones, but it is the keeping of a BALANCE—by the touch—between the sympathetic and cerebrospinal system! THAT is real osteopathy!

With the adjustments made in this way and manner, we will find not only helpful influences but healing and an aid to any condition that may exist in the body—unless there is a broken bone or the like!

1842-3   M. 36   5/10/44
Q. What treatment is recommended in lieu of osteopathic treatments?
A. If there has been one found we haven't it yet!

5211-1   F. 51   6/13/44
. . . for this particular body we would continue with the present chiropractor. We would ordinarily give that osteopathy is more vital, but there are chiropractors and there are chiropractors. This is a very good one; don't lose him! He understands this body.

Massage

Massage is a therapeutic modality which has traditionally been used as an adjunctive therapy (i.e., used in manual medicine or physical therapy). Only in recent years has it become established as a recognized profession in this country (in other parts of the world massage has a long-standing professional stature). Massage was frequently recommended in the Cayce readings for a wide variety of problems. In analyzing the readings in which massage was suggested, Joseph and Sandra Duggan (1987) concluded that one of the main benefits of massage in the readings was to coordinate the nervous systems (note the similarity to Cayce's definition of osteopathy in reading 1158-24). Their book, *Edgar Cayce's Massage, Hydrotherapy & Healing Oils,* provides an excellent review of the use of massage in the readings and contains important insights into the subtle variations in technique and massage oils which Cayce recommended.

Roger Jahnke's article on body therapies (1986) makes a strong case that many of the innovative body therapies being used today (e.g., reflexology, connective tissue reflex massage, shiatsu, polarity, applied kinesiology, Trager, Reiki, etc.) fit well into the Cayce approach. He notes, "The autonomic nerve-balancing mechanism of neuroreflex techniques and the reprogramming of the body/mind brain feedback loop through neuromuscular release also are verified, although not named in the readings" (p. 42).

Massage may be particularly helpful as an adjunct to chiropractic, a combination becoming increasingly common in the chiropractic profession (Calvert, 1989). In view of Cayce's emphasis on soft tissue manipulation and relaxation, massage would appear to be useful in this role—particularly when suggestive therapeutics are deemed appropriate (to be discussed later in this chapter).

Excerpts from the Cayce Readings
386-1   F. 20   8/9/33
The massage would be not so much of the osteopathic or adjust-

ment nature, but more of the neuropathic—or a gentle quieting of the nerves.

386-2   F. 20   9/28/33
Q. How often should the massages be given?
A. As suggested, it would be best that the massages be given just before the application of the active forces from the low electrical vibrations [Wet Cell Battery] that carry the stamina in the body that acts with the activities of the nerve impulses themselves.

1789-8   F. 33   4/17/40
About three times each week, preferably as the body is prepared for rest of evening or night, we find it will be most helpful to gently massage into the system all the body will absorb of an equal combination of Olive Oil and Peanut Oil; especially across the sacral and the lower portion of the spine. This should extend, of course, UP the spine to the 9th dorsal, but more in the sacral, lumbar, than in the upper portions of the body. We find this should be done not hurriedly, not as something to be gotten through with, but take twenty or thirty minutes to give such a massage. This will be helpful in keeping better equilibrium and activities to portions of the body, and make for more regularity with the activities of the organs of the system.

3075-1   M. 24   7/2/43
Follow this with a gentle massage, that stimulates or relaxes by the stimulation of each of the ganglia along the cerebrospinal system; more specifically in the areas where the cerebrospinal and sympathetic coordinate—in the larger forms of the ganglia. These we find the 1st, 2nd, and 3rd cervical, 1st, 2nd and 3rd dorsal, 9th dorsal, and in the lumbar axis and coccyx center.
Q. Should the massage be osteopathic, or could it be given by someone other than an osteopath?
A. Anyone that understands the anatomical structure of the body, in knowing how to coordinate the sympathetic and cerebrospinal systems in the areas indicated. These are not merely to be punched or pressed, but the ganglia—while very small—are as networks in these various areas. Hence a gentle, circular massage is needed; using only at times structural portions as leverages, but not ever—of course—bruising structure.

3223-1   M. 31   9/19/43
Each day when the Appliance is removed, give a light massage—
not attempting to make corrections but massage along the spine
and also along the sympathetic area; that is, on the spine itself and
then about an inch-and-one-half of the spine centers on either side
particularly in the lumbar and sacral areas and from the first dorsal
to the first cervical, with this combination of oils—all the body will
absorb:

> Olive Oil .... 1 ounce
> Peanut Oil .... 1 ounce
> Lanolin .... ¾ teaspoonful.

Hydrotherapy

Hydrotherapy is a form of physical therapy which involves the
use of water in a variety of ways such as Epsom salt baths, sitz baths,
hot and cold showers, douching, cabinet sweats, steam baths, fume
and vapor baths, enemas, and colonics. Hydrotherapy was frequently recommended by Cayce to stimulate circulation and pro-
mote elimination of waste products. For a brief summary of the use
of hydrotherapy in the readings, see Karp (1986).

Hydrotherapy has been used extensively in the psychiatric treatment of mental illness and was an important modality in the approach advocated at Still-Hildreth Sanatorium.

> Hydrotherapy is another valuable aid for which we are
> equipped. Baths and hot packs are used to quiet the nerves, to
> induce sleep, and especially to stimulate elimination through
> kidneys and skin . . . Many patients have a history of long con-
> tinued constipation with evidence of resulting autointoxica-
> tion . . . some assistance is necessary. For it our main reliance
> is colonic irrigation, by which the colon is thoroughly cleansed
> by large quantities of normal salt solution . . . The value of this
> is obvious. (Hildreth, 1929, p. 519)

Hydrotherapy was also used effectively at the Forest Park Sanitarium.

> The patients we care for are not responsible . . . few, if any of
> them will take enough exercise to get the proper amount of
> elimination through the skin . . . If there is a toxic condition,

which we have found to be in almost every case, the treatments given in our hydrotherapy department are very effective. They are especially beneficial in violent cases, because of the relaxation produced. (*The Chiropractic Psychopathic Sanitarium News*, undated, p. 25)

Excerpts from the Cayce Readings

257-254   M. 50   12/18/43
Q. How often should the hydrotherapy be given?
A. Dependent upon the general conditions. Whenever there is a sluggishness, the feeling of heaviness, oversleepiness, the tendency for an achy, draggy feeling, then have the treatments. This does not mean that merely because there is the daily activity of the alimentary canal there is no need for flushing the system. But whenever there is the feeling of sluggishness, have the treatments. It'll pick the body up. For there is the need for such treatments when the condition of the body becomes drugged because of absorption of poisons through alimentary canal or colon, sluggishness of liver or kidneys, and there is the lack of coordination with the cerebrospinal and sympathetic blood supply and nerves. For the hydrotherapy and massage are preventative as well as curative measures. For the cleansing of the system allows the body forces themselves to function normally, and thus eliminate poisons, congestions and conditions that would become acute through the body.

440-2   M. 23   12/12/33
Q. Do you advise the use of colonics or Epsom salts baths for the body?
A. When these are necessary, yes, For everyone—everybody— should take an internal bath occasionally, as well as an external one. They would all be better off if they would.

2524-5   M. 43   1/13/44
Set up better eliminations in the body. This is why osteopathy and hydrotherapy come nearer to being the basis of all needed treatments for physical disabilities.

1863-1   F. 44   11/28/42
The blood supply indicates that there are the effects of toxic conditions through the body, and a subluxation in those areas from which the nerve impulse contributes to the activity of the liver and

gall duct . . . first we would have a series of at least five or six of the hydrotherapy treatments. These would include mild sweat baths, with the fumes of Witch hazel added; with a massage following same . . .

3440-1   F. 29   1/4/44
During the rest period from the osteopathy, take at least two hydrotherapy treatments—letting the body be thoroughly relaxed in a Pine Oil Bath; that is, with Pine Oil in the Bath in which the body would lie for twenty to thirty minutes every day. The two hydrotherapy treatments (colonic irrigations) should be about ten days to two weeks apart.

Hot Packs

Hot packs were a common treatment in the Cayce readings and were also frequently used at Still Hildreth Sanatorium. The readings recommended packs to "facilitate the absorption of beneficial elements into the system, relax the patient, ease pain, stimulate circulation, and break up congestion" (Karp, 1986, p. 544). Castor oil was probably the most common pack suggested by Cayce and was especially useful for assisting in the elimination of wastes. Olive oil was usually recommended in conjunction with castor oil packs to improve eliminations. William McGarey's book, *The Oil That Heals* (1993), is a complete source of information on all aspects of the therapeutic use of castor oil.

Excerpt from the Cayce Readings
2465-1   F. 28   3/17/41
There has been a lesion in the lacteal duct and that as coordinating with the organs of the pelvis.

Hence at times such a state is produced as to almost become obsession, but possession in same.

The reaction to the pineal becomes so severe as to short-circuit the nerve impulse; carrying or producing a fluttering or an engorgement in static waves to the base of the brain.

Thus periods are caused when there is lack of self-control.

These would be the applications:

For an hour each day for three days in succession, apply the hot Castor Oil Packs over the lacteal duct and the caecum area . . .

On the evening of the third Pack—that is, at the end of the three-day series, you see—take internally two tablespoonfuls of Olive Oil.

Exercise and Activity

Exercise and activity play an important role in physical therapy and may also contribute to mental rehabilitation due to their mood-altering characteristics (Greist et al., 1979) and the opportunity they provide for social interaction (Seilheimer & Lee, 1987). Exercise and activity may also be conceptualized as nonspecific stress management techniques. As such they may make a significant contribution in the rehabilitation of persons suffering from schizophrenia (Li, 1981; DeBenedette, 1988).

Cayce provided some important guidelines for structuring exercise and activities for persons suffering from schizophrenia. Activities should be specific and constructive. In other words, do something that is useful so that the person engages both mind and body in a balanced manner. Don't engage in make-work or activities where it makes no difference how the activity is done. Outdoor activities in the sun and fresh air were most often recommended with specific references to activities such as tennis, golf, swimming, horseback riding, etc. Each individual was encouraged to do some physical exercise where the person would "break a sweat." Sweating may have been suggested because it provides a natural means of detoxification.

Excerpts from the Cayce Readings
271-1 M. 34 2/13/33
The exercises should be specific, and as much as possible both of a physical and mental nature, that are constructive—or that are building in their activity.

271-4 M. 34 4/17/33
In the matter of the physical activity, this should be that which makes the body physically tired of evenings. And early to retire, in most occasions, is better for the body.

And as soon as the body awakes of mornings, it should be required to begin some sort of physical activity; rather than the mental—which is that which will make for the introspection of self. Hence suggestions and a good deal of talk regarding what the activities of the day will be, should be the beginning of the day.

271-5   M. 34   5/1/33
Well that there be reactions for the physical activity, or exercise in the open. Not too strenuous, to be sure; but there must be very constructive forces.

638-1   F. 72   8/21/34
Keep the body in the open as much as possible, with as pleasant surroundings as possible. Never allow the body to condemn itself, nor have anyone condemned or disturbed by overanxiety in the presence of the body. But continue to make as much as possible of dependency as possible, and look to the body as being depended upon for certain activities—specific activities, in walking and in doing definite things. See?

1513-1   M. 47   1/7/38
Q. On his return home, what kind of exercise would be best?
A. Keep in the open as much as practical, but NEVER alone . . .

3223-1   M. 31   9/19/43
Keep in the open quite often. Keep the body active at some definite activity.

Electrotherapy

The Cayce readings recommended the use of several appliances and techniques which utilize electrical energy for healing. Some of these modalities fall within the electromagnetic spectrum (i.e., violet and ultraviolet rays) and others were described as utilizing vibrational energy of a low electrical nature (i.e., Wet Cell Battery, Impedance Device, magnetic healing). The low electrical energy was said to be the life force or creative force within the body.

1800-4   7/27/25
The human body is made up of electronic vibrations, with each atom and element of the body, each organ and organism of same, having its electronic unit of vibration necessary for the sustenance of, and equilibrium in, that particular organism. Each unit, then, being a cell or a unit of life in itself, has its capacity of reproducing itself by the first law as is known of reproduction—division. When a force in any organ, or element of the body, becomes deficient in its ability to reproduce that

equilibrium necessary for the sustenance of the physical existence and reproduction of same, that portion becomes deficient through electronic energy as is necessary. This may come by injury or by disease, received from external forces. It may come from internal forces through lack of eliminations produced in the system, or by lack of other agencies to meet the requirements of same in the body.

Cayce's description of this force closely parallels the various Oriental traditions (e.g., acupuncture, Qigong, etc.) which recognize the biophysical dimension of healing:

> Oriental medicine is completely consistent with the supposed "new" idea in a rational science that a person is more of a resonating field than a substance . . . Qigong, simply stated, is the cultivation of Qi or vital life energy. Stated in a more modern and scientific language, Qigong is the practice of activating, refining and circulating the human bioelectrical field. Because the bioelectrical field maintains and supports the function of the organs and tissues, Qigong can have a profound effect on health. (Jahnke, 1990, pp. 3-4)

McGarey's *Acupuncture and Body Energies* (1974) provides an excellent introduction to the similarities between Cayce's portrayal of vibrational healing and Oriental approaches. *Vibrational Medicine* by Richard Gerber, M.D. (1988), and *Energy Medicine Around the World* by T. M. Srinivasan, Ph.D (1988), are also useful prefaces to the field of vibrational healing. The International Society for the Study of Subtle Energies and Energy Medicine (ISSSEEM) is an organization founded to explore the various aspects of energy medicine. Interested readers may contact the society at: 356 Goldco Circle, Golden, CO 80401.

In conjunction with electrotherapy, Cayce also emphasized the use of gold (and occasionally silver) to rebuild the nervous systems of individuals suffering from schizophrenia. In some individuals, the body was apparently unable to assimilate these elements naturally due to genetic defects or injury. In these cases, the appliances usually served as a conduit for providing these elements "vibratorily."

The most frequently suggested appliances and techniques will be briefly discussed. Some excerpts from the readings will follow to give the reader a sense of how the appliances were to be used. Circulating Files which provide an in-depth examination of most of these modalities are available. Interested persons should contact the A.R.E. for further information.

Wet Cell Battery

This was the most commonly recommended appliance for the regeneration of nerve tissue in cases of dementia praecox (see Table 5.5). Although the battery delivers a very minute direct current voltage, Cayce maintained that the therapeutic benefit was due to vibrational energy generated by the device. The readings stated that the battery, when used in conjunction with various therapeutic agents (such as gold), acted indirectly upon the nervous system via the glandular system. Presumably, the glands were not secreting properly for the maintenance of normal neurotransmission. Therefore, electrotherapy was required to restore normal glandular activity.

Excerpts from the Cayce Readings

271-1   M. 34   2/13/33

. . . yet—as we find—from the activities in many portions of the system—if there are added to the system those elements [gold] that would produce stamina in the tissue of the nerve cords in cerebrospinal, in the association of the cerebrospinal and sympathetic in varied plexus and the muscular forces . . . much better conditions may be brought for the body . . .

For the first three to five weeks we would apply each day the Wet Cell Battery . . .

271-8   M. 34   6/12/33

With the sun and sea baths continued there may be the less amount to make for activity, but without the vibrations—or any of the vibrations from the low electrical forces [Wet Cell Battery], with those supplies of the minerals [gold] necessary to be active in constructive influences in brain tissue and nerve elements of the system, as we have indicated, these of the sun rays are hardly efficient or sufficient in keeping constructive forces.

271-9   M. 34   6/26/33

But, we would insist that there be applied those vibrations [Wet Cell Battery] for the correction of the activities in that assimilated by the system for the replenishing of nerve energy cooperation between the cerebrospinal and sympathetic and brain centers themselves.

386-1 F. 20 3/9/33
. . . using also the Wet Cell Battery (Plain, see? but carrying the Gold). The positive anode should be of the copper, and attached to the 4th dorsal plexus. The negative anode carrying the Gold would be attached to the right and up an inch from the umbilicus plexus, or over the assimilating ganglia—from the lymph reaction in digestive system, so that the foods that are assimilated will create a constructive force in the blood supply, responding to the cells of the glands in the body.

1068-1 F. 40 11/26/35
Use the electrical forces, as indicated, of the plain Wet Cell Appliance . . . these passing through the system create a nominal or normal balance, for they become effective with—or attune the atomic vibrations of the body to their normalcy. Just as one would attune an instrument to accord or coordinate its chords with other portions, producing the vibrations that become harmonious; just so do they become harmonious in the body.

1428-1 M. 30 9/2/37
Also we would add the vibratory forces of the Wet Cell Appliance that would clarify or purify the activity of the glandular system; and through these low electrical vibrations we would carry the vibrations from Chloride of Gold . . .

1513-1 M. 47 1/7/38
But we find, if there will be the administration of the elements [vibratory gold] that are the basic reaction of nerve impulse and plasm itself carried into the system in such a manner as to make for a revivifying of the energies through the creating in the glandular forces of the body the elements necessary for the replenishing of the impulses, these may be brought yet to an active service for the body in such measures that there may be a restoring of the mental forces and a better coordination.

This would necessitate also then the supervision of a sympathetic physician that would make adjustments in the coccyx and the lumbar centers; and the application through the low electrical vibratory forces that carry gold into the system—in the low electrical vibratory manner . . .

And there would be applied the Wet Cell Appliance carrying the Chloride of Gold . . .

1789-8   F. 33   4/17/40

However, as we have indicated, that there may be better coordination, better activities in the actions between the impulses of the mental and the physical self, the low electrical forces [Wet Cell Battery] that will carry the strengthening impulse to the nervous system will be most beneficial.

Thus we will find that the body will not tire so, and there will be more animation to the activities of the body; with less periods (that arise at times) when there is needed a stimulation from others concerned about the body . . .

2721-2   F. 19   9/23/42

With the rest of those applications made, we find that if there were a more consistent use of the Wet Cell Appliance that carries the Chloride of Gold to the body—which with the glandular system will supply the tissue that supplies nerve and brain tissue—we would bring better conditions for this body.

Impedance Device (Radio-Active Appliance)

The Impedance Device (also referred to as the Radio-Active Appliance) was also frequently recommended by Cayce for the treatment of a wide variety of problems. It was said to function strictly at the vibrational level, working directly with the low electrical energy of the body (the "life force"). The readings state that the Impedance Device works with the same vibrational energy as the Wet Cell but is less powerful. Its application was often suggested to relax and coordinate the systems of the body.

The term "radio-active" in no way signifies atomic radiation of a toxic nature. In fact, the vibrational energy associated with this appliance cannot be measured with current empirical technology. The original designation was intended to describe the interaction of the appliance and the subtle energy involved (i.e., like a radio and radio waves). The name was changed to Impedance Device to avoid confusion as to the nature of the energies involved.

Excerpts from the Cayce Readings

444-2   F. 43   11/18/33
... the lowest form of electrical energy is the basis of life.

552-2   F. 15   6/13/34
The vibrations that are to be set up by the application of low electrical vibration will create more and more the ability for the suggestive forces to reach to the nerves of consciousness in the body itself, see?

1110-4   M. Adult   7/11/36
The Appliance [radio-active] will aid in relieving nervousness ...

1158-11   F. 47   11/19/37
As given respecting the use of the Radio-Active Appliance, the vibrations created by same are NOT curatives—these are EQUALIZERS. If the body is tired, if the body grows weary, mentally or physically, this will be found to be MOST beneficial—it is for ANY body, and it would be extremely well then for this body. If there are periods when there is weariness, if there is the tendency for an overnervousness, use same. This only stimulates the activity of the nerve or vibratory forces of the low electrical energies in the system to UNIFY their purposes.

1173-8   M. 28   7/30/36
... they are as one—body, mind, soul—as the effective activity of a low current of electrical reaction or radiation is created in the active forces of the Radio-Active Appliance—it brings to the system just those influences; the tendency to make the body-physical, the body-mental, and mental-spiritual forces more and more in accord by a unison ... Let these be some considerations: If there is the constant dosing or constant application of synthetic influences [drugs], these become at times hindrances to the body. But if there are those activities from nature's storehouse, then we find these work with the Creative Energies and impulses of an organism to create and to bring about coordinating influences in the system.

1472-2   F. 57   11/6/37
Restlessness, insomnia and irritation will disappear [with the use of the Radio-Active Appliance].

1800-28   12/7/36
And this will be . . . a type of appliance [radio-active] for bringing rest to the weary, rest to those who have been inclined to depend upon sedatives, and narcotics for rest; to those who have been under great periods of stress and strain; to those who seek to find an equalizing influence that will assist them in producing a coordination in their physical and mental spirituality upon the body-physical.

3440-1   F. 29   1/4/44
Each day following the Pine Oil Bath, attach the Radio-Active Appliance for one hour—and go to sleep. This will put the body to sleep. This will regain a great deal of that rest which the body in the last ten years has lost. This will make better coordination between the extremities of the body, through the circulation—the lymph and deeper circulation.

5428-1   M. 31   6/2/44
Just as a battery may be charged or discharged, so may the human body be recharged by the production of coordination [by the Radio-Active Appliance].

Violet Ray

The Violet Ray is a high-voltage, low-amperage source of static electricity which was invented about 1920 and was in common use during the 1920s and '30s.

> Its frequency of over one million cycles per second makes a mild form of diathermy, a treatment providing therapeutic heating of tissues beneath the skin. The Violet Ray consists of a hand-held base into which a vacuum-glass applicator or "electrode" is inserted. The electrical current is diffused into rapidly vibrating sprays of deep violet color, giving the appliance its name . . . The primary function of the appliance was to stimulate the superficial circulation. In the process, according to Cayce, additional beneficial effects could be obtained, including more restful sleep, greater physical stamina, improved eliminations, relief from nervous complaints, and a better balance through the system. (Karp, 1986, pp. 517-518)

The Violet Ray was often recommended by Cayce for cases involving possession (see Table 5.5 and Appendix E).

Excerpts from the Cayce Readings
263-13   F. 29   12/16/40
. . . the Violet Ray. This is a high voltage, stimulating all centers that are as the crossroads, the connections between the various portions of the physical-body functioning, the mental attitudes and attainments . . .

1572-1   F. 50   4/18/38
. . . use the Hand Machine Violet Ray . . . These treatments will tend to make for the raising of the vibrations of the body, disassociating the effects of repressions in the system; producing better coordination throughout.

Ultraviolet Ray

Short-wave ultraviolet light was also recommended by Cayce in a few cases to aid in the assimilation of gold (when taken orally to rebuild the nervous systems).

Excerpt from the Cayce Readings
5690-1   M. 27   3/6/31
The defects in the elements within the body itself, as we find, may be added to system through a gold treatment, either taken vibratorily into the system [electrical appliance] or taken in a soluble form, so that the reactions with the vibrations set up with electrical forces will have the desired effect of producing that stamina necessary in the nervous energies and plexus themselves, as to produce coordination—provided, the cerebrospinal centers are made in accord one with another . . .
Q. How should the gold be applied?
A. Either through the vibratory forces of a low electrical vibration, as in wet battery, or it may be taken [as] soluble solution, see? soda and gold into the system. That, when taken, would necessitate the use of such vibrations as of the ultraviolet ray to make same become active in the system for resuscitation of those elements necessary to create. It may be taken either way. See?

Vibratory Metals

The Cayce readings assigned a crucial role to the use of vibratory metals (gold and silver) in the treatment of schizophrenia. Gold was by far the most commonly recommended of these metals (see Table 5.5) and will be the primary focus in this discussion.

The electrical appliances which have been discussed provided the most frequently suggested means for the assimilation of gold. Apparently, taking the gold orally without vibrational energy was not sufficient to guarantee its proper assimilation.

In contemporary medical practice, gold is used in the treatment of rheumatoid arthritis (Hardin, 1989). Taken orally or by injection, gold can produce toxic reactions in some individuals. When utilized in these forms, its use should be monitored by a physician.

The Cayce readings recommended gold for the treatment of numerous conditions, including rheumatoid arthritis. As noted, the readings generally preferred the gold to be administered "vibratorily" and stated that the use of electrotherapy increased the assimilation of the mineral. In consideration of the possible toxicity of gold for some individuals, perhaps the suggestions for vibratory gold were also related to safety factors.

Excerpts from the Cayce Readings
173-1 M. 59 9/10/26
This [osteopathic adjustments] will remove strain, yet would not enliven tissue in itself. We begin, then, giving internally, and through a vibratory force, those forms of soda and gold, internally, that rejuvenate the whole system, as to repropagation of nerve energy. Stimulating same, see?

281-27 6/11/36
. . . gold, that is a renewal; while silver is a sustaining cord, a renewer of the energies as applied between the physical forces and the energies of activity of life itself upon nerve and brain forces as well as the very essence of the glandular secretions of the body.

849-27 M. 31 6/4/38
Hence we would add those influences that are the lowest form of electrical vibration that will carry with same the elements which in their final analysis are the bases [basis?] of the association or connection with mentality, consciousness and matter in activity; that is, gold and silver.

915-2   M. 62   6/15/35

As we find, the application of the Radio-Active Appliance in the experience in the present would be most helpful for this body: also those vibrations through the same activity carrying the Chloride of Gold into the system.

Or the Gold may be taken internally in very minute doses, for the stimulation of those gland secretions that make for creative energies and forces through the activity of all the glands in the body; thus making coordination between the reproductive forces or glands and the pineal and the adrenal. These would be the more helpful in the present.

988-7   M. 25   11/19/35

Not only does the activity of the gold, then, make for this vibration in the body, but it produces in the endocrinals—through its associations of the metallic force . . . through the electrical charges, the low form passing through the system—the stamina, as it were, to the plasm of the nerve forces themselves.

5405-1   M. 22   8/22/44

There is within the nerve centers that which, in the elements of material, contributes to the white and gray matter of the nervous system, and, as has been indicated, this may be in patient, in gentleness, rebuilded, even when destroyed much more than is indicated here. But with the use of these elements—silver and gold—to the body in such measures and manners as to supply those necessary influences to re-establish in the physical forces of the body those necessary channels along which impulses run, we may replenish, we may supply those forces, for even this body.

Medicine

The powerful neuroleptic drugs currently in use have profoundly affected research into the etiology and treatment of schizophrenia. Although it is impossible to say with certainty how Cayce would have viewed the use of these drugs (they came into use several years after his death in 1945), one can draw some reasonable conclusions by studying the the readings' perspective on medications in use during that era. A general principle in the readings was to avoid drugs as much as possible and use natural substances when medication was essential. This approach is in keeping with the notion that the body is a "medicine chest" capable of supplying whatever is needed to maintain health. Disease can result when the body is unable to perform this vital function. Treatment is directed at re-establishing the body's innate ability to rebuild itself.

Cayce insisted that some of the drugs being used to treat schizophrenia (particularly the bromides) actually accelerated the degenerative processes taking place in the brain. Even so, in some instances where the illness was so acute as to endanger the patient or attendants, he recommended the use of bromides to quiet the body (e.g., 5715-2).

Insulin coma was another frequently used treatment for schizophrenia before the advent of neuroleptics (and during Cayce's career as psychic diagnostician). Although the therapeutic mechanism was unknown, it had been found that the inducement of a transient hypoglycemic coma, which was quickly reversed by infusions of glucose, was essential for therapeutic efficacy. In a controlled study, Fink et al. (1958) compared insulin coma to chlorpromazine and concluded:

> Chlorpromazine was found to be as effective in modifying psychotic behavior as insulin coma therapy. There was no difference in the improvement rating on discharge, incidence of complications, or effects on the psychotherapeutic relationship for either therapy . . . In comparison to insulin coma, chlorpromazine is safer, easier to administer, and lends itself to long-term management. No evidence has been educed that either therapy has altered the basic schizophrenic process, nor is there any evidence that there is greater specificity of either form of therapy for schizophrenic illnesses. (p. 1850)

Lozovsky, Koplin, and Saller (1985) report that the therapeutic effectiveness of insulin coma may be related to "the modulating effect of insulin on brain dopamine receptor sensitization" (p. 190).

> Thus our studies indicate that two seemingly completely different treatments of schizophrenia, i.e., neuroleptics and insulin coma therapy, could affect the same target, DA receptor, and might have an essential common mechanism, normalization in dopaminergic transmission. Therefore this effect of insulin is consistent with and supports the dopaminergic hypothesis of schizophrenia. (p. 192)

McCall (1989), while recognizing the disadvantages of insulin coma, speculates that this modality may benefit the large subgroup of schizophrenic patients who are not responsive to neuroleptic treatment.

Although insulin coma was widely used at mental institutions during Cayce's era and was occasionally noted in the readings (or in correspondence from relatives), its use was not condemned in the readings. Case [3905] provides an example of the readings' flexibility in suggesting a range of therapeutic interventions, including insulin coma.

Thus one can surmise, based upon the readings' judicious recommendations for bromides and insulin coma, that Cayce would have been agreeable to the discreet use of antipsychotic medications—perhaps reserving them for acute cases. The insidious and irreversible side effects of these drugs (such as tardive dyskinesia) are well documented. Cayce would likely have insisted that the use of manual medicine be pursued along with the other modalities documented in this book. It is probable, however, that he would have suggested the use of neuroleptics during acute stages or cases where the individual would not respond to other interventions. Research on low dosage or intermittent schedules is presented in the discussion section of Chapter Six and should help clarify this subject.

Excerpts from the Cayce Readings
386-2 F. 20 9/28/33
When unusual conditions arise, as the activities where there are the supersensitive influences of outside forces upon the body, and these reactions take the form of hallucinations (from the normal reactions), then the quieting of the body through suggestions will be found much better than with the use of influences [drugs] that would deaden the nerve reactions and tend to increase (as time goes on) those influences from without.

173-5 M. 28 7/29/36
The less medications, as medicines, the better it will be for the body: provided these are not necessary to add stimulation to some depleted or defunct activity of an organ or for the strengthening of the body in some way or manner. But these are rather as tonics and stimulants than as medications, as we find. For nature should be the healer.

886-1   F. Adult   4/11/35

In the present, as we would find, there had best be kept the hypnotics rather than narcotics, to keep the body the more quiet; but this should at all times be under the direction of a physician, see?

1428-1   M. 30   9/2/37

In the bodily functions there have been those effects of activities to allay an infection that acted upon the organs of the body as related to the higher or the more emotional nervous systems and forces of the body through the genitive system.

These with pressures, while the conditions have been allayed or eliminated, pressures left in the coccyx, the lumbar and lower dorsal area, continue to make for the effect of these highly active forces upon the system.

These are from the serums and the medicines taken, rather than the dis-ease or disturbance itself.

This, then, is not a true dementia praecox condition. While there is incoordination between the cerebrospinal and the sympathetic nervous system, this arises rather from the conditions that have been indicated [use of medications].

1452-1   F. 38   10/9/37

In the approach then, first as we find, from the very nature of the reactions, medications—as medical reactions, in the form of any bromides, or those that would make for a degeneration of the feelings to the system—would only allay; but produce those conditions where softening of the reflexes from brain forces to the activities through the system would set up in such natures as to become WHOLLY destructive to the physical body and its reactions.

1969-1   M. 38   7/28/39

In the present environs (this is not meant to be as a disputation), it is not thoroughly understood. For here we have a condition that is as much POSSESSION as a weakening of the nerve forces in the system; and the general nerve breakdown will NOT be eliminated by the administering of drugs nor by the mere activity of suppression.

1969-2   M. 38   8/19/39

For it is as a split personality in the present, with the reflexes forming that which has been indicated—that causes the incoordi-

nation in the mental and spiritual and physical forces of this body.
Then keep the entity as far as possible from that which mitigates
or subjugates the body-forces with the spiritual influences—or from
sedatives or bromides. For these will only add to the confusion of
the reactions . . .

2721-1 F. 18 4/6/42
The administration of sedatives, while keeping down the ravings
(because of the pressures upon the nerve system) has destroyed
more than it has aided. For, it has added to the inabilities of some of
the organs of the physical forces to assimilate or eliminate properly . . .
The administrations of the various natures have in the main only
aggravated. While there have been times when seemingly there were
calm periods for the body, these were very temporary.

3905-1 F. 21 3/20/44
In considering that which may be helpful for this body, we find
that the physical body, the mental body and the spiritual body must
be taken into consideration; and not applications made that would
permanently make a dissociation of the oneness of the entity's purposes in the earth . . .
We find that it will be well to give the entity . . . the shocks with
overdoses, even of insulin; to cause reflexes in the brain reaction to
the emotions of the body.
But when these have been given it will be well to coordinate these
by the osteopathic correction of subluxations existing in the body-
forces.
At the time of birth there was a pressure brought about in the areas of the coccyx and the lower end of the spine that makes, even
yet, a dissociation in that area of the coccyx and the end of the cerebrospinal nerve segments. Correct these.
Give the shocks first, yes; else the body-mind will not be controlled in relation to these . . .
Don't give so many of the shocks as to upset the pancrean reaction entirely.
As to the number of these that should be given before beginning
the osteopathic corrections, this should be determined by the response. For remember, as indicated, the physical, the mental and
the spiritual body should be considered in making the applications.
Consider it as an entity, not merely as a physical body.

3964-1 F. Adult 6/29/22

[Thus she] . . . will be able to sleep easily without those harrowing expressions that come at times to the body when trying to sleep. Do not force sleep through drugs, as this will show its effect in the digestion, and is very much worse for the body.

4186-1 M. Adult 11/4/22

To relieve, or to give the proper incentives to the body, to remove this condition, must come through a twofold treatment; that of medicinal properties in the system to give correct incentives to the body in its circulation and functioning proclivities, and also a correction of the physical defects at the 3rd lumbar by manipulation or adjustment. The medicinal properties we would take into this system would be these:

> Tincture of Valerian .... 3 ounces
> Bromide of Potash, or Potassium ...... 2 ounces
> Elixir of Calisaya .... 2 ounces
> Sufficient simple syrup to make 7 ounces

The dose would be [one] tablespoonful every 2 hours while the body is in this nervous state or tension, as it shows at present. One tablespoonful at night just before retiring at other times.

4432-1 M. Adult 11/25/28

. . . these may be kept continually so, until we would find within six months to sixteen months a response that would bring bettered conditions, provided there were not the continuation of those narcotics in the system . . .

Continue with these until we are able to reduce the amount of the narcotic . . . or this may be changed to a capsule that would assist in relieving the pain or the depression, and which would be easier removed, though of necessity there will have to be those of common judgment used, else we will find self-destruction coming to the front in same. In these capsules we would use this, as a liquid, and this in each dose:

> Eucalyptol, Oil of .... 1 minim
> Creosote .... ½   "
> Turpentine, Extract of ... 1   "
> Canadian Balsam 1   "

Needn't make more than two or three of these, for they will not last. These should not be given more than one every other day, see? This will of necessity not be begun until the dosage of the hypnotic is reduced to a very nominal or normal . . .

4545-1   F. Adult   "Prior to 1923"
. . . through the mental action of the impressions to the body from causes of the blood supply to the brain, she cannot carry reason to her other faculties. She is without reason . . . There is something needed to rebuild the nerve forces . . . The brain in action uses the specific part prepared by the system to be used by the brain in its action. It takes from certain organs and functions through that which is carried in the system to carry out its action. There is something lacking to be carried to the brain and it should be supplied by medicinal properties . . .

> Iodide of Potassium .... ¼ grain
> Iodide of Soda .... 2 grains
> Red Prusate of Potassium ..... ½ grain
> Powdered leaves of Elder ...... 1 grain

[Mix] all of this together with three grains of Senna. This is a dose and should be given every other day . . . it will be acted upon and carry the stimulus and incentive to the nerves and brain . . . Softening of the brain has not yet begun in this body . . . This will act on the nerves and as a stimulant to the splenic force and to the dorsals, which controls the splenic action of the body.

5467-1   M. 45   6/21/30
Give, then, these internally—not changing from some that are being given at present, but give as this:
First prepare as a carrier, this: Take 2 ounces of wild cherry bark and 6 ounces distilled water, add together, reduce by slow boiling to 2 ounces. Strain and add to same lactated pepsin 1 ounce. Then prepare as this:
Take 1 dram Indian Turnip, 2 drams Wild Ginseng—add to 4 ounces distilled water. Reduce by simmering, not heavy boiling, to 2 ounces. Strain and add to the carrier. Then add to this solution, Tincture of Capsici 2 minims. Cut ½ dram Balsam of Tolu in 1 ounce 85% alcohol and add to solution.
Give the dosage of this every 4 hours, 10 to 20 drops, see?
Each day, also, at eventide, give Chloride of Gold to the distilled water, 1 to 15 ounces of water, 15 grains Chloride of Gold—distilled water, see? Also prepare 6 ounces distilled water with 10 grains Bromide of Soda. The dose at eventide will be, 10 minims Chloride of Gold and 5 minims Bromide of Soda.

Atomidine

Atomidine was occasionally suggested in the readings as a stimulant for the glandular system. William McGarey states:

> It can be seen that—from Cayce's source of information—Atomidine used internally in cycles such as have been suggested earlier produces results which benefit the internal secreting glands, produce coordination between the endocrines, aid in balancing the functioning of other glandular tissue throughout the body, and aid in the process of elimination and assimilation. Atomidine Circulating File, p. 13; available from the A.R.E.)

Atomidine is to be taken on an empty stomach and under a physician's supervision. It is to be used in cycles which vary for each individual's needs and in relation to the other interventions suggested.

Excerpts from the Cayce Readings

294-130   M. 54   1/14/32
. . . or, to put it in common parlance, most glands function as machinery would under oil. The iodine being the oil for the glands—see?

1787-2   M. 48   2/2/39
These properties [Atomidine] as we find add to the system not only the healing but purifying of the glandular system and STRENGTHENING through the ability of the blood supply for coagulation . . .

3104-1   F. 56   7/21/43
. . . the Atomidine acts as a gland purifier—causing especially the thyroids and the glands in the stomach, particularly the pyloric portion of the stomach and throughout the duodenum, to change in the form of secretions thrown off—and this affects directly the circulation.

Diet/Nutrition

Diet recommendations were included in most of the readings for individuals suffering from schizophrenia. Usually the suggestions were of a general nature and sought to provide a balanced supply of nutrients with consideration for a normal acid/alkaline balance. There are numerous books available which can introduce the reader to the Cayce approach to nutrition (e.g., Reilly & Brod, 1975; Bolton, 1969; McGarey, 1983, etc.) and it is not necessary to dwell at length on this topic presently. The A.R.E. publishes a handy one-page condensation of the Cayce suggestions entitled *Basic Diet* (Edgar Cayce Foundation, 1971) which can be conveniently located in the kitchen area to provide guidance in the choice and preparation of foods.

In several cases, a blood- and nerve-strengthening diet was recommended for individuals suffering from dementia praecox. In no cases were there suggestions for extreme diets or the use of megavitamen supplements. Although Cayce occasionally recommended the use of dietary supplements in cases of extreme malnourishment, these supplements were to be used in cycles to stimulate the body's own natural assimilative abilities.

Excerpts from the Cayce Readings
271-1   M. 34   2/13/33
The diet should consist of those foods that are well balanced, but keep away from meats; only that necessary to give strength or vitality to the body. Rather would this be as an outline, though it may be altered or changed to meet the varying needs or to supply that necessary, for much may be added and much may be taken away at times—but this would be as a general outline:

Mornings—citrus fruit or cereal (whether dry or cooked—change them about for the body), or stewed or fresh fruit in their season with a little cream and sugar. But do not mix the citrus fruit and cereal at one meal; either use one or the other.

Noons—preferably either soups or broths from vegetables; or vegetable salads of the green nature, with which there may be taken any of the dressings that make same more palatable to the body. (But do not feed the body differently from the one who waits on him, or eats with him, or the companion. Have them eat the same thing!)

Evenings—Whole vegetable diet of all characters and natures. Prepare these preferably with fats of butterfat or vegetable oils, rather than meats. At the same time, of course, there may be included fresh fruits; as pineapple, or the like. Not bananas, nor raw apples. Occasionally there may be taken the breast of chicken, but never fried meats; either stewed, boiled or roasted would be better—but keep as far away from the meats as possible.

271-4   M. 34   4/17/33
It is preferable that the diet be an alkaline one, rather than acid. For, in an alkaline diet all constructive forces are enabled to work much better for the recuperation of physical as well as mental activities of the body.

271-5   M. 34   5/1/33
Keep the diet in the order that there may be the proper reactions. It is necessary that there be the proper balance towards a rebuilding and replenishing, or a normally balanced diet. For each vegetable taken that is grown under the ground, there should be at least two or three of those that grow above the ground. Those of every nature that may be constructive. Nuts are harmful at times, but small quantities—especially of almonds—are good for the body. Not black walnuts, not English walnuts. Pecans, almonds, filberts, and the like, are very good—in small quantities. Beef, properly prepared (but not with greases), may be taken occasionally; broiled (but, remember, not broiled in its own grease; preferably in oils of vegetables, or the like—see?).

2022-1   F. Adult   10/9/39
Not a heavy diet, and not wholly a liquid diet; but semi-liquid, and those foods that are blood and nerve strengthening. Have a great deal of celery soup, or celery extracts with the soups; broiled liver, and those things of such natures. Plenty of fruits, and raw vegetables if possible.

3440-1   F. 29   1/4/44
In the diets, don't overcrowd with sweets nor starches. Keep these well balanced with vegetables, fruits and the like.

Surgery

Mentioning surgery in a discussion of therapeutic techniques for treating schizophrenia might conjure up images of "icepick surgery" and scenes from *One Flew over the Cuckoo's Nest*. Although very little psychosurgery is currently performed on psychiatric patients (McCall, 1989), perhaps 20,000 patients received this treatment between 1936 and 1951 (Flor-Henry, 1975).

In contrast to psychiatry's preoccupation with brain pathology as the basis for mental illness, the Cayce readings emphasized systemic interactions—particularly in respect to surgery. Consistent with the readings' frequent association of pelvic disorders with psychosis, surgery on the reproductive tract was occasionally suggested. Only in cases of brain insult, in which tumors or other blatant forms of pathology were present (e.g., [5167]), did the readings recommend brain surgery.

Excerpts from the Cayce Readings

2197-1   F. Adult   3/12/24

Those organs of the pelvis function abnormal, there having been suppression through the functioning of the genital organs, producing first obstruction in the gland, and to bring the normal to this body would be necessary by operation, to remove those glands in the pelvic organs of gentation.   This will remove pressure, and with the submerging of the whole sensory system the control over the physical may be brought to the normal functioning.

Do that. The sooner the better. This may be accomplished by Gilbert in Baltimore.

3589-1   M. 21   1/25/44

There may be the necessity eventually of operative measures here, to do away with those tendencies for inflammation to the organs of the genital system; for these are sources, but these conditions will necessarily have to be quieted a great deal and the corrections made of those pressures in the 1st, 2nd and 3rd cervical and in the coccyx end of the spine.

4179-1   F. Adult   7/11/22

After this has been used to gain control of the body [hypnosis], we will find we will produce the clotting of certain cellular forces along the spine, notably along the lower dorsals. This will of necessity have to be removed. See, operate. That will be done from the frontal side.

4285-1   F. Adult   10/27/22

But when the body is in the hypnotic state, the body should then be treated, and not in its normal state, by deep manipulation and vibration to the body itself, see?

These we would do to bring the most relief to this body. By this mode we may gain control, or we can by operative force bring the body to a better condition; that would be by the removal of the fallopian tube and genital glands themselves. See?

5167-1   M. 30   1944

As we find, the better place for this . . . (where there may be used operative measures, also a brain specialist and with those specializing in dementia cases), would be Macon, Missouri [Still-Hildreth Sanatorium]. There we may find help. Ready for questions.

Q. Is the brain itself injured or is there a brain tumor?

A. It is a tumor. As has been indicated, the seams cause pressure in the casement and these run crosswise, as well as downward. Hence all of the reflexes are abnormal. This is the reason why most diagnoses are: dementia praecox. It isn't true dementia, but a gradual wasting of gray matter. X-ray should indicate it. These have been made, but fluids form, you see, and these do not show in X-rays. Flouroscope would be the better manner of examination, or infrared X-rays, or shadowgraph.

Q. Are there any glandular defects or malfunctioning of glands underlying this condition?

A. No glandular disturbance.

COGNITIVE THERAPIES

The expression "mind is the builder" is one of the most frequent declarations in the Cayce readings. This phrase encapsulates the realm of the mental, which the readings portrayed as intermediate between physical and spiritual.

Contemporary psychology has made considerable progress in researching mental processes and developing clinical models which address the reality of mind. The designation of "cognitive" was chosen as the heading for this section for three reasons: (1) it is a term which is familiar to researchers and clinicians and therefore provides access to the ideas and literature in this area, (2) "cognitive" is sufficiently broad to include all the various "mental" techniques suggested by Cayce, and (3) the numerous clinical models which utilize cognitive theory often incorporate behavioral techniques (hence the advent of "cognitive-behavioral" therapies) and thus emphasize the dynamic, interactive quality of mind portrayed in the readings.

Hypnosis

Hypnosis can be defined as "an induced sleeplike condition in which an individual is extremely responsive to suggestions made by the hypnotist" (*American Heritage Dictionary*, 1984). Although Edgar Cayce occasionally recommended formal hypnosis for persons experiencing mental problems, more often he advocated a "naturalistic" approach which was used in conjunction with other therapies. Cayce referred to this form of hypnosis as "suggestive therapeutics." For example, he often recommended that the persons administering massage and osteopathic treatments give positive suggestions during the treatments. Similarly, during electrotherapy, suggestions were to be given for the rebuilding of the nervous systems. Cayce also advised that the hypnogogic state be utilized by giving hypnotic suggestions during the early stages of sleep.

The induction of a hypnotic trance is a common consequence of various physical treatments. It is quite common for individuals receiving a relaxing massage to enter an altered state of consciousness resembling (or identical to) a hypnotic trance. This is likely due to the muscle relaxation produced by the massage and the rhythmic patterns of the strokes.

Milton Erickson, perhaps the most famous hypnotherapist of this century, often referred to trance as a state of relaxed self-awareness. Therefore, getting people to physically relax and feel comfortable is an important preliminary step in most hypnotic inductions. Erickson regarded body stillness as a reliable indicator of trance (in Havens, p. 245). Stephen Gilligan (a student of Erickson's) reiterates this theme by associating conscious mind activities with muscle tension: "As we will discuss further, it [the conscious mind] arises from and is maintained by muscular tension" (1987, p. 23). Gilligan specifically mentions massage as a naturalistic means of achieving trance in which there is a "balancing of muscle tonus" and "the strong skin-bounded differentiation between self and other is dissipated by muscle tone shifts, thereby enabling the person to synchronize with complementary biological rhythms and align with unitary psychological processes" (p. 42). Gilligan suggests a cultural link between conscious mind activities and the types of trances utilized by a particular society.

Hypnotically entranced individuals often do not feel like moving or talking in any elaborate fashion. To reiterate, this lack of movement partly reflects a value implicit in most hypnotic rituals . . . The point to be made is that trance can be developed and maintained via inhibition of movement or rhythmic (circular and repetitive) movement, i.e., an absence of irregular and arrhythmic orienting responses (and muscle tension) that give rise to the conscious mind. The relative immobility of the hypnotic subject may have developed as a needed complement to the incessant movement (goal-oriented action) occurring in the waking-state style favored by Western culture; it may also reflect the dissociation from the physical self (man dominating nature, including his body) that generally occurs in our culture. (p. 54)

Immobility and lack of muscle tension on the part of the subject and the use of rhythmic and repetitive movements by the massage therapist are very descriptive of the massage process. Participation in the massage process quickly leads one to agree with Gilligan that massage can be a powerful, trance-inducing experience.

If the electrical therapies advocated by Cayce have the calming effects which he described, it makes sense that subjects receiving these treatments would also be induced into a hypnotic trance and would be amenable to direct suggestion. The Radio-Active Appliance (Impedance Device) was noted as being particularly effective in this respect.

Furthermore, Cayce recommended that the period immediately preceding sleep, and the first few minutes of sleep, be utilized to provide presleep suggestions. Using the presleep period as a naturalistic hypnotic induction makes virtually every client a potential hypnotic subject.

Henry Bolduc (1985) provides an excellent orientation to the use of hypnosis in the Cayce readings. As a professional hypnotist, he provides through his insights and practical suggestions for applying the Cayce suggestions (particularly regarding self-hypnosis) a useful introduction to this topic which are highly recommended.

In a broader sense, Cayce viewed environment as a powerful suggestive force that must be utilized in therapy. This aspect of suggestion will be dealt with in a later section addressing the role of therapeutic milieu.

The role of suggestion cannot be overestimated in the treatment of schizophrenia. Persons suffering from this disorder are often resistant to treatment due to lack of motivation, cognitive deficits, intrapsychic confusion, and defective interpersonal skills. The readings insist that "suggestive therapeutics" is the best way to encourage compliance to the therapeutic agenda.

A quick review of the principle, "all healing comes from within" (Chapter Four) may be useful to emphasize the necessity of tapping the healing potential of the divine force within. In cases of chronic schizophrenia (i.e., dementia praecox) the readings consistently advocated the use of suggestive therapeutics to access this resource and thus stimulate the healing process.

Excerpts from the Cayce Readings
271-1   M. 34   2/13/33

The treatments also that should be included by the same attendant, or the same one with the body, would be—when the body is put or is ready to go to rest of evening—to massage gently but thoroughly all along the whole cerebrospinal system, and during such periods (for most often we would find the body would gradually fall into that state of near between the waking and sleeping state) make gentle suggestions that QUIET, REST, PEACE, HAPPINESS, JOY, DEVELOPMENTS IN EVERY MANNER THAT ARE CONSTRUCTIVE PHYSICALLY AND MENTALLY, will come to the body through its rest period! Or, the suggestion to the deeper portion of the subconscious forces of the body.

271-3   M. 34   4/3/33

In the administering of those suggestions that have been outlined, as indicated, it is presumed that all will be adhered to in the manner given; and one activity becomes then dependent upon another. With the revivifying of urges from physical to mental, through those reactions in the activity of the forces from the [Wet Cell] appliance to the brain's activity, unless the suggestions are carried with same it may be made more harmful than beneficial. If these are carried together in their activity, then they will produce those reactions—as given—for the betterments of the body. These, as we find, should be adhered to more in the manner that has been outlined for the body, and there may be expected to be the better reactions from same. For, without this there comes that of not knowing what to do with the impulses; and the body then becomes at times irresponsible for the activities of the mental reactions. Then, we would carry out more closely those suggestions that have been given and will bring for this body the better physical and mental reactions . . .

Q. Are we doing everything possible for him in his present state of mind?

A. If the whole of the suggestions given had been adhered to, there would not be the recurrent conditions that are apparent in the present! The suggestions must be made; else leave off, or change, or do without the whole thing! . . .

Q. Why did he seem to lose the cheerfulness of the past ten days?

A. As we have just given, when there is that application for the body that will make for reactions in nerve impulse to a tempered condition in brain's reaction—and the suggestions not adhered to for those activities as outlined, there may be expected these results!

Either DO it, or don't try to do it!

271-4   M. 34   4/17/33

However, for these suggestions to be more effective, they should not be given in merely a singsong manner; nor said just once. But take at least the time to repeat same (the suggestion), positively, three to five times; that there may be the full response in the positive forces of the suggestion to the mental activities of the body.

And we would, for the time being, use the same suggestion; or the same affirmation. And by affirmation we mean that it should be an affirmation!

271-5   M. 34   5/1/33

Then, in the suggestions that we would make when the body is sleeping, resting, there should be had those that will make for the better creative forces; for to reach the subconscious self it must be without the physical-mental self. See? Yet in the waking state, in the activity, there will be seen those reactions occasionally; at first possibly once a week, possibly once a day, possibly several times a day, dependent upon how persistent the suggestions are made with the active forces that are being set out in the system from the physical angle. See?

Change the suggestions, then, in this manner, or to this:

THERE WILL BE, IN THE WHOLE OF THE PHYSICAL AND MENTAL BODY, THAT RESPONSE TO THAT CREATIVE ENERGY WHICH IS BEING CARRIED INTO THE SYSTEM. PERFECT COORDINATION WILL COME TO THE BODY. THERE WILL BE NORMAL REACTIONS IN EVERY WAY AND MANNER THROUGH THE CREATIVE FORCES OF DIVINE LOVE THAT IS MANIFEST IN THE HEARTS AND MINDS OF THOSE ABOUT THE BODY.

This should be repeated three to four times, until it has gradually reached the subconscious, or the unconscious, or the consciousness of the living forces that are impelling activity in a distorted condition, as to the balance in the mental forces of [271].

386-2   F. 20   9/28/33
Q. What suggestion should be given the body?
A. That the application of those influences in the system is creating a normal balance, and will surround the body, its functioning, its activities, with those forces that will prevent the recurrence of the conditions that have disturbed the body; and normalcy will ensue.

386-3   F. 20   10/25/33
Then, to keep these in balance and to guide these impulses, so that there may be a controlling of the impulse to the nerve system, we would—with the manipulations and the applications made [electrotherapy]—give the suggestions for the body to respond in a normal manner in the impulses created by the vibrations that are set up from the elemental forces in the body. Such suggestions as this:
NOW THERE IS BEING CREATED IN THE IMPULSES FROM THE GANGLIA IN THE SYSTEM THE NORMAL REACTION TO THE SENSORY AND SYMPATHETIC SYSTEMS OF THE BODY. AND THE REACTIONS WILL BE A PERFECTLY NORMAL BALANCING IN THE MENTAL, PHYSICAL AND SPIRITUAL BEING ON THE BODY.
Q. When should the suggestions be given?
A. As the outline has been. When the manipulations and battery actions are being given. That means at the same time!

1513-1   M. 47   1/7/38
Q. What can be said to him to assist to regain full confidence in his ability?
A. There must be the PHYSICAL reactions and the suggestions as the applications are made. And hold to the SPIRITUAL portions of such suggestions.

1553-17   F. 72   10/30/39
As to the suggestions that should be given—when there are the administrations of ANY of the influences for aid, whether the rubs or the packs or whatnot, the suggestions should be of a very positive nature, yet very gentle, and in a constructive way and manner; expressing hope always that there is a creating, through the hope, the

expectancy for certain activities to the body that it desires to do—much in the manner as would be given to a child in its promptings for an aid to itself.

And let the suggestions be constructive in the spiritual sense, when the manipulations or adjustments are given, as well as when there are the periods of the rubs and other applications. These would be well in this manner, though each individual should construct same in his or her own words:

"Let there be accomplished through the desires of this body, mentally and physically, that which will enable the body to give the better, the truer, the more real expression of its own self; as well as that in which the entity or body may influence itself in relationships to others for greater physical, mental and spiritual attitudes towards conditions" . . . if the suggestions are followed in the manners as indicated for the body, it should be done not as something just to be gotten through with—by the body or the one making the application for the body, but for PURPOSEFUL experiences; and it will make it much better. It will not require so LONG a period, but of a more definite nature . . .

Q. Should suggestions be made by BOTH the doctor and those taking care of her?

A. Just as indicated, these should be made whenever any applications are made—whether for the rubs, the adjustments, or the packs. The BODY desires attentions—but in a manner in which there are, as indicated, the suggestions that it is to become not so reliant upon others, but so—because of the very nature of the applications—that it may do more and more for itself.

Whenever there is the suggestion, it should be not as "There WON'T be," but "You WILL do so and so," see?

Q. What can we do for the crying—nervousness and her refusing to drink?

A. This can only be met through the suggestions—for, as has been indicated, these periods come and go; and, as has been outlined heretofore, it is a lack of the coordinating between the cerebrospinal and sympathetic impulses or reflexes.

2129-1   F. 35   2/29/40

Then, as we find—under the supervision of one who would be gentle, kind, and apply constantly suggestive therapeutics (not hypnosis but a constant influence by suggestions)—we would have these applications . . .

2248-1   F. 24   5/27/40
After each application of the Wet Cell Appliance, allow the body to rest—as it will be inclined to sink into slumber—and during such periods make POSITIVE suggestions for coordination and helpful activity to the body, in a prayerful, meditative manner; not as routine to be gotten through with, but as positive suggestions that are to be helpful to one of God's children.

3075-1   M. 24   7/2/43
Hence we have here conditions that at times approach near to that of possession of the mind by external influences, or that very close to the spiritual possession by disincarnate forces.

Owing to those conditions which existed in the manner in which coordination is established in the physical reactions between impressions received through sensory system and the reactions upon the reflexes of brain, we find these at times become very much disassociated. And those impressions received sympathetically, or through vision, through hearing, through sensing by impressions, become the motivative force in the reaction.

At such times possession near takes place.

Select some good hypnotist . . . and have the body put under influences.

3996-1   F. Adult   12/26/24
As the mind becomes longer distance between the hallucinations, when treatments are given, keep the suggestions until it reaches the inmost being of the body, correcting itself from within, through the Divine in self.

4097-1   M. Adult   9/16/22
We would stimulate the functioning of the spleen forces to an extent of taking, or calling forth from the blood and circulation from the brain to the spleen, so that we would supply a new force to the circulation entirely and give off its force to the brain itself. This we will find will necessarily have to proceed through the action of the sensory system, or by impressions the body is to receive from other minds more powerful than its own at the present time. This would be accomplished by the body being subjected to extreme heat so that all centers of the nerve system become perfectly relaxed. When under this condition the body would be put into a subnormal state, that is hypnosis or mesmeristic forces applied to the body itself when in this state.

4506-2   F. 55   5/21/26

This subjugation should be made by one that gives the massage and adjustments of the centers in the cerebrospinal system, or by one who gives the nerve centers the incentive for normal action.

This may be begun by the one so manipulating, insisting that the body (during the time of treatment) keep entirely quiet, and the operator talk continually, with the suggestion necessary for the improvement in the body, physical and mental, see? for, with these conditions, this would gradually bring about this subjugation with the centers where the cerebrospinal and sympathetic are at junctures with each other, as [are] seen in the cervical, the dorsal, and in the whole of the sacral and lumbar region.

5014-1   M. 11   4/8/44

Even through the period of giving the massage, as well as the Appliance [Wet Cell Battery], let there be suggestions given to the body in that way not merely of speculation but as to positive activities of the body; planning, as it were, its activities for the next day. As an illustration: On the morrow, or in the morning there will be certain activities. This should be very thoroughly outlined, very consistently suggested.

Thus, we will find a change in the activities of the body, bringing the reflexes to the brain centers with the nervous system in the ganglia where there are the closer associations with the sympathetic and suggestive nerve forces of the body.

5598-1   M. 23   8/8/30

. . . and this, as we find, would require one very strong in character, in purpose, in application; one who may subjugate through hypnosis, or through that of the power of suggestion over the physical body. There will be found that this will require time, patience, and persistence . . . It will be found necessary to make many of the suggestions in the beginning as the body goes to normal sleep. While it will make same become flitful at times, and make for many struggles from within, these—as we find—offer the only manner for even prospective aid . . . This, as is seen, must be builded within the mental being of the body.

Routine

The development of a daily routine represents a behavioral utilization of suggestion. Constructive activities repeated in a daily sequence produce habitual behaviors which lay the foundation for a healthy lifestyle.

Excerpts from the Cayce Readings
271-4   M. 34   4/17/33

As to the general activities of the body, there should be those things, events, happenings, that will make the tendencies for the body-mind and body-consciousness to use the mental forces. Not only in reconstructing, in the mental abilities of the body, those conditions that have transpired in the past; but there should be such questions and such conversations as to require the answers to show constructive forces in the activity of the mental body or mind—see?

These should not be made tiring, nor so as to cause overanxiety; but patience—patience and persistence on the part of those that give the suggestions, both in the subconscious (or during those periods when the body is in rest or repose) and in the waking state . . .

Make for constructive creative activity; the necessity for the mind to put this and that construction on those things that are spoken of.

And let the conversation ever be of creative forces, life—life's activities! Not any that is of a destructive nature, in any way or manner!

In the matter of physical activity, this should be that which makes the body physically tired of evenings. And early to retire, in most occasions, is better for the body.

And, as soon as the body awakes of mornings, it should be required to begin some sort of physical activity; rather than mental—which is that which will make for the introspection of self. Hence suggestions and a good deal of talk regarding what the activities of the day will be, should be the beginning of the day.

271-7   M. 34   5/29/33

Q. Can you suggest anything that will keep him busy and contented?

A. The varied activities in which the body may be engaged. As we have given, it requires a classification of various activities. A portion of time should be set for each thing, as a budget would be made up. So many hours of rest, so many hours of physical activity, so many hours of recuperation in varied activities, so many hours for this, that and the other—and keep persisting in these until they are a matter of routine, which makes for the power of suggestion to be active in the replenishing and rebuilding mental force of a body; and it doesn't necessarily become a machine, for the reactions will be in the mental balance that is created.

271-8   M. 34   6/12/33
Q. Is it wise to let him sleep in the mornings as long as he wants to?
A. If the hours are changed, or reversed—and he goes to bed early enough, be better that he rises earlier. This would naturally have to be gradually changed now. You couldn't send him to bed, or make him go to bed early, since he is sleeping until ten and eleven in the morning!

Bibliotherapy/Videotherapy

Cayce recognized the power of mass communication in shaping the thoughts and behaviors of individuals. Furthermore, he emphasized the importance of constructive influences upon a person recovering from psychosis. Given the prominence of violence in movies, television, and even the daily newspaper, one would likely find it difficult to follow Cayce's advice of maintaining a constructive environment unless the mass media were monitored and censured to a substantial degree. One has to wonder about the effects of "television therapy" in many institutions where the chronically mental ill are allowed (and encouraged) to watch television to keep them preoccupied.

Excerpts from the Cayce Readings
271-4   M. 34   4/17/33
When matter for reading is desired, do not give the body reading matter other than that which is constructive. No gang land. No underworld. Not a great deal of animosity or excitement in the reading matter. See?
Q. Are movies occasionally well for the body?
A. Provided they do not carry that same element of reaction to the mental body as we have indicated [violence and destruction]. Those that present reactions of a constructive nature are well.

Behavioral Modeling

Behavioral modeling is a potent means of changing and maintaining a desired behavior without resorting to simplistic reward/punishment techniques often associated with behavioral approaches. Persons undergoing rehabilitation need to learn appropriate behaviors in a therapeutic context. Behavioral modeling is based upon a social learning theory model which provides a realistic explanation of how complex behaviors are learned in social situations. Bandura (1977) is a leading proponent of "observational learning from competent examples":

> Because mistakes can produce costly, or even fatal consequences, the prospects of survival would be slim indeed if one could learn only by suffering the consequences of trial and error. For this reason, one does not teach children to swim, adolescents to drive automobiles, and novice medical students to perform surgery by having them discover the appropriate behavior through the consequences of their successes and failures. The more costly and hazardous the possible mistakes, the heavier is the reliance on observational learning from competent examples. Apart from the question of survival, it is difficult to imagine a social transmission process in which the language, lifestyles, and institutional practices of a culture are taught to each new member by selective reinforcement of fortuitous behaviors, without the benefit of models who exemplify the cultural patterns. (p. 12)

Obviously, persons suffering from a major mental illness such as schizophrenia cannot be expected to learn from trial and error. Nor can reinforcement contingencies for all the important behaviors necessary for a high level of social functioning be maintained to produce these desired behaviors. Cayce recognized that a competent model could help provide an environment in which the recovering schizophrenic could learn how to function normally by following the therapeutic program. Cayce repeatedly insisted that "mind is the builder" and that mind needed a constructive model as a pattern. The use of a companion as a model was often recommended by Cayce and will be discussed in detail in a later section.

Excerpts from the Cayce Readings
271-5   M. 35   4/2/33
Q. Is there any way in which we may get this body to eat any form of fruit?

A. Gradually. Listen at just what has been given! The body assumes activities and acts by suggestion of everyone around the body! If all around the body eat fruit, the body will gradually eat fruit itself! Isn't that just what we have been saying?

Q. Should I [L. J. Hesson] insist upon his getting up in the morning, or does it antagonize him?

A. As given, it is best that the body arise as soon as it awakes. Do not antagonize, but suggest! Do so yourself, and the body will get up too!

Thought Monitoring

Thought monitoring is a cognitive technique for reprogramming mental processes. Cayce often stated that "mind is the builder" and inferred that aberrant thinking could produce an unhealthy body and discordant social relations. Therefore, it was considered therapeutic to consciously monitor and eliminate "negative" thoughts or thoughts which were unrealistic (i.e., "out of touch with reality"). Obviously, this process would only work for a relatively high functioning individual who was capable of conscious processing and self-reflection.

Excerpts from the Cayce Readings

1513-1   M. 47   1/7/38

And keep the body-mind active in constructive thinking, expectancies for building up of energies for the restoration of the mental and physical abilities of the body of [1513].

1789-5   F. 33   7/26/39

Q. Why am I so retiring when I meet people?

A. Do as has been indicated and find a relief—rather than questioning self. For such questions build resentment in the inner self, because of the not understanding of a nervous breakdown.

Positive Attitude

The Cayce readings emphasized the role of positive attitudes in the treatment of schizophrenia. Positive attitude was considered important in both the person providing treatment and the individual being treated. It is easy to become discouraged and "burned out" in this field since the rehabilitation process is often lengthy and uncertain. Persons working in this area must find means of renewal to maintain a positive attitude and utilize appropriate ways to convey this attitude to the patient.

Excerpts from the Cayce Readings

271-7   M. 34   5/29/33

These, to be sure, are as yet very slow, and may be considered by some as very slight; but if that attitude is still held by those about the body that there is no improvement, that there is no change, that he still remains stubborn, that he still remains in the inactive forces that have existed, he'll remain that way—to himself and most to others . . .

1513-1   M. 47   1/7/38

Q. Should he be told that he has been put on the retired list of the Post Office department and will have to apply for reinstatement to active work or what should be done under the circumstances considering his mental condition at present?

A. As has been indicated, to give the body the impression that it has been left entirely out, without there being some adjustments and some reconstructive forces done to make for a correction, will make for a greater derangement through the mental incapacities of the body and will cause violence.

Then it will be necessary to make the applications and gradually build up the expectancy of the body for its abilities to gain an equilibrium necessary for active service in that department of the Service.

SPIRITUAL THERAPIES

The spiritual dimension of therapy pertains to issues involving purpose, meaning, value, intentionality, and wholeness. In the simplest terms, spirituality addresses the problem of how to manifest love through the various therapies which have been described.

What are the techniques which provide an avenue for the expression of compassion? Is it really necessary to address spiritual issues in the treatment of a major mental illness such as schizophrenia? These are important questions which will be addressed in this section.

Therapeutic Milieu

Cayce maintained that the environment acts upon an individual in a suggestive manner through the sensory and sympathetic systems (271-5). Therefore, a supportive, constructive milieu was considered essential for reprogramming the nervous systems of persons undergoing treatment.

Therapeutic milieu was an important factor in the treatment program at Still-Hildreth Osteopathic Sanatorium and other progressive institutions of that era. Cayce referred several persons to Still-Hildreth who were suffering from major mental illness and couldn't receive proper treatment locally. The premise upon which Still-Hildreth was founded was stated by the founder of osteopathy, A. T. Still. "Dr. Still had said to me time and again that when our profession could have property of its own, with proper surroundings and environment, a large percentage of the insane could be cured through osteopathic treatment." (Hildreth, 1938, pp. 247-248)

The Still-Hildreth model comes as close to a holistic model as one can find in the literature of mental illness. The property of nearly four hundred acres contained a lake and bathhouse and afforded excellent facilities for walking, swimming, skating, fishing, baseball, tennis, and croquet. Indoor recreation consisted of reading, dancing, cards, checkers, chess, billiards, moving pictures, and music.

> Each patient is given the largest degree of freedom that his condition allows. Every effort is exerted to make him feel at home and realize that the sole purpose of his residence here is to get well. Kindness and gentleness in dealing with patients are rigorously enforced. (*Still-Hildreth Guide and Explanation,* undated)

The chiropractic mental hospitals of the same era used a similar approach. The practice of manual medicine was combined with a therapeutic milieu.

As for Clear View, there were factors which this writer believes contributed to its success between 1926 and 1951. First, although the environment was austere, offering no more than marginal comforts, the institution was managed with a firm hand within the limits of its economic resources by its matron, Mrs. Marie Hender. There existed a tight control over patient management along with a no-nonsense atmosphere which translated into a strong and positive therapeutic milieu. Patients knew they were there to get well and not to spend a useless life.

By contrast, state hospitals were then not much better than prisons . . . Overcrowding, neglect and often brutal treatment in an environment of despair made state hospitals places to avoid like the plague. By contrast, a clean, well-managed facility in which there was considerable individual attention offered a refreshing refuge to those who could afford private care for their loved ones. (Quigley, 1983, p. 71)

The use of therapeutic milieu in these institutions echoed the moral treatment movements of the nineteenth century. These movements protested the horrible treatment of the insane and demanded that programs based upon the humane treatment of patients be implemented. Moral treatment was conceived of as:

. . . a system based upon the theory of corrective experience, and implemented by molding the physical and social environment of the hospital. The goal of moral management was the reconstruction of damaged brain tissue by resocialization, by influencing the physical organ through the medium of the mind. The pivot of this system was education and the imposition of regular habits of life and work, appropriate mental stimulation, orderly thinking, and correct values . . . By regulating the milieu in order to impose absorbing tasks and civilized social intercourse, it was hoped that pernicious habits and associations would be broken while correct and socially acceptable patterns of thought and behavior would be fostered . . . it is here that modern psychiatrists find some of the earliest examples of therapeutic milieus. (Caplin, 1969, pp. 26-30)

In these early attempts at "socioenvironmental therapy," the physical setting was considered so important that the internal design of the asylums was a highly specialized area of expertise. The therapeutic effects of light, spatial arrangement, and temperature on the patients were given a high priority.

Bockoven's definition of moral treatment includes a discussion of the "spiritual" dimension of this approach:

. . . [moral treatment] meant compassionate and understanding treatment of innocent sufferers. Even innocence was not a prerequisite to meriting compassion. Compassion was extended to those whose mental illness was thought due to willful and excessive indulgence in the passions. (1963, p. 12)

The Cayce readings insist that compassion, as manifested in gentleness, kindness, patience, and caring, is a profound expression of spirituality and an essential aspect of therapeutic milieu. A therapeutic milieu should be considered more than just a clean facility with adequate programs for exercise and recreation. Spiritual qualities, as manifested by the staff, provide the basis for the therapeutic process. This can be demonstrated by comparing the rather opulent facilities at Still-Hildreth with the relatively plain facilities at ClearView. Both institutions insisted upon close supervision by caring attendants combined with manual medicine. The stated therapeutic efficacy of each institution (in terms of published cure rate) was essentially equal, suggesting that fancy facilities were not essential in providing an effective therapeutic milieu.

The stated objective of founding the Forest Park Chiropractic Sanitarium coincides so closely with Cayce's suggestions about the importance of spiritual ideals in maintaining a therapeutic milieu, a direct quotation from *The Chiropractic Psychopathic Sanitarium News* (1925) is appropriate to emphasize the role that spiritual values played in these institutions.

Business is analogous to the human body. The chemist may analyze every atom of the human body . . . but there is still something which the chemist cannot analyze, and which cannot be perceived by any of the senses. It is this something that puts life into the various elements and makes of the otherwise dead materials a living body. In the human body we call this something the Spirit, Life or Soul. In business we call it a principle, or ideal, and sometimes an OBJECTIVE.

As in the human body, we may have in business all of the necessary elements for success. There may be ample buildings, sufficient machinery, plenty of capital, markets for the product, together with the demand for additional quantities of the product, plenty of laborers to do the work, and yet unless there is that something which we call an OBJECTIVE, an Ideal, or maybe a Soul, lacking, the business will not succeed . . .

The ideal which leads to success is basically and fundamentally—SERVICE. By this we do not mean Service selfishly and doggedly rendered, but Service that to all outward manifestations and purposes is rendered for its own sake and none other. Of course, in every case of Service there is always a corresponding return, which may or may not be measured in dollars and cents, but which is in practically all cases of business measured in this manner . . . Our OBJECTIVE, then, is not the building of a great business that will amass for us fortune, as individuals, but it is the building of a great institution that will offer hope, health and happiness to the thousands of people now suffering from mental trouble, and also to the many thousands who may yet become afflicted.

To the accomplishment of this OBJECTIVE we have dedicated our lives.

A. G. Hildreth's account of the founding of Still-Hildreth Sanatorium is in essential agreement with the spirit of the objective just quoted. A reading of his book, *The Lengthening Shadow of Dr. Andrew Taylor Still* (1938), will provide the reader with a sense of the altruistic nature of the founder of osteopathy and the deeply spiritual foundation of this profession.

The primary physical considerations for a therapeutic milieu as outlined in the Cayce readings are cleanliness and access to fresh air and sunshine (a rural setting was often recommended). The therapeutic value of being close to nature is a theme often repeated in the readings. Sitting quietly in a pine grove or walking along a beach at the ocean were specific activities mentioned in the readings. The spiritual experience of relating directly to nature should not be underestimated when these activities are integrated into a holistic model. The interpersonal requirements for a therapeutic milieu are explicitly stated in the excerpts which follow.

Excerpts from the Cayce Readings
271-1   M. 34   2/13/33

. . . in an environ that is as growth—and the body physically and mentally treated as an individual, a unit, rather than as a class or a mass consideration, much better conditions may be brought for the body . . .

First, as we would find then, it would be necessary that there be a change in the environment and surroundings of the body; to a clean atmosphere, in plenty of sunshine and out-of-door activity . . .

Q. Please suggest name of best place for him to go for these treatments.

A. In the country somewhere, with an attendant, where the environment may be made such as we have outlined! One that would be with him at all times!

271-2   M. 34   3/27/33

Q. When he is depressed or moody, which would be the most successful way to cooperate or help him?

A. The most successful way is to accomplish this through the suggestive forces of the body, as we have indicated.

As for material meeting of conditions, these are in accord with that given: Patience, lovingkindness, and the like. Not too positive, as to create that of animosity. Not too sympathetic, as to make for pitying of self. But rather that which makes for constructive influences for the surroundings of the body.

271-4   M. 34   4/17/33

And let the conversation ever be of creative forces, life—life's activities! Not any that is of a destructive nature, in any way or manner! . . .

Remember, you are dealing with mental recuperative forces; and conditions act upon the mind just as would be experienced in the development of a six- to eight-, to twelve-year-old child!

But the mind is being rebuilt! Give it the proper things to build upon! Else there will be found that the reactions and tendencies will be towards those things destructive, or whatever is taken in the mind.

Speak, act, think constructively about the body! Some may consider it a hard job, but it's worth it—and it's worth it to themselves, because it'll make 'em live better, if they'll do it!

271-5   M. 34   5/1/33

Now, in the cerebrospinal system there are centers, or ganglia, where there are those connections with the cerebrospinal that go more directly to the brain. And we find that all the sensory system are more sympathetic with the activities of the sympathetic, or the sensory and sympathetic nerve system—see?

Hence by speech, by vision, by odor, by feeling, all make a sensitive reaction on a body where there is being electrical stimulation to ganglia to make for connections in their various activities over the system.

Hence it may be easily seen how careful all should be, how much precaution, patience and persistence must be had in making every suggestion; by speech, by sight, by feeling, by vision, by eating, by sleeping, by all senses of the body; to coordinate with the proper balance being made in the system. See?

All suggestions about the body should be of constructive nature; the love influence that comes from within every heart, mind and soul, that would build for creative forces without selfish motives in same.

271-10   M. 34   7/10/33

We would still, in a gentle, sympathetic manner, insist upon those material applications that will be helpful and beneficial in maintaining, in a physical sense, the suggestions that are received by the mental body in its environment and surroundings. Hence the necessity of conditions being kept in an even, harmonious manner as much as possible; not condoning or allowing the body to have its own mental way, and react to same, but in an even, gentle tone and manner, but positive in regard to those things that would be for the betterment of the body in its physical and mental reaction. And whatever is promised, fulfill. Do not promise one thing to gain a point and then abuse the promise.

386-1   F. 20   8/9/33

We would change the surroundings, and the environs. And let them be as near to nature as is possible. And while the body should not be left alone at any period, until there is an equal balance in the mental and physical activities, it should be so—in its surroundings—that is not only near to nature but has to depend UPON itself for the necessities of its activity; in the preparation of foods, in the preparation of rests, and in the activities of the body . . .

And the environs should be where the body would not only be as near to nature as possible, but the sun, the sea, the sand, the pines or the woods, should all be a part of the surroundings—or nature itself, see? and wear as few clothes as possible; yet making for physical activities throughout the change.

In the surroundings there should be suggestive forces that are constructive and spiritual, and creative in their activity for the body.

915-2   M. 62   6/15/35
Q. Any further suggestions for the body's welfare, now that he is under changed environs?
A. Keep those conditions of quietness about the body, yet gradually—with the conversation and activities—make for interests of a more general as well as specific nature. These are the better relations.
Q. Any advice or counsel that will be of help to his wife in taking care of him?
A. Keep the same attitude of helpful hopefulness.

1158-24   F. 50   5/20/40
Let's describe this for a second, that the entity or body here may understand, as well as the one making the stimulation:
Along the cerebrospinal system we find segments. These are cushioned. Not that the segment itself is awry, but through each segment there arises an impulse or a nerve connection between it and the sympathetic system—or the nerves running parallel with same. Through the sympathetic system (as it is called, or those centers not encased in cerebrospinal system) are the connections with the cerebrospinal system.
Then, in each center—that is, of the segment where these connect—there are tiny bursa, or a plasm of nerve reaction. This becomes congested, or slow in its activity to each portion of the system. For, each organ, each gland of the system, receives impulses through this manner for its activity.
Hence we find there are reactions to every portion of the system by suggestion, mentally, and by the environment and surroundings.

1784-1   M. 21   1/6/39
Let the attitudes of those about the body, and those making the applications, be NEVER those of censure, but rather that there is given each the opportunity for ministering to a soul seeking its course to its Maker.

1789-4   F. 33   5/4/39
Only remove the body from the hospital, then, under the supervision of a sympathetic physician, BUT IN CHARGE of the SISTER, IN the environs NOT at home, but on Long Island somewhere.

2200-1 M. Adult 1/20/31
Keep as much sunshine as possible, and companionship of a nature that makes for the uplifting and brighter side, creating within that mental impression of the whole replenishing and building body that which lives within, that may aid self most.

2721-1 F. 18 4/6/42
We find that we may bring help if there will be the changing of the body to those environs such as in Macon, Missouri [Still-Hildreth Osteopathic Sanatorium] . . .
This will necessitate some changes as conditions develop, but under such environs we may find help. There will NOT be any under the present environs or surroundings [Rochester State Hospital] . . .
These treatments must be done in a cooperative, coordinative influence with those who would supervise or administer help for this body.

2967-1 M. 27 4/18/43
It is necessary that the body be kept in the open activity, rather than being too closely confined—when the weather and the outside conditions permit. For, these will make for reactions that will improve this lack of impulse and physical reactions, as well as the coordination between cerebrospinal and sympathetic forces.

5467-1 M. 45 6/21/30
. . . and this may be accomplished best by those who will be in accord with that as is attempting to be created and brought about in the physical conditions of the body, and unless those in charge of the applications are in accord, in sympathy with, do not attempt it . . .
Q. Is it all right to treat him at home, or would it be necessary to take him to the hospital?
A. As given, would be best to be treated in the home in the beginning, for we will find reactions and changes as will come about, and after the beginning of the change for the betterment, we will then make changes as to the surroundings.

Companion Therapy

The importance of companionship and friendship in the maintenance of mental well-being is a vastly underrated area of human activity (Rubin, 1985). Cayce often recommended the use of a companion (he also used the terms attendant, sympathetic nurse, etc.) to help in the maintenance of a therapeutic milieu for the patient. Spiritual qualities such as kindness, gentleness, patience, etc., were important in the selection of a companion. Professional counseling skills were not considered essential.

The companion's job was to keep the therapeutic process on track and adhere to the suggestions provided by the readings. The companion modeled the behaviors required of the patient and provided assistance in the use of the various appliances.

Companions were not suggested for all cases—only those where the illness was acute or had progressed to the point of dementia praecox (brain degeneration). A rule of thumb presented in the readings was that a companion was necessary "until there is an equal balance in the mental and physical activities" (386-1). In other words, if the individual was able to maintain a relatively high level of functioning (and adherence to the suggestions), a companion was usually not recommended.

Excerpts from the Cayce Readings
271-1   M. 34   2/13/33
. . . with a companion constantly that would make for those engagements mentally and physically in activities that are constructive and yet, with patience and persistence, have those activities carried on in such a way as to make for constructive thinking, constructive activity, both as to the association and as to the speech, and as to the environment.

With such there must necessarily go patience, lovingkindness, grace, mercy, and patience with those activities that make for little of fear, yet positive in the speech, in the associations, and yet giving place and vent to those periods when there may be seen those reactions from the physical and mental that are not—as yet—wholly under the submerged activity of these repressions created in an incoordinating system.

386-1   F. 20   8/9/33
. . . the body should not be left alone at any period, until there is an equal balance in the mental and physical activities . . .

Q. Would her aunt, Mrs. [760], be a good person to be with her?
A. Excellent!

383-3   F. 20   10/25/33
Q. How can I prevent myself from becoming blue and depressed at times? And how can I prevent myself from crying so easily?
A. By not remaining alone! Be joyous! Whistle, sing, holler, anything that makes for activity! Just don't allow it to come on! Put it on someone else! Be with someone else!

1789-1   F. 32   1/13/39
To be sure, it will require that there be a constant attendant; and one physically able to handle the body, but NOT in a manner of other than kindness, patience, and with LOVING care—rather than the attempts to further break down the self-expression . . .
The impulses of the imaginative system [sympathetic system] must be quieted through gentleness and kindness, yet positiveness.
And let such an one, who has the care of the body, be one not lacking in prayer and in love for the fellow man.
Q. What environment would be suggested, where these directions might be followed?
A. As indicated, where there is care; an attendant, constantly and where there is a loving and not a HORRIBLE environment!

1513-1   M. 47   1/7/38
Q. On his return home, what kind of exercise would be best?
A. Keep in the open as much as practical, but NEVER alone—until there is at least the opportunity for better equilibrium to be gained by the releasing of pressures and the building up to the glandular forces and to the activities from the electrical forces through the Gold Chloride in the system.

1789-2   F. 32   3/10/39
As we find, if there would be the better influences or forces, there would be those manners followed as indicated—under the supervision of a sympathetic nurse, that would be always close with the body . . .
Q. Is the body in a condition to be moved from the hospital?
A. Only if it is under the careful supervision of one competent to handle the situations.
Do not attempt to move until some one has known all the details and is willing (not merely for the money but because of the sympathy, the Christian spirit) to ASSUME the responsibility and care for this body.

And that will be the manner in which one may be chosen for such an office—to see, to know ALL the situations, see? Not just to be hired, but one that would give of self for the aiding of someone . . .

Q. If Hanser is willing, would it be a good place for the body to remain instead of present hospital?

A. This depends upon just what has been given. It isn't merely the willingness that is necessary—it should be one that is DESIROUS, see?

Willing for hire is one thing—willing because of the love and the human element is another—willing because of the physical, mental and spiritual experiences is still another . . .

But if those who are desirous of being of help will pray ABOUT it, they will receive direction!

Do that.

This is not merely for show, not merely for sympathy—but that there may be the will, as indicated, for the recovery of the abilities of this body.

2248-1 F. 24 5/27/40

Then, we would put the body under the supervision of a sympathetic nurse, in pleasant environs, where more liberties may be had and yet less incoordinated activity accorded for the physical body.

The requirements for such a nurse would be, first: One of a sympathetic nature; not merely desiring a job of care, but one versed in psychological aspects of human reaction, ESPECIALLY in a SPIRITUAL way and manner . . .

This one—the nurse—must be spiritual-minded, and not merely seeking a material occupation.

2465-1 F. 28 3/17/41

We find that this condition may be better attended to not in an institution; while it will require care, close observation, and for a time at least there should be had a close companion with the body . . .

Do these—and as we find the environ of the home will be much more satisfactory; for the body as well as for the mother; but do have the companion in the first few weeks anyway.

2614-1 F. 37 11/7/41

Keep about the body congenial companionship, or MAKE self express congeniality in whatever environ or sphere of activity the period may carry the body.

5405-1   M. 22   8/22/24

This would require, to be sure, that the body be released to a competent nurse, and the care would preferably be where there will be the ability for the entity to apply itself in some useful activity. The more out-of-doors, the better.

This can be accomplished, if there is first obtained such a caretaker for the body . . .

Q. Just where should these treatments be followed?

A. As has just been indicated, where there would be some individual who would care for this body, and in the attitude of doing it not for the money, but for love of the fellow man. Yes, there are many who will do so. These can be obtained, as we find, should there be the desiring to change to the farm for such, in Massachusetts.

Q. In what way can his mother best help him?

A. By the act of the life itself, as indicated, and by assisting those who will aid those in assisting this boy.

5598-1   M. 23   8/8/30

. . . and this, as we find, would require one very strong in character, in purpose, in application . . .

Q. Where can such a nurse be found?

A. It will require many searchings out, but there be many that may be found. Seek if ye would find.

Prayer and Meditation

Edgar Cayce was a man of prayer and meditation and it is not surprising to find suggestions for these activities in the readings. The readings state that there are objective, demonstrable effects of prayer and meditation in the physical bodies and day-to-day lives of persons practicing these disciplines.

Of course, meditation would not be feasible in acute cases of schizophrenia. The type of meditation mentioned in reading 3440-1 is a form of visualization and [3440] was functioning at a relatively high level at the time of the reading.

Excerpts from the Cayce Readings

2967-2   M. 27   4/18/43

Then, with care, with prayer—these would be the applications as we would suggest for this body . . .

3440-1   F. 29   1/4/44

Do not use the Appliance [Radio-Active] for more than an hour and a half, and sleep through most of that period—do use the period for rest and meditation, to meditate on making self into those activities which it hopes to accomplish (and that it may!) in relation to art and music. Meditate on these. For, you can even learn to sing and play the piano and never sing a note or touch a piano—in the mind! And then you can put it into practice when the body is better attuned. For music and art must come from the soul, to be worthwhile.

"Fruits of the Spirit"

In keeping with the spiritual emphasis of this section, it might be helpful to consider some excerpts from the readings which deal directly with the role of spiritual qualities which Cayce referred to as "fruits of the spirit" (e.g., patience, kindness, service to others, hopeful attitude, etc.). The importance of applying spiritual values by the companion or staff in a therapeutic milieu cannot be overemphasized. Cayce maintained that these values would be internalized by the patient and provide a direction for the therapeutic process. When the patient was functioning at a sufficiently high level, the patient should be encouraged to apply spiritual values by being of service to others.

Excerpts from the Cayce Readings
386-3   F. 20   10/25/33

Q. Any other advice at this time?
A. Be joyous. Be happy at all times, and apply in the daily experience that which is not only a desire to be of help to someone else, but physically help others and it will help self the more—mentally and physically!

1513-1   M. 47   1/7/38

. . . that the activity may become such where the body mentally and physically may be not only active for itself but as a help for the surroundings—and not as a dread to the family and the connections thereof.

1789-1   F. 32   1/13/39

Now as we find, there may be help brought to this body, if there can be—under changed environs—the application of that which is the fruit of the spirit of truth, of helpfulness, of gentleness, of kindness, of patience.

As we find, many changes will be necessary in making applications that may be helpful.

The first, this change of environment [this woman was in the Manhattan State Hospital].

1789-7 F. 33 11/24/39

Thus to have friends, be friendly; to find that which is love, beauty, joy, MAKE these in the experiences of others. Not those that attune or give expression only for the body-forces or self-indulgences or appetites, but those that are as the pearl of great price—a smile, a loving touch, a tender word—which are worth much more than all those influences or forces of MATERIAL things . . .

This does not indicate that the entity is to be a recluse, nor one that shuts self away from associations with others; not the goody-goody individual, but one that is joyous in its relationships with others.

And give—give—give of self in activity, in thought, and in the relationships which bring harmonious and hopeful influences in the experiences of others . . .

Yet in the MENTAL SELF it has made rather the inclination to shut self away. Keep this out of the experience in the present. See life, know life, experience life, through the associations with others.

1789-8 F. 33 4/17/40

Keep the attitude of helpfulness and hopefulness to others. Put away hate and malice, suspicion of others. Trust in the LORD! for thy strength cometh from Him.

3365-1 F. 17 11/11/43

No one is to be condemned, though many might be for what has happened. But spiritually the body is not at a standstill.

If more kindnesses are shown, more love, greater peace may be brought to this body.

There is such an advanced state of lack of coordination in the reflexes. It is not possession, it is deterioration [dementia praecox] that prevents there being coordination in the mental forces. For the reflexes nominal in brain have been broken down.

All that may be done in this particular experience, then, as we find, is to persuade those whenever possible who have the care, and those who were and are responsible, to create, to make for friendships, showing patience and love and thought—by being as oft with the entity as possible. For, remember, it must ever be not just as a duty to perform, something to be done. For, one day there will come to those that have asked help here, "I was imprisoned and ye have visited me not—I was imprisoned, in body, in mind, and ye visited me not."

It is with that thought, then, that those close to the entity should consider it a privilege to give such care to this body. With such there may come help. It is not impossible, but is it probable? The probability is with those who care—care!

Just think in self, "somebody cares!" it is the greatest thought that comes to the mind of man—"somebody cares." For what? As to whether ye are this or that, or that they may use you for this or that? No! That they would like to give, like to be, like to supply thy every thought, thy every need of every nature.

It is with that spirit, if these are applied, that there may be brought a change entirely. For it is not possession.

Then there may be given peace, in the quietness. For as He gives, "When ye do My biddings, I will give thee peace." That is what is needed in the mind of this soul.

5380-1   M. 54   7/20/44

Then apply self in just being helpful, just being kind, just being patient, just being long-suffering with others, as ye would have thy Maker be with thee, and we will bring relief.

5405   M. 22   8/22/44

The giving of sedatives, the giving of certain classes of treatment, has destroyed the ability in the physical self to respond to kindness. For, as may be found in the experience of every human soul, the soul responds to all the fruits of the spirit of truth, when even the mind and body may not. But know that mind, in the material, is the builder. Thus, with the correct—or a direct-spiritual application of the tenets of truth—patience, long-suffering, gentleness, kindness, brotherly love—there may be help . . .

Let those responsible for the body live the prayerful life. Not merely hoping, but in their likes and dislikes. Put away all of anxiety, all of animosity, all of hate, all of holding others responsible. For know in Whom ye believe, and know that He is able to keep that ye commit unto Him against any experience, be it spiritual, mental, or physical.

Color and Music Therapy

Cayce often commented that art in all its various forms was spiritual in nature and possessed vast therapeutic value. A couple of reading excerpts are cited which point out the healing potential of color and music. One can easily imagine numerous examples of how this potential could be fulfilled in relation to the therapeutic milieu just discussed. Of particular interest is the reference to the use of music to "set the electrical forces in the physical body" (933-2). In other words, the use of music in conjunction with electrotherapy would be a natural combination of these therapies.

Excerpts from the Cayce Readings
933-2   M. 20   6/7/35
. . . the RHYTHMIC vibrations of the body, as to music, set the electrical forces in the physical body. As: An activity of the brain upon the nervous system makes for the releasing of vibration. Hence the study of music as related to electrical vibration and electrical applications for the human body, or as a technician in same, brings BOTH to bear upon that which will make for the greater understanding by the entity.

For many an individual that has had a brain wreck might be aided by electricity and music to a revivification of those cells, of those atomic forces that need their coercion and their regeneration by their absorbing one into another—rather than being separated and fighting its own self, or lack of proper coagulation of the cellular forces in the blood and brain forces; as in some forms of dementia, strained by great religious fervor or excitement that makes for the separation of that which is the SPIRITUAL and the MATERIAL applications THROUGH the vibratory forces of a physical body.

2712-1   F. 22   3/26/42
Keep about the body the colors of purple and lavendar, and all things bright; music that is of harmony—as of the Spring Song, the Blue Danube and that character of music, with either the stringed instruments or the organ. These are the vibrations that will set again near normalcy—yea, normalcy, mentally and physically, may be brought to this body, if these influences will be consistently kept about this body.

4501-1   F. 22   2/17/41

... for, as is seen, the body mentally—and the body in its nerve reaction—would respond as quickly to color forces as it would to medicinal properties ...

6

Therapeutic Model

◆

THE PURPOSE OF this chapter is to develop a therapeutic model which incorporates the principles and techniques advocated in the Cayce readings. It is hoped that by transposing the ideas presented in the readings into a format which is compatible with contemporary mental health resources, headway can be made in the application of this progressive therapeutic model.

There have been drastic changes in the mental health system since the time of the Cayce readings. Community programs and rehabilitative models (both psychosocial and psychoeducational) provide resources not available during Cayce's lifetime. Since many of these resources are compatible with the Cayce model, they have been included when appropriate.

The model presented in this chapter will have two primary applications which parallel the current mental health system: (1) a private practitioner format and (2) an institutional format. It is interesting to note that Edgar Cayce used both of these formats during his career as psychic diagnostician. For most of his life he served as a private practitioner—a consultant. He furnished information, advice, encouragement, and constructive criticism. As a rule, he did not personally perform the therapies or arrange for treatments. In his role as consultant, he furnished the names of professionals who could perform the therapies recommended in the readings and gave suggestions when problems or questions arose during the course of treatment.

For a brief period of time, Mr. Cayce was affiliated with an institution which offered the full range of services recommended in the readings. One of his most cherished dreams was the building of a hospital where all the suggestions in the readings could be faithfully carried out. With the help of a financial backer who was interested in promoting the work, a hospital was built and operated for a short time before financial calamities produced by the Great Depression led to its closing. To a large extent, the institutional application of Cayce's readings in the medical domain has been carried out through the A.R.E. Clinic in Phoenix, Arizona.

Regardless of the format, the basic model is the same and consists of five stages: stage one is a general orientation, stage two consists of adjunct therapy, stage three involves integration of the client into the community, stage four focuses on case management, and stage five is an evaluation at the end of one year from the date of entry into the program. The two formats will be presented and a brief discussion will follow.

Since there is considerable variability in the level of functioning and the therapeutic requirements for individuals suffering from schizophrenia, the therapeutic model presented in this chapter will be based upon a "worst case scenario." The hypothetical client is assumed to be functioning at a relatively low level (i.e., "chronic" course with preponderance of "negative symptoms"). Obviously, such is not always the case. However, this assumption is useful because it subjects the model to the most difficult therapeutic demands. Clients with more resources may benefit from an abbreviated version of the model (e.g., they may not require companion therapy).

The Private Practitioner Approach

This application of the model is an extension of the approach developed by Charles Thomas Cayce (1978). In this format, a mental health professional (such as counselor, psychologist, social worker, psychiatrist, etc.) serves as a consultant by providing leadership and guidance to the therapeutic process. This consultant should have a working knowledge of the Cayce material regarding mental health and some clinical experience with schizophrenia.

Stage One

Stage one is an orientation in which the consultant becomes acquainted with the client and does the initial assessment. Assessment consists primarily of an intake interview and a medical examination. The client's history is taken and the client's mental status is assessed (Walker, 1981). The client's history should include all psychiatric treatment received and a list of medications prescribed. If possible, relevant charts from previous facilities are provided by the client to facilitate this process. A Quality of Life Scale (QLS) or some other assessment tool may be administered so that the patient's progress in the program can be evaluated by comparing initial scores with those obtained at a later date (stage five).

Ideally, the medical exam is performed by an osteopathic psychiatrist who is well versed in the traditional form of manual medicine. This exam should investigate the possibility of somatic dysfunctions (i.e., spinal injury, lesions, subluxations, adhesions, etc.) as noted in the Cayce readings. The traditional physical exam should, of course, be completed with special attention to glandular imbalances and kidney functioning. Blood work and other medical assessment procedures (e.g., brain scans) are left to the discretion of the physician. If the client is currently taking antipsychotic medication or is deemed an appropriate candidate for such, the attending physician should prescribe and monitor medication appropriately.

It is important that the assessment procedure be open to the possibility of intuitive information about the client. This may occur in a variety of ways.

The most obvious is to follow the lead of Edgar Cayce and obtain a psychic reading from a reliable source, if one is available. Another possibility is for the interviewer to structure the assessment procedure to follow the format used most often in the Cayce readings. This format usually included some brief general remarks about the nature of the problem, a review of the major physical systems involved in the production of the symptoms, suggestions for treatment, a brief prognosis, etc. Familiarity with the Cayce readings contained in Chapter Three should enhance one's ability for recognizing patterns of pathology. Whether this occurs intuitively or as a matter of conscious cognition really doesn't matter if the information is useful.

It is important to keep in mind that the intuitively produced insights provided by Edgar Cayce were usually verified by subsequent physical examination by a health care professional. This is a good policy to follow in the assessment procedure. Do the interview, utilize any intuitive information that is available, but by all means obtain a physical examination by a qualified health care professional before beginning treatment.

Stage one also presents the opportunity for the consultant to provide the client with some basic information about schizophrenia. There is considerable support in the literature for the use of psychosocial and psychoeducational interventions during this phase. The degree to which the consultant wishes to utilize these approaches is a matter of personal preference and professional expertise. These interventions will be discussed briefly later in this chapter when the institutional format is presented.

The final requirement of stage one is the selection of a companion who will serve as an adjunct therapist by establishing and maintaining a therapeutic milieu for the client. This individual should be a contemporary of the client and could be described as an "advocate, companion, counselor, and advisor" (Anthony and Liberman, 1986). Cayce seemed to prefer the word companion although he used other terms occasionally such as attendant, sympathetic nurse, and caretaker. The companion need not be a trained professional but must possess characteristics which have been shown to have therapeutic significance. The primary requirements are that the adjunct be well adjusted and capable of empathy, nonpossessive warmth, and genuineness (Rogers, 1957). In other words, the main requirement is for a relatively healthy, mature person interested in helping another human being suffering from a chronic illness.

Cayce emphasized that the companion should be motivated by the desire to help a fellow human rather than simply seeing it as a way to earn money. This altruistic quality is associated with one who is "spiritually minded." Cayce recommended working with ideals as an excellent way to develop this attitude.

Finding a suitable companion for a client could be a challenge for the consultant. One approach is to ask the client's family for assistance in locating such a person. In at least two readings, Cayce suggested that family members could fill the role (an aunt for [386] and a sister for [1789], however he suggested that the mother not become directly involved in case [2967]. The assessment process could be structured to determine family resources in this regard (a family interview might be utilized).

Another potential source of adjuncts would be college students interested in practical experience working with the mentally ill. This program could provide valuable experience which could help students decide if they wish to pursue careers in the mental health field. It is not unreasonable to expect that universities could offer credit for such experiences, particularly psychology programs which provide applied study courses for undergraduates and practicums for graduate students. Organizations with a holistic frame of reference (such as the A.R.E.) may also be a good source of companions. Finally, a simple notice stating the requirements for the position and the benefits of service may suffice to provide suitable companions to operate a private practice.

It is important that the consultant do an assessment of each companion. This may include a review of personal references, an interview, and the use of psychometric instruments such as the M.M.P.I. If the consultant does not possess the expertise to perform these assessments, the services of a qualified professional should be obtained. It is extremely important that the companion is a stable, well-adjusted individual who can contribute to the therapeutic process.

Stage Two

Stage two is where the bulk of therapy occurs. The consultant has arranged for living quarters (probably an apartment or cottage) in which the companion and client will live for a period of two to three months. The principles and techniques presented in Chapters Four and Five form the basis for treatment. The consultant oversees the establishment of a routine which incorporates these therapies.The routine consists of a regulation of sleep patterns, balanced diet, exercise, recreation, electrotherapy, manual medicine, massage, suggestive therapeutics, and appropriate vocational opportunities. The companion models adherence to the routine and maintains a supportive milieu for the client.

The consultant should monitor progress and intervene if troubles arise. Counseling for the companion and/or client may be appropriate. Fine tuning of the treatments may be required or alternate modalities may be suggested.

Stage Three

After several weeks of companion therapy, the consultant determines if the client has benefited from treatment sufficiently to be fully integrated into a community setting. If the present housing situation is appropriate, the client may simply continue living there following the same routine that has been well established. If desirable, a roommate may be sought to share the living arrangement. This will largely be determined by the choice of the client and existing resources (such as the cost of maintaining housing). An alternative approach might be to relocate to a specific setting with significant others (e.g., living with relatives, friends, or mate). In this case, the companion and client could make the move together. They might spend several days maintaining the routine established in stage two. If family members or friends are involved, the companion and consultant can educate them to the specifics of the program and provide problem solving and coping skill training as required. The consultant may need to provide counseling at this time to insure that the client is integrated into the community successfully. When stage three is successfully completed, companion therapy is concluded.

Stage Four

Stage four involves case management by the consultant and requires regular follow-up sessions to monitor the client's progress. For most clients, one session each month should provide sufficient monitoring to insure that the client is progressing. If decompensation is evident, the consultant should provide remedial interventions as required. This may involve reinstatement of an earlier stage of the program or hospitalization in extreme cases.

Stage Five

Stage five provides an opportunity for client and program evaluation. The assessment procedure from stage one is repeated in regards to interview, administering of psychological instruments, and physical examination. These procedures provide direct information about the effectiveness of the treatment for each individual.

On a larger scale, these evaluations provide collective data which can be used to evaluate the effectiveness of the treatment in relation to other current approaches. The program is designed to provide a simple pretest/posttest experimental design for research validation. This aspect of the model will be discussed in Chapter Seven when research implications of this approach are considered.

An Institutional Application of the Therapeutic Approach

Because there is considerable overlap between this format and the private practitioner approach just presented, only the variations between the two formats will be discussed in this section. Keep in mind that this is only one of numerous possible formats of implementing this model.

Stage One

The most obvious difference in stage one is the setting. Whereas the private practitioner utilizes an office or the client's home for stage one, the institutional model provides a facility with considerable resources. For example, a group home could be utilized. It might consist of a building such as a large house which has been constructed (or remodeled) to provide living arrangements for about ten adults. Such facilities are fairly common in most mental health programs (so called "half-way houses").

Another major difference between the institutional and private practitioner model is the presence of staff in the group home setting. Having immediate and regular access to professionals such as a massage therapist, dietician, psychologist, or physician creates a reassuring atmosphere which is helpful during the orientation process.

This setting provides a supportive environment in which the assessment can be accomplished and the daily routine established. Psychosocial training in coping skills and psychoeducation regarding the therapeutic program can be incorporated into this orientation period so that the transition to adjunct therapy can be made smoothly. Peer pressure associated with group living can provide a powerful motivational tool for maintaining the daily routine. Because some of the therapies recommended by Cayce are not standard for the treatment of schizophrenia (e.g., massage, electrotherapy, etc.), introducing these modalities in a supportive atmosphere where everyone is using them would help to create a positive initial experience which facilitates the adoption of the treatment plan. The group home also makes the job of matching client and companion easier. These individuals can get to know each other and develop rapport in a relatively supportive environment.

The companion can also be integrated into this setting and receive valuable experience using the Cayce principles and techniques. In fact, the group home setting can be considered an excellent training ground for companions. Persons wishing to become companions can spend a brief period as "interns" at the group home and become familiar and comfortable with the program before they have to use it on their own. An institution specializing in the Cayce approach to the treatment of schizophrenia may wish to develop a formal internship program for the training of future consultants and the various professionals required in this approach. If some form of certification were provided, the task of obtaining qualified and motivated companions could be simplified because there would be a demand for persons possessing the skills and experience developed in this program.

Stages Two Through Five

These stages closely follow the patterns developed in the private practitioner model. Because the group home offers training in the various coping skills found to be effective in the treatment of schizophrenia, clients and companions may wish to avail themselves of these services on a regular basis (perhaps two or three times a week). This can provide some constructive diversion from the daily routine and afford opportunities for social interaction.

Vocational training and job opportunities can also be provided more easily in an institutional format since such an organization has more resources and contacts within the community. During vocational training, the companion can assist in the rehabilitation process by insuring that the client will be at work and able to accomplish the assigned tasks.

Case management is a standard process in any institutional setting and should pose no special problems in this model. Similarly, evaluation is a common procedure in many mental health programs. The documentation process required for collecting and maintaining accurate records is fairly standard.

Discussion

Although the therapeutic model has been presented in two formats, there is considerable overlap between these two applications. Just as in the current mental health system, the two formats can coexist and complement each other. It is quite likely that a number of private clinics would naturally evolve from successful private practices.

It is encouraging to note a trend toward the acceptance of some of the ideas presented in the Cayce material by the mental health establishment. For instance, Hyde (1985) proposes a private practitioner approach in which the clinician acts as a consultant and is called a "schizophrenia counselor." Hyde's emphasis on planning and maintaining a low-stress, balanced lifestyle with attention to diet, exercise, rest, and appropriate medication closely parallels the suggestions of Edgar Cayce. Hyde is not alone in suggesting that a progressive approach to the treatment of schizophrenia is long overdue. In the section which follows, a brief review of the literature relevant to the Cayce model will be discussed.

Supportive Milieu

The holistic approach suggested in the Cayce material is a milieu model in its broadest sense. The environment surrounding the client is designed to be constructive and supportive twenty-four hours a day for a period of several months. The institutional format emphasizes environmental support both in the form of a group home and a shared apartment with an adjunct therapist. In an excellent review of the support literature, Anthony and Liberman (1986) recognized two forms of support: supportive persons and supportive settings.

A "support person" might reduce a person's disability and handicap through a number of different roles (e.g., advocate, companion, counselor, and advisor). Attempts at making the setting more supportive focus on the programs or resources within the environment rather than on support persons, per se (e.g., sheltered work and living settings, and special discharge programs). The distinction between supportive persons and supportive settings simply highlights the different ways in which environmental modifications occur. In practice, these modifications often occur simultaneously. (p. 552)

The proposed therapeutic model incorporates both aspects of support by providing sheltered living and work opportunities and an adjunct therapist to live with the client for an extended period of time. The effectiveness of support persons has been demonstrated in studies by Katkin (1971, 1973) and Cannady (1982). Cannady's study is particularly important since the support persons were citizens from the patient's neighborhood and not professional mental health practitioners. The selection criterion for these support persons was simple—they were to be "relatively healthy people." No other criteria were assumed significant. Support persons were assigned one-on-one to the clients. More than one worker was assigned in certain cases for short periods when deemed necessary. All supportive care workers and supervisors were under contract and all were paid.

During 1980 there were 46 clients in the program, 46 supportive care workers, and 5 supportive care supervisors. Total program expenses were $56,886, or an average cost of $1,237 per client . . . In contrast to these dramatic reductions in costs and inpatient treatment needs, there was one client at one of our state hospitals whom we have not been able to get into our community supportive care program. This one client now costs the state $140 per day, or $51,100 per year. (pp. 15-16)

This support program was monitored from 1978 to 1980. During this three-year period, inpatient psychiatric treatment days decreased 97%, 74%, and 92%, respectively. This study suggests that support persons can provide cost-effective rehabilitation for chronic populations.

Stickney, Hall, and Gardner (1980) studied the effects of utilizing both a support person and a supportive environment at the time of a patient's discharge from a hospital. The study population (n = 400) was treated with degrees of support varying from little support to a combination of personal and environmental support. The results demonstrated that increased levels of support produced dramatic increases in referral compliance and decreases in recidivism.

In an analysis of various milieu approaches, Gunderson (1980) has found several key factors which are present in therapeutic milieus:

. . . a high patient/staff ratio with relatively small (10 or less beds) units. Moreover, the staff members were predominantly youthful contemporaries of the patients . . . there was a distribution of responsibility among all staff members, and a high premium was placed upon the involvement of all members of the community—including the patients . . . (p. 67)

The Earth House Model

Although the integrated model that has been proposed is designed to fit into the rehabilitative programs used by many community health centers, the basic principles have been utilized by a variety of other programs. Earth House was founded in 1970 by Rosalind LaRoche as a prototype structured home for recovering schizophrenics. The program combines an orthomolecular orientation with psychotherapy and compassion. The program emphasizes education, hence the client is referred to as a student rather than patient. Students are encouraged to "learn about the nature of their illness, the nutrients, diet, exercise and life habits which will assist their recovery" (Fitch & LaRoche, 1984, p. 36). This education includes classes in "wellness management" and "responsible patienthood." The use of "operatives" (support persons) provides around the clock supervision of students who are having problems adjusting to the routine or are experiencing acute symptoms. The operatives may assist the student at Earth House or at a later stage in the student's home. The exercise program is a rigorous one and includes aerobics, hatha yoga, swimming, and sports games. Students are required to jog a minimum of one mile twice a week and encouraged to take long walks. They must also do household chores, volunteer jobs, and part-time jobs as soon as they are capable. Academic and art classes are offered to assist the students in developing a high level of functioning in all areas. The program has four stages: arrival, adaptation, advanced, and graduate. At the graduate stage, the student lives in supervised housing in the general vicinity of Earth House where medications, nutrients, diet, and exercise can be monitored. Upon completion of this final stage, the student is ready to return to live alone or with relatives.

Earth House completed a study over a three-year period to evaluate the program (n = 82). At the end of that time, 45% of the students had "graduated from Earth House (i.e., were able to work and live in sheltered or independent living situations), 16% had voluntarily withdrawn, 21% were asked to leave, and 18% were still in the program.

The Fountain House Model

Fountain House is another example of a progressive approach to the treatment of major mental illnesses such as schizophrenia. Fountain House is an intentional community which operates as a club with persons suffering from mental illness as its members. The primary purpose of Fountain House is to assist its members to function at the highest possible level by providing a supportive milieu. Staff and members do all the work required to maintain the club. Staff do not ask members to do work that they do not also perform themselves. The program components include: a prevocational day program, a transitional employment program, evening and weekend social programs, apartment program, and medical assistance (monitoring medications, psychiatric consultation, general health issues).

The clubhouse model as represented by Fountain House can be considered the good news in schizophrenia rehabilitation.

The clubhouse model is justifiably popular because it meets patients' (they are always referred to as "members") needs in an integrated and humane manner. Clubhouses are first and foremost precisely that—a house where members can gather, socialize, feel comfortable, and be with friends. Since all members have had some kind of serious mental disorder, no stigma enters there; the clubhouse is a stigma-free island set in a community awash with stigma. (Torrey, 1988, pp. 263-264)

There are many clubhouses around the country and clinicians interested in the Cayce model would do well to become aware of such resources in their local communities.

Vocational Rehabilitation

Work is an important activity in the rehabilitation of persons suffering from schizophrenia. Providing a work environment which minimizes stress is crucial to this phase. The Fountain House model recognizes the problems inherent in providing appropriate work opportunities for the chronically mentally ill and deals with this dilemma by offering two levels of work. A prevocational day program provides training for entry level employment which leads to a transitional employment program. The Fountain House model views work as essential to the rehabilitative process: " . . . work, especially the opportunity to aspire to and achieve gainful employment, is a deeply generative and reintegrative force in the life of every human being" (Beard, Propst & Malamund, p. 47). Fountain House guarantees its members the right of employment in commerce and industry at regular wages in nonsubsidized jobs. A cooperative relationship exists between the clubhouse and participating employers. This is not a charitable act on the part of the employers. No adjustments or lowering of work standards are made and replacement workers are provided in case a worker is unable to work on any given day. Employers can count on the contracted work being done every day at competitive wages.

Floyd (1984) studied the patterns of employment in a group of schizophrenics (n = 150) during a twelve-month period and found that the high rate of unemployment "appeared to be primarily due to their failure to remain in jobs rather than their difficulty in finding them" (p. 93). Stress was a major factor in the subject's failure to remain employed and could be reduced by jobs with "high objective quality" (feedback on work performance), good supervision, good social climate, organization so that they were not working on their own all the time, and work that was interesting. Skilled jobs are more likely to provide work situations with these stress-reducing characteristics. Subjects doing skilled work tend to be unemployed for significantly less time than semiskilled or unskilled workers. The implications for rehabilitation are that clients should be given the opportunity to develop the highest level of vocational skills possible in areas that they find interesting. Job placement in supportive, highly organized environments are desirable. Floyd notes that these job characteristics are identified as desirable by the large body of research on "normal" workers.

In a thoughtful article on vocational rehabilitation, Mackota and Lamb (1989) comment that work may provide an excellent activity in which social skills are of less importance than in other interpersonal situations. They note that certain schizophrenics may do better in jobs which are relatively isolated but relapse in jobs requiring higher levels of social interaction. They cite stress as the key factor in these cases and recommend that vocational assessment address the client's ability to deal with social stress in the work environment.

The authors reiterate the beneficial effects of work in regards to self-confidence and a sense of empowerment. The patient is encouraged to discard the role of dependent patient and assume the role of productive worker. Realistic expectations play an important role in this transition.

> If the patient is given a clear, consistent message that a certain kind of performance is expected and that craziness, apathy, or rationalization such as, "I can't do that, I'm handicapped," are not acceptable, then the patient is likely to perform better. Work therapy is directed to the healthy part of the person. The aim is to maximize the individual's strengths rather than to focus on psychopathology. (p. 550)

The structure resulting from an integration of social support with realistic expectations yields a vocational opportunity with low stress and increased rehabilitative potential.

King (1983) has proposed a biochemical contribution of work therapy. Work which involves gross motor activity is viewed as metabolizing stress hormones which have been associated with schizophrenia. From a historical perspective, the 18th-century treatment of "the work cure" in which patients were encouraged to do supervised, homely labor may have been effective to the extent that it provided structured activity which reduced stress at a fundamental biochemical level. King particularly favors outdoor activities such as gardening and farming.

Somatic Interventions

Medication

Neuroleptic medication clearly represents a powerful somatic intervention in relieving the florid symptoms of acute psychosis. Therefore, issues related to schedule and dosage of medication and negative side effects are important and should be closely scrutinized in any therapeutic model.

The negative side effects of such medications are numerous and vary in severity from annoying to life threatening. "These drugs can affect virtually every organ of the body from the skin to the liver" (Lickey & Gordon, p. 121). The most serious and disruptive side effects include: tardive dyskinesia, dystonia, akathisia, dry mouth, blurred vision, cardiovascular hypotension, and sleepiness.

There is considerable research data which suggests that levels of medication can be safely reduced or eliminated during rehabilitation (e.g., Kane et al., 1985; Marder et al., 1987). "In summary, low dose and intermittent dose strategies seem to offer great promise for an as yet undetermined percentage of stable schizophrenic outpatients who are closely followed by their psychiatrists and who have a relative or friend available to collaborate" (Herz, 1986, p. 53). The supportive milieu proposed in the holistic model provides an ideal situation for monitoring and adjusting medication to the lowest possible therapeutic levels. Since the deficit symptoms of schizophrenia are often exacerbated by medication, diminishing drug levels would tend to facilitate client participation in rehabilitation. Decrease in drug levels also relates to "quality of life" issues which are important if rehabilitation is to result in the highest level of functioning possible for each client (Schulz & Pato, 1989). Kane et al. (1985) concluded that patients on low dose levels had fewer symptoms of tardive dyskinesia and were rated as functioning better socially than standard-dose patients.

Antipsychotic medications were not available during Edgar Cayce's lifetime, so naturally there is no mention of them in the readings. Generally speaking, Cayce recommended that the body's natural healing potential be utilized and stated that this natural potential was often diminished by drugs. On several occasions, however, he did recommend the use of powerful medications in moderate doses to stabilize a person's deteriorating condition. This is the approach advocated in the therapeutic model and is consistent with the literature just cited.

Massage

The physiological effects of massage in health promotion and stress reduction are well documented. Massage has been shown to increase blood flow (Severini & Venerando, 1967), reduce pain (Cyriax, 1980), decrease muscle fatigue (Cyriax, 1977), and reduce stress (Kreamer, 1986). Woody (1980) has used massage in his clinical practice to treat anxiety and tension in his patients. In addition to the physiological benefits of massage, Woody acknowledges psychological effects. "Psychologically, massage is known to soothe through tension reduction and to facilitate positive relationships (such as trusting and caring)" (p. 14). In a controlled study (n = 183), Weinberg and Kolodny investigated the psychological effects of massage and concluded that massage "consistently produced positive mood enhancement with significant decreases in tension, confusion, fatigue, anxiety, depression, and anger while maintaining high levels of vigor, which is representative of mental health" (p. 202).

There are many systems of massage available today, as there was in Cayce's time. Cayce frequently recommended a gentle, soothing type of massage as exemplified in the Swedish and neuropathic approaches. When he suggested osteopathic massage, the instructions frequently included comments aimed at keeping the massage gentle. It can be noted that the type of massage most frequently recommended by Cayce would also have stress-reducing qualities. Cottingham (1987) has studied the effects of various types of massage and concluded that the type of massage does indeed produce varied autonomic response and stress-reducing potential.

In summary, the studies suggest that slow, deep manipulative pressure to the muscles or abdominal viscera produce parasympathetic reflex responses that include a decrease in blood pressure and heart rate, a synchronizing of EEGs, and a decrease in baseline EMG activity. Light touch to the skin appears to induce a similar vagotonic response. In contrast, painful touch to the skin or musculature induces an arousal, or sympathicotonic response, that includes an increase in blood pressure and heart rate, an arousal EEG pattern, and an increase in EMG activity. Finally, various rates or patterns of stimulation appear to evoke different autonomic responses. (pp. 154-155)

The relatively gentle techniques employed in Swedish massage are ideally suited to stress reduction. This traditional approach is readily accessible because it is taught at most massage schools.

The systematic use of massage as a treatment for schizophrenia has been pursued in various clinics in Europe and the Soviet Union. Figueiredo, Goncalves, and Mota Cardoso (1980) reported favorable results in a study designed to assess the potential for massage as a treatment for schizophrenia. Cott (1971) cited the use of massage in the USSR as part of a holistic program emphasizing body cleansing through controlled fasting. Glielmi, Greco, and Piazza (1972) studied the effect of massage therapy on the affective-cognitive content of psychiatric patients. All subjects showed improvement in affective-cognitive content following massage therapy although schizophrenics produced less improvement than other psychiatric groups.

Successful Institutional Applications

Fortunately there exists an abundant literature on clinical successes using institutional programs closely resembling the proposed model. The most obvious example is the Still-Hildreth Osteopathic Sanatorium which operated in Macon, Missouri, from 1914 to 1969. Cayce often referred persons to this institution for the treatment of major mental illness. The precision of diagnosis and treatment at this facility was exemplary and equaled or exceeded the standards of the state hospitals of that era (Gerdine, 1919; Hildreth, 1942). Accurate records were maintained and provided the basis for an evaluation of therapeutic effectiveness. F. M. Still (1933) reported a cure rate of 35% in cases of dementia praecox (n = 1002). This population represented all cases of dementia praecox which were at the Sanatorium long enough to be diagnosed. Since some of the cases were of a chronic nature, the cure rate was considerably higher for cases with early intervention (68% when treated within the first 6 months of onset). Still stated that the osteopathic cure rate compared favorably with cure rates at state hospitals of the same era (7% average cure rate for total dementia praecox populations).

The chiropractic profession, in that same period, produced a number of institutions which specialized in the treatment of mental illness. Two of the most successful were the Forest Park and Clear View Sanitariums located in Davenport, Iowa. W. Heath Quigley (1973) was the director of Clear View from 1951 to 1961 and maintained extensive records for the purpose of evaluating treatment efficacy. He reported significant improvement in most cases of schizophrenia—70% of the patients were "released and socially restored." Although he attempted to use empirical methods to provide a longitudinal study of his population, his work was "plagued by the inability to have a control population for study and adequate follow-up methods" (p. 116). Quigley placed emphasis upon the long-term status of his patients in evaluating their treatment. "It is clearly evident that the condition of the patient as he leaves a mental hospital is not as important as how long he can remain in society in useful performance" (p. 116). To his credit, Quigley did publish numerous case studies which provide useful information about the clinical results of his work (1958). Still (1933) echoed Quigley's emphasis on long-term social adjustment as a criteria for program evaluation by stating, "We didn't consider them as being well unless they were able to return home and resume their former place in society, unless their family thought they were normal, and this at least from the economic standpoint differentiates the sick patient from the well person" (p. 4).

Although the claims of success put forth by the osteopaths and chiropractors are not endorsed as representing conclusive empirical evidence for their treatments, at the very least one must concede that such evidence is supportive of the therapeutic model presented and invites further consideration. In a field in which useful empirical evidence is extremely difficult to obtain, these findings support the position that a combination of therapeutic milieu and manual medicine can be effective in the treatment of schizophrenia.

Some Alternative Applications

There will likely be many individuals reading this book who are interested in this approach but unable to apply it within the framework of the private practitioner or institutional models proposed. Numerous alternatives exist and these possibilities will be briefly explored.

The most obvious alternative is direct application of the suggestions by family and friends without the assistance of a mental health professional. In a sense, these persons would serve as "general contractors" and obtain professional services on their own. This would be the most practical route if consulting professionals were not available. Financial considerations may also affect the appropriateness of the various therapeutic options. It is important that a qualified professional be involved in some manner to monitor medication levels (if they are being used) and also to serve as a resource if serious problems arise. It may be difficult to find a psychiatrist (M.D.) who is sympathetic to this approach. The assistance of an osteopath who is board certified in psychiatry may prove more useful. Unfortunately, D.O.s with this expertise may also be difficult to locate.

Another alternative application of the Cayce suggestions would be to revive the models created at Still-Hildreth and Clear View. This would be an institutional application with great potential for treating the full range of major mental illness, including schizophrenia.

Such a program would overlap considerably with the Cayce model and may provide a useful format in cases of treatment of resistant schizophrenia.

Basically, there were two therapeutic modalities suggested by Cayce which were not employed at Still-Hildreth and Clear View: suggestive therapeutics and electrotherapy (i.e., vibrational medicine). These two treatments are important because they provide the basis for regeneration of the nervous system in chronic patients. These interventions are compatible with the philosophy and clinical application of manual medicine and could easily be incorporated into such a program.

Likewise, many of the Cayce suggestions could be utilized directly into numerous community mental health programs around the country. Most of the somatic treatments fall under the heading of "stress management." The literature on support persons (companions) is substantial and deserves more widespread application. Since osteopaths (D.O.s) are legally recognized health care providers in the United States, it might be advantageous to use a D.O. (who practices manual therapy) to perform physical examinations on mental health clients. Somatic dysfunctions could be diagnosed and treated as a result of routine physical examinations. The financial savings to the mental health system could be substantial. As chiropractic becomes more widely accepted, it could also play a significant role in the treatment of major mental illness.

Understandably, there are few if any public institutions in this country which would be open to a therapeutic model based upon the work of a psychic diagnostician. However, most of the principles and techniques advocated in the readings did not originate with Edgar Cayce. Therefore mental health workers should feel free to incorporate principles and techniques which are helpful, regardless of the source. Reference to Edgar Cayce is certainly not essential. It really doesn't matter what the model is called or whom a therapeutic technique is attributed to, so long as it is helpful to those persons devastated by the effects of mental illness.

7

Research Implications

◆

THE PSYCHIC READINGS of Edgar Cayce indicate a preference for applied research. "In the application comes the awareness" is an oft-repeated phrase in the readings which conveys this partiality. The therapeutic model presented in Chapter Six provides an excellent opportunity for applied research since the model lends itself to empirical validation in numerous ways. The assessment criteria were designed to provide data on relapse rate so that the model could be compared to other approaches which use that criteria as a measure of effectiveness (see Hogarty's review, 1984). The Quality of Life Scale (see description by Heinrichs, Hanlon & Carpenter, 1984) was selected as a means of monitoring level of functioning—an important consideration when evaluating a therapeutic model which offers the possibility of addressing deficit symptoms.

The view advocated throughout this work has been that the Cayce material is not self-validating. It should be subjected to scholarly inquiry and empirical testing. The approach taken has been that the Cayce information is *plausible* and deserving of further consideration. The preceding chapters have provided evidence that the Cayce suggestions for treating schizophrenia are not outlandish or dangerous. To the contrary, they are in general agreement with much of the current literature. Although there is no certain knowledge of the precise mechanisms by which the various interventions recommended by Cayce may have a therapeutic effect, the same can be said of many common contemporary psychiatric interventions. The "discovery" of many of these treatments can best be described as serendipitous, if not outright accidental (e.g., phenothiazines for schizophrenia, lithium for bipolar, ECT for medication-resistant depression, etc.). In all these instances, treatment efficacy led to research and not the other way around. The apparent success of the Cayce approach in the few cases where it was applied consistently, combined with the anecdotal reports of hundreds of similar cases in the literature of manual medicine, support the proposition that this model is deserving of further consideration in a research format.

In addition to an investigation of the Cayce approach at the global level of a therapeutic model, researchers may wish to pursue specific lines of inquiry related to more traditional research questions. In the following sections, some of the research implications inherent in the Cayce material will be discussed and suggestions for further research proposed.

Variability

Variability is a major problem in schizophrenia research and must be addressed if significant progress in the understanding of this illness is to be gained. Heterogeneity and nonspecificity are two of the most frequently cited sources of variability.

Heterogeneity

If the diagnostic category of schizophrenia actually represents numerous subgroups of various etiologies (as current research and the Cayce readings suggest), identification of the various subgroups should be a high priority for researchers and theoriticians.

Identifying possible subtypes is of great importance in the search for the underlying pathophysiology and etiology. If a diverse group of disorders is pooled together in studies of biological correlates, important findings may be lost because fundamental differences have been averaged out. Only a broad spread of variance is left behind as a clue to suggest the possible heterogeneity of schizophrenia. This variance is perhaps one of the most consistent observations in research on schizophrenia. (Andreasen, 1987, p. 15)

Horrobin recognized the potential effects of heterogeneity in his discussion of the possible role of prostaglandin as an etiological factor in schizophrenia.

I have discussed only the positive evidence for the various concepts because careful scrutiny of the negative evidence shows that in each case it only rules out the concept concerned as a full explanation for all types of schizophrenia and not as a partial explanation for some types. Since my purpose is reconciliation, the positive evidence is more important. (Horrobin, 1979, p. 530)

Horrobin was not advocating sloppy research or uncritical acceptance of uncontrolled studies. He simply acknowledged the reality of heterogeneity in schizophrenia and suggested that researchers stop looking for the cause of schizophrenia.

The kidney dialysis research discussed in Chapter One provides another example of this principle. Technical considerations aside, even when such studies overcome inherent logistical difficulties and impose a fair amount of experimental control, results do not preclude uremic poisoning as an etiological factor in *all* cases diagnosed as schizophrenia. Such research can only eliminate uremia as *the* single cause of schizophrenia. The occasional diagnosis of various forms of autointoxication (including uremia) in the Cayce readings suggest that such factors should not be summarily dismissed because of negative findings in studies which do not adequately address the issue of heterogeneity.

Furthermore, simply acknowledging heterogeneity is not sufficient to eliminate it as a source of variability. One must develop a conceptualization to understand the nature of the problem. Kirkpatrick and Buchanan (1990) offer three possible conceptualizations of heterogeneity:

1. All schizophrenics suffer from a single pathophysiologi-

cal process, but there is individual variation relative to the brain areas involved by this process; other examples of such a situation include syphilis and multiple sclerosis.

2. Schizophrenia is a syndrome consisting of a number of different diseases (e.g., "process" schizophrenia), each with its own pathophysiology. A similar situation exists in the syndrome of mental retardation.

3. The clinical heterogeneity of schizophrenia is due to a number of pathophysiological processes. These processes may coexist in some individuals, i.e., some schizophrenia patients may suffer from more than one such process. (Kirkpatrick & Buchanan, 1990, p. 545)

These proposed models are not necessarily mutually exclusive; for example, "individual variation" (proposal #1) may be a significant factor even though a number of pathophysiological processes may be involved (proposal #3). Such combinations closely parallel the information in the Cayce readings. For even within the relatively specific subgroup of dementia praecox (which closely resembles Crow's Type II schizophrenia and Kirkpatrick and Buchanan's deficit syndrome schizophrenia), the readings did indicate various pathophysiological processes such as deficit glandular secretions, brain toxemia, and faulty neurotransmission. Also, considerable variance in developmental course and cross-sectional manifestation of symptoms was noted as resulting from individual differences.

Although there are numerous possible approaches to reducing heterogeneity, Kirkpatrick and Buchanan's emphasis on identifying pathophysiological processes is perhaps the most appropriate since it offers the possibility of understanding the relationship between etiology, physiology, clinical presentation, and developmental course. With this in mind, an attempt will be made to establish an understanding of pathophysiology based upon the Cayce readings. Specifically, the concept of dementia praecox, as elaborated by Kraepelin and described by Cayce, will form the basis of this effort.

Kraepelin viewed dementia praecox as a somatic disorder linked to pathological metabolism resulting in brain degeneration and chronic course (Kraepelin, 1919). The Cayce readings were in general agreement with this conceptualization, but went further by elaborating the pathophysiology involved. Three of the most common patterns will be described and defined by the designations of

glandular deficiency, toxemia, and *pineal involvement.*
These three patterns of pathophysiology were viewed as variable in regard to etiological factors and developmental course. For example, an individual with an inherited tendency toward glandular *deficiency* could also suffer from *toxemia.* The course of the disorder was also variable in that the pathological processes did not necessarily lead to actual brain degeneration in all cases. Table 7.1 provides a visual representation of these patterns so that they can be compared to current criteria of subgrouping. Less frequent patterns of pathology are also cited in the readings and readers may wish to study cases in Group IV (Chapter Three) to become familiar with some of these patterns. Table 7.1 represents the author's attempt to translate the Cayce information into a format familiar to contemporary researchers. As such, it is a preliminary construction intended to serve as a catalyst for further investigation rather than a finished, "concrete" diagnostic structure.

Dementia praecox resulting from *glandular deficiency* was probably the most common form cited in the readings and may be viewed as representing a core subgroup. The deficiency was often linked to the reproductive system: " . . . there are those glands that secrete fluids which in the circulation sustain and maintain reaction fluid [neurotransmitters?] in the nerve channels . . . [pressures] have destroyed gland functioning for the creating of these fluids" (271-1). The deficiency could be produced from various forms of pressure (i.e., lesions, subluxations, adhesions, etc.) resulting in glandular dysfunction or, alternatively, it could be produced by hereditary factors. Dementia praecox resulting from pressures was cited as having better outcome than the genetically linked variety if treated before extensive brain degeneration occurred. Presumably, the pressures could be relieved by treatment with manual medicine. Or perhaps the body's own self-corrective tendencies could compensate by relieving the pressures and allowing some degree of homeostasis to occur. The hereditary dimension of this syndrome will receive further consideration in a later section. At this point the reader need only keep in mind that these two etiological factors could operate in tandem—a genetic predisposition could be exacerbated by somatic dysfunction during the life span (diathesis/stress).

The precise nature of the *glandular deficiency* was not stated and this could prove to be an important area for future research. Dehydroepiandrosterone (DHEA), an adrenal androgen, has been reported to be significantly lower in medication unresponsive in chronic schizophrenics than in acute schizophrenics and normal controls (Tourney & Hatfield, 1972; Tourney & Erb, 1979; Erb et al., 1981). This finding is consistent with the *glandular deficiency* pattern of dementia praecox noted in the Cayce readings (i.e., chronic course with preponderance of "deficit" symptoms and resistance to dopamine-blocking medications which would not address glandular deficiency as the major etiological factor).

The author is not suggesting that DHEA is *the* glandular deficit cited in the readings. Rather, this particular finding should be viewed as an example of the type of research that could be extremely productive if the Cayce readings provide an accurate perspective on the pathophysiology of a major subgroup of schizophrenia. Interestingly, such a discovery could lead to dramatic advances in the pharmacological treatment of chronic schizophrenia.

Although current research has focused on brain biochemistry as the most likely area of pathology in schizophrenia, such has not always been the case:

> The possibility of a link between schizophrenia and gonadal activity was perhaps first suspected by Kraepelin in 1881 . . . During the period from about 1910 to 1930, there were a number of reports reflecting a popular conviction that various endocrine systems played an important role in the pathogenesis of schizophrenia. In an evaluation of these reports, Hoskins regarded the observations implicating the gonadal system as the most credible, considering the relatively crude research methods of that period. (Mason, Giller & Kosten, 1988, p. 357)

Hemphill, Reiss and Taylor (1944) reported degenerative changes in testicular biopsy samples from patients suffering from chronic schizophrenia. Note that this study preceded the use of antipsychotics and therefore would not reflect neuroleptic medication effects.

In summary, *glandular deficiency* may be closely associated with a primary pathophysiological process resulting in brain degeneration, deficit symptoms, and chronic course. This pattern may be viewed as a primary or core subgroup within the larger population of persons diagnosed as schizophrenic.

A second form of dementia praecox was said to be produced by *toxemia.* There were two common patterns of this type: (1) spinal lesions would be noted as affecting the flow of blood to the brain, thus restricting nutrient flow and preventing the evacuation of metabolic wastes; and (2) the toxemia could result from systemic toxicity related to failure of the emunctory system (e.g., kidneys, liver, etc.). The first of these processes was said to leave "impurities" in the brain which produced hallucinations:

4097-1   M. Adult   9/16/22
. . . we find the action of the brain itself to be that of dementia praecox—that is, the softening of the tissue used to present the reaction of impressions to the centers as distributed from the action of the sensory system in itself . . . [pressures in the cervicals affected] the flow of blood through the brain, that can absorb from the system those impurities that have been left and caused the hallucinations of the body at the present time . . .

The systemic variation of this form of toxemia was said to have similar effects:

3996-1   F. Adult   12/26/24
. . . blood forces not eliminating properties brings pressures on centers that deviates the sensory system in such a manner that the expression as found in the body gives those hallucinations that become so detrimental to self and self's satisfactions, and to others seeing these manifestations.

Generally speaking, the *toxemia* pattern was acknowledged by the practitioners of manual medicine (see the discussion in Chapter Five regarding hydrotherapy and other forms of detoxification used by osteopathic and chiropractic institutions) and conceptualized theoretically as the "poisoned brain" model of dementia praecox (Hildreth, 1929, p. 519).

The third major pattern of dementia praecox which the readings discussed was associated with *pineal involvement*. To appreciate Cayce's perspective of the pineal, readers are encouraged to read the discussion section of Appendix B where the concept of the "pineal system" is delineated.

294-141   M. 55   4/23/32
[The pineal is that] . . . which makes for—or known as—the impulse or imaginative body. Hence one that may be called

demented by others, who has hallucinations from a pressure in some portions, may be visioning that which to him is as real (though others may call him crazy) as to those who are supposed to have an even balance of their senses . . .

281-24   6/29/35
      Then, through pressure upon some portion of the anatomical structure [i.e., the pineal system] that would make for the disengaging of the natural flow of the mental body through the physical in its relationships to the soul influence, one may be dispossessed of the mind; thus ye say rightly he is "out of his mind."
      Or, where there are certain types or characters of disease found in various portions of the body, there is the lack of the necessary *vital* for the resuscitating of the energies that carry on through brain structural forces of a given body. Thus disintegration is produced, and ye call it dementia praecox—by the very smoothing of the indentations necessary for the rotary influence or vital force of the spirit within same to find expression. Thus derangements come.
      Such, then, become possessed as of hearing voices, because of their closeness to the borderland. Many of these are termed deranged when they may have more of a closeness to the universal than one who may be standing nearby and commenting: yet they are awry when it comes to being normally balanced or healthy for their activity in a material world.

Involvement of the pineal system was frequently associated with altered states of consciousness lending a transpersonal quality to the psychosis (Appendix B). Paranormal experiences, identical in many respects to DSM-III-R criteria for psychosis, were associated with pineal activity and have been designated "kundalini crisis" at various points in this book.
      Cayce viewed the pineal system as including the endocrine glands. Therefore, activation of the pineal system may be reflected in abnormal endocrine secretion. The clinical manifestation of this pattern bordered on manic psychosis, perhaps best represented by the diagnostic label of schizoaffective mania (Spitzer et al., 1978). Lower spinal injury resulting in pathology in the pelvic region was a common etiological pattern in these cases.
      There is considerable evidence of endocrine abnormalities in

schizophrenia and particularly in the overlap with mania (e.g., Whalley et al., 1985; Whalley et al., 1989; Mason, Giller & Kosten, 1988; Kiriike et al., 1988). Psychosis associated with reproductive system activity has been reported (Brockington et al., 1981; Nott, 1982; Dennerstein, Judd & Davies, 1983; Gitlin & Pasnau, 1989) and may shed light on the consistent findings of gender differences in schizophrenia (see Chapter One). Disturbance of steroid hormone levels can produce a psychosis resembling schizophrenia and schizoaffective mania (Judd, Burrows & Norman, 1983; Isaac, 1978). Widespread anabolic steroid use by athletes has resulted in cases of steroid psychosis resembling schizoaffective mania (Pope & Katz, 1988).

It is conceivable that in some of the cases where Cayce noted *pineal involvement,* a form of endogenous steroid psychosis was producing clinical features identical to schizoaffective mania. This possible overlap of schizophrenia with affective disorders is an example of *nonspecificity* and will be discussed further in the following section.

Nonspecificity

"The diversity of medical pathologies that leads to schizophreniclike syndromes suggests the multiplicity of possible biological derangements that could induce the clinical presentation of schizophrenia." (Garza-Trevino et al., 1990, p. 971) This apparent overlap of schizophrenia with other disease processes and diagnostic categories has produced a source of variability labeled nonspecificity. Although there are a multitude of diseases and syndromes which could be examined for the presence of nonspecificity, bipolar (manic-depressive disorder) and epilepsy have been chosen for the present discussion due to the relatively large body of research and clinical data relating them to schizophrenia. They also have historical significance due to Kraepelin's original nosology of the psychoses:

Seizure disorders have always been of interest to psychiatrists. Kraepelin noted that there were three types of psychotic conditions: dementia praecox, manic-depressive illness, and the psychoses associated with epilepsy. As psychiatrists have become more aware of the multiple medical conditions that can cause behavior change, and particularly psychosis, they have become increasingly aware of the behavior changes associated with seizure disorders. For psychiatrists, the study of seizure disorders not only is important for diagnosis and treatment of psychiatric disorders but also has many theoretical implications for the understanding of behavioral disorders in general. (Neppe & Tucker, 1988a, p. 263)

Prior to the development of EEG by Hans Berger in the 1930s, seizure disorders were regarded as mental disorders (Neppe & Tucker, 1988a). The recognition that certain subgroups within epilepsy present with a schizophrenia-like psychosis at a higher rate than the general population has led numerous researchers to investigate this relationship (e.g., McKenna, Kane & Parrish, 1985; Perez & Trimble, 1980; Slater & Beard, 1963). Oyebode (1989) has gone so far as to designate a category of *epileptic schizophrenia:* "The clinical features of schizophrenia with epilepsy are reported as being indistinguishable from the pathognomonic features of functional schizophrenia" (p. 327). Roberts et al. (1990) view temporal lobe epilepsy as a "mock up" of schizophrenia and Trimble (1977) has reviewed evidence linking dopamine neurotransmission to both disorders. Some researchers regard schizophrenia and epilepsy as being inversely related (see Trimble's review, 1977), a view based largely upon the occurrence of psychosis after forced normalization of the epileptic process (Schiffer, 1987). Csernansky, Holman and Hollister (1983) discuss the role of neurotransmitters in schizophrenia and epilepsy and suggest that homeostasis of the brain may be a key factor:

> The dopamine hypothesis of schizophrenia is usually presented in a static, rather than dynamic fashion. We propose that increased dopaminergic activity may represent a stage of a dynamic schizophrenic process rather than its cause. Dopamine, as well as other neurotransmitters, responds in an adaptive fashion to stimuli that perturb the homeostasis of the brain. One such stimulus could be an epileptic focus in the temporal lobe. Other such stimuli undoubtedly exist. (p. 325)

The Cayce readings provide an interesting perspective on the relationship between schizophrenia and epilepsy. The involvement of the *pineal system* was often cited as a significant factor in both disorders (see Appendix B for a discussion of the concept of the *pineal system* and excerpts on epilepsy from the readings). The readings note the variability within epilepsy (a subject to be discussed shortly) and maintain that there is a core group which the readings regard as representing "true" epilepsy (i.e., *ideopathic epilepsy,* Circulating Files 1-9 on epilepsy provide an excellent source of data for those interested in this subject).

Readers should keep in mind that the *pineal system* may represent the "consciousness system" and thus would naturally be involved in disorders resulting from alterations in consciousness. The important point here is that the "positive" psychotic symptoms exhibited in certain cases of epilepsy may be produced by the same pathophysiological processes that lead to "positive" psychotic symptoms [i.e., Schnieder's (1959) first rank symptoms] in schizophrenia; hence, nonspecificity. Understanding the process in one disorder could lead to a breakthrough in the other. Trimble's attempt to use the "dopamine hypothesis" as a connecting link is an example of one such attempt. The Cayce readings suggest that an understanding of the pineal system could accomplish the same end—a position that does not discount the role of dopamine since this neurotransmitter may play a significant role in the pineal system.

A close look at epilepsy may provide more than an understanding of the pathophysiology of a subgroup within schizophrenia. A consideration of current models of epilepsy may lead to a reconceptualization of schizophrenia. Progress in research has led clinicians to view epilepsy as a symptom: "Epilepsy is not a disease; it is a symptom of something wrong with a part of the body—the brain—just as deafness is generally a symptom of something wrong within the ears" (McGowen, 1989, p. 14).

Part of the difficulty in understanding about epilepsy is a hangover from the ideas of the great physicians of the last century. "Diseases" were described, for example, Addison's disease, Bright's disease, and Grave's disease . . . With these comments in mind, the reader will find it helpful to think of an epileptic seizure as a symptom—an event that is just one of the few ways that the brain has of reacting to untoward internal processes. The continuation of such reactions constitutes epilepsy. It is the doctor's task to disentangle, if at all possible, the factors in the equation that result in seizures. (Hopkins, 1981, pp. 7-8)

The utilization of the approach is premised on an understanding of the etiology and developmental course of schizophrenia. Epilepsy is certainly not "understood" in any definitive sense, but at lease some of the factors involved have been recognized. Epilepsy is currently conceptualized as consisting of two major groups:

> In general, doctors think of epilepsy in two ways. If they are able to find out what it is that has caused a person to have epilepsy they say that the person has "symptomatic epilepsy." Symptomatic means "a sign, or indication." If doctors can't tell what is causing the epilepsy in a person, they call it "idiopathic epilepsy" . . . (McGowen, 1989, p. 51)

Symptomatic epilepsy may be produced by injury to a baby's brain before or at birth (PBCs), infectious disease during childhood or head injury at some point during a person's life. Since only about one-third of all persons suffering from epilepsy are diagnosed as symptomatic (McGowen, 1989), there is much work to be done in this field.

One can easily imagine a similar approach to schizophrenia—but only if etiological and developmental factors are better understood. This is where the Cayce material can make a contribution to schizophrenia research. If the readings are a valid glimpse into the various etiologies and subgroups within schizophrenia, a shift in emphasis in basic research is imperative. As important as the brain is to the manifestation of schizophrenic symptoms, the readings indicate that a broader consideration of somatic factors is important if the mysteries of schizophrenia are to be resolved. Many of the various forms of somatic dysfunction (e.g., spinal injuries) which, the readings cited, are assessible by history and physical examination. Information concerning birth complications, childhood injuries, complaints of subclinical back discomfort, etc., may provide valuable clues to *symptomatic* subgroups of schizophrenia. These clues should not summarily be noted on charts and dismissed as peripheral to the manifestation of psychosis.

With a recognition of these somatic factors, other patterns with heavy genetic loading, chronic course, and brain degeneration might be differentiated as *ideopathic* schizophrenia (a classification quite similar to Kraepelin's original perspective). If, as the readings noted, the patterns with heavy genetic loading are associated with specific glandular dysfunctions, even this *ideopathic* designation might eventually fall within the *symptomatic* domain (i.e., the domain of *known* causes). Jablensky's discussion of this subject portends this possibility:

Schizophrenia can occur as a symptomatic disorder in association with a variety of cerebral and physical diseases. Disorders with schizophrenic features occur in association with no less than 12 major groups of neurological, endocrine, and infectious diseases; intoxications; and intracranial lesions. Epilepsy is the most notable example, but recent additions to the list include ideopathic basal ganglia calcification and aqueduct stenosis . . . Unfortunately, the search for cerebral or somatic pathologies associated with schizophrenic symptoms has not been systematic . . . However, if the clinical characteristics of psychotic illness secondary to cerebral or physical disease eventually prove to be indistinguishable from "true" schizophrenia, then a number of discrete entities linked to specific genetic or exogenous causes eventually may be identified, resulting in a fragmentation of the nosological group and a progressive shrinkage of the share of idiopathic forms. (Jablensky, 1989, p. 522)

Whereas the apparent overlap between schizophrenia and epilepsy is interesting, it is most generally viewed as peripheral to the mainstream of schizophrenia research. In contrast, the interface with the affective disorders has a long history of heated debate and proliferation of theoretical postulations. Pope and Lipinski (1978) provide a sample of this dialogue by proposing that schizophrenic symptoms are nonspecific and that many persons diagnosed as schizophrenic are actually suffering from bipolar disorder.

It will be seen that all studies found their good-prognosis "schizophrenics" indistinguishable from "pure" bipolar MDI [manic-depressive illness] cases on virtually all demographic, treatment-response, family history, and other indices, but significantly different from strict schizophrenics on most of the same indices . . . Rigorously speaking, every study of "schizophrenia" in the literature that does not make some reference to prognostic, family history, or treatment-response criteria must be considered, until shown otherwise, to be contaminated with up to 40% cases of MDI. This, in turn, raises a broader conjecture: if the "schizophrenic" symptoms are as noncontributory as they are illustrated to be in the particular case of schizophrenia vs. MDI, it follows that they may be so generally nonspecific as to be almost unusable for many research purposes . . . The nonspecificity of "schizophrenic" symptoms call into question all research that uses them as the primary method of diagnosis. (pp. 822-826)

For an alternative perspective on this controversy which emphasizes the dominance of schizophrenia in this nosological borderland, readers are directed to Welner, Croughan, and Robins (1977). At any rate, the end result of this controversy seems to be the uneasy acceptance of a middle ground classification designated schizoaffective disorder (Kasanin, 1933). The situation is further complicated by the possibility that this diagnostic category is heterogeneous (Tsuang & Simpson, 1984) and may represent a section of a psychotic continuum between schizophrenia and the affective disorders (Meltzer, Arora & Metz, 1984).

The Cayce readings may shed some light on this dilemma. Again, the pineal appears to be involved and the nonspecificity of symptoms may result from involvement of this system (see 480-3, 964-1, 1452-1 for case examples of manic depression in the Cayce readings; the involvement of the pineal in bipolar disorder is briefly discussed in the literature review in Appendix B). As noted by Pope and Lipinsky, a major source of nonspecificity is the clinical presentation of mania (specifically the acute manic psychosis occasionally found in bipolar) which is troublesome because it can be indistinguishable from acute schizophrenia. It is probably not a coincidence that this same clinical picture applies to the previously discussed subgroup of epilepsy. Significantly, the same medications (e.g., anticonvulsants) are effective in all three subgroups (i.e., individuals suffering from schizophrenia, bipolar, and epilepsy with manic psychosis features) while some standard medications for mania (i.e., lithium carbonate) are often ineffective (Wise, 1989; Prien & Gelenberg, 1989; Post, 1990; Chouinard, 1988; Ballenger, 1988; Keats & Mukherjee, 1988).

The significance of this apparent overlap is not that schizophrenia, bipolar, and epilepsy are really the same process. Rather, it is that they contain subgroups which share common systemic interactions manifesting as similar symptom clusters. There is apparently considerable variability in these systemic interactions. To the degree that there may be certain patterns which are more common than others, one may postulate the existence of "diseases." But as is the case with current models of epilepsy, perhaps the diagnostic categories of major mental illness should be viewed as *syndromes* rather than *diseases*. Unfortunately schizophrenia is often referred to as a "brain disease" resulting from faulty dopamine neurotransmission—there are many such examples to be found in the literature as is evident by the citations in this book, particularly Chapter One. With this in mind, a greater understanding of the pathophysiological processes involved in schizophrenia may lead to future designations of *symptomatic* and *idiopathic* schizophrenia, or some such distinction.

One is led to wonder whether much of the variability which plagues schizophrenia research is a product of a misconceptualization. The variability may be a product of attempts to oversimplify the disorder by viewing schizophrenia as a single *disease* while simultaneously seeking to maintain an unreasonable degree of specificity on its manifestations. This criticism is not new to the field, as numerous researchers have complained about the failure of diagnostic criteria to clearly define schizophrenia. Such efforts at reformation have often focused on biological factors as the ultimate criteria. However, research in this area has failed to resolve the problem.

The "dopamine hypothesis" represents one of the most significant of the biological approaches to understanding schizophrenia. A brief consideration of this model may shed further light on the problem of nonspecificity. Dementia praecox and schizophrenia, as defined by Kraepelin and Bleuler, respectively, emphasized "negative symptoms" and chronic course with little regard for "positive" or florid presentation. This emphasis was shifted to a pathonomonic approach with the advent of Schneider's first-rank symptoms, a conceptualization producing greater diagnostic *reliability* by defining schizophrenia in terms of "positive symptoms." The observation that neuroleptics were relatively successful at alleviating these symptoms by blocking dopamine receptors in the brain led to the conceptualization of schizophrenia as a *disease* produced by faulty dopamine neurotransmission. The question of the *validity* of defining schizophrenia by positive symptoms has been addressed by Mackay:

> Kraepelin and Bleuler recognized most of Schneider's first-rank phenomena as superficial and variable accompaniments of schizophrenia, and indeed most contemporary research has shown that the presence of positive symptomatology is a singularly weak prognostic indicator. It is perhaps unfortunate that most modern biological attention has been attracted to

an arbitrary set of clinical phenomena which stand in no established relationship to the defining characteristics by which the disease was originally categorized. Moreover it is ironic that, in his belief in a metabolic aetiology, Kraepelin placed great store by chronicity and irreversible deterioration—features which most clinicians still feel are central to any valid definition of schizophrenia, but which correlate so poorly with positive symptoms. The most widely held neurochemical hypothesis for schizophrenia suggests that the disease is associated with relative overactivity of central dopamine (DA) systems . . . It seems to be a strange turn of events that neurochemical thinking about schizophrenia has been governed by an inference from acute pharmacological effects on a set of symptoms whose relationship to Kraepelin's disease is questionable. (MacKay, 1980, pp. 379-380)

Mackay has identified the major contributor to nonspecificity in schizophrenia—the equation of positive symptomology (and presumably faulty dopamine neurotransmission in the brain) with schizophrenia. As noted, these symptoms occur in many other syndromes, and the drugs which address dopamine hyperactivity are effective in relieving these positive symptoms regardless of diagnostic label. The solution, as stated in a previous section, is to understand the pathophysiological processes which are driving the symptom clusters. The concept of dementia praecox, as defined by Kraepelin and described by Cayce, represents a plausible model for unraveling this nosological knot. The key is to focus more attention on the systemic abnormalities so frequently acknowledged yet so easily dismissed and overshadowed by undeniable functional and organic brain pathology typically associated with schizophrenia.

The Cayce material may provide additional information and insights into psychopathology in all its manifestations. While the present discussion has focused on nonspecificity in regards to certain positive symptoms associated with schizophrenia, bipolar, and epilepsy, it is important to realize that the Cayce readings (especially the 9,000+ "physical readings") may provide insight into the broader consideration of all of the various manifestations of psychopathology. The readings contain many examples of mental illness (e.g., unipolar depression, anxiety disorders, personality disorders, etc.) as well as "organic" illnesses which often present with mental symptoms (e.g., multiple sclerosis, cardiovascular disorders, etc.). Thus, the relatively comprehensive perspective of the Cayce readings may provide a means of understanding and constructively addressing heterogeneity and nonspecificity with the ultimate goal of reducing variability at all levels.

Manual Medicine

The potential contributions of manual medicine to schizophrenia research fall into two general categories: (1) direct involvement in clinical assessment and treatment and (2) theory and basic research which offer a unique perspective on how the body works, resulting in alternative interpretations of anomalous research findings in the schizophrenia literature.

The first of these contributions is self-evident. If the Cayce readings (and the osteopathic and chiropractic literature) are correct in asserting a predominant role for various forms of somatic insult in the etiology of schizophrenia, it is reasonable to expect that manual medicine could make a significant contribution to the assessment and treatment of these dysfunctions. As an example, the Still-Hildreth lesion study (Table 5.1) comes to mind as a possible aid to subgrouping, if the study were modified to include additional information such as case history, medication response, genetic loading, symptoms, etc. Subgrouping would thus reduce variability by attenuating heterogeneity.

At the level of basic research, manual medicine could provide alternative interpretations of previously anomalous findings. The ANS (autonomic nervous system) literature cited in Chapter One may serve as an example of this type of contribution. Since the prevailing view is that schizophrenia is a *brain disease,* researchers have tended to view peripheral indicators such as ANS reactivity as a convenient avenue for investigating underlying brain pathology. As the Cayce readings and manual medicine literature have indicated, such a view is not entirely without merit because a substantial number of the persons diagnosed as suffering from schizophrenia do have significant brain pathology. However, the work of physiologists such as Irvin Korr suggests that such a simple model may not suffice to explain all of the anomalies associated with the ANS literature. Readers are directed to the extensive work of Korr addressing the phenomenon of "segmental facilitation." A few examples of Korr's thinking are presented here to familiarize the reader with this perspective:

... the osteopathic lesion represents a facilitated segment of the spinal chord maintained in that state by impulses of endogenous origin entering the corresponding dorsal root. All structures, receiving efferent nerve fibers from that segment are, therefore, potentially exposed to excessive excitation or inhibition. (Korr, 1947, p. 197)

In a large percentage of patients segmental relations were established between the pathologic organ or structure and the areas of low ESR. Segmental relations between the pathologic tissue and the skin resistance pattern were by no means always clear, but the relations were especially sharp in those entities in which there was a pain component . . . we were able to demonstrate that new and prominent areas of low electrical skin resistance could be induced experimentally by acute stresses and myofascial irritations and accidentally as a result of trauma.

These observations were strong assurance that the persistent area of low electrical resistance, whatever its basis, is a functionally and clinically significant sign and that is marked, at least in some cases, physiologically abnormal and relatively vulnerable segments of the body. (Korr, 1955b, p. 268)

What does facilitation mean, functionally and clinically? In general, it means that the tissues innervated from the lesioned segment, and therefore the individual as a whole, are sensitized to all the influences operating within and without the individual. Facilitation of the sensory pathways in the disturbed or lesioned segments means that there is easier access to the nervous system—including the higher centers—through these segments. The lesioned segment is one through which environmental changes—especially noxious or painful stimuli—have exaggerated impact upon the man. (Korr, 1955a, p. 277)

That portion of the cord becomes dominated by this noisy input, and in that portion of the cord the "picture" of the periphery which the CNS steadily watches is garbled and distorted by the high noise-to-signal ratio. Reports from the various proprioceptors may be so conflicting that the cord is presented with "pictures" of impossible situations . . .

The central excitatory state at the corresponding level (and side) of the cord is exaggerated, leading to the establishment of an "irritable focus," described in recent years in terms of facilitated segments. In the portions of the cord that are receiving the noisy, garbled input, all kinds of neurons become susceptible to "facilitation," making exaggerated responses to incoming impulses from any source. (Korr, 1976, p. 41)

It should not be surprising, in view of these diverse organ and tissue responses, that sympathetic hyperactivity, sustained over long periods of time, may tend to produce pathological changes in the target tissues, the clinical impact varying with the tissue and its role in the body. (Korr, 1978, p. 240)

Because a structural defect, an osteopathic lesion, sensitizes a segment to impulses from all sources, and for reasons previously given, the lesioned segment is to be considered not a radiating center of irritation, but rather a neurological lens which focuses irritation upon that segment. Because of the lowered barriers in the lesioned segment, excitation is channelized into the nervous outflow from that segment. (Korr, 1947, p. 197)

Considering the fact that as many as half of the persons diagnosed as schizophrenic exhibit abnormal ANS response which may be interpreted as being hyperaroused (see discussion of ANS anomalies in Chapter One), one must wonder if this is a potential subgroup displaying a peripheral marker of a "facilitated segment" (i.e., spinal lesion) rather than a primary brain pathology. A reevaluation of the schizophrenia ANS literature with a consideration of the osteopathic philosophy and research literature may be a practical means of resolving some of the anomalies in this area.

One other important concept from Korr's research is relevant in this discussion of neuropathology in schizophrenia. Korr did considerable research exploring the "trophic" function of nerves.

Flowing down every single nerve fiber is a stream of nerve-cell cytoplasm in a volume so great that the nerve cell is said to "turn over" its material completely three or four times a day and this flow is essential to the continual nourishment of the fibers themselves along their entire length. And so we asked ourselves: Is it possible that the innervated muscle or organs share this trophic dependence on the nerve cell and that at least certain components of the axoplasm are transferred from nerve cells to body tissues? (Korr, 1970, p. 83)

The trophic influence of nerves was demonstrated by injecting radioactive solutions onto hypoglossal and vagal neurons of rabbits and measuring the axonal delivery to the tongue (Korr, Wilkinson & Chornock, 1967). Since trophic processes represent nonimpulse neuronal influences, this complicates one's understanding of the Cayce readings. When the readings use the term "nerve plasm," is it a reference to neurotransmitters in the traditional sense, or could it be a reference to cytoplasm in the trophic sense? When the readings refer to a "lack of stamina" in the nerve cells, could this be referring to a breakdown in trophic processes? And finally, do the frequent references to the nervous system's inability to "replenish" itself due to glandular dysfunction refer to pathological neurotransmission or a failure of the trophic process? These questions emphasize the complexity of the systems of the body and suggest alternative perspectives on possible mechanisms of neuropathology in schizophrenia. In a larger context, the underlying philosophy of osteopathy may be useful in understanding the manifestation of illness such as schizophrenia.

As our survey has made quite clear, the degree of fullness of expression of the pattern behind the lesion complex is greatly influenced by a large variety of factors. These obviously include all the factors that distinguish one individual from another: the constitutional factors (another generic term behind which we vainly try to conceal ignorance), age, environment, past history, nutrition, emotions, personality, and many others. A given structural defect may produce no clinical manifestations in one individual and a serious one in another. A relatively quiescent lesion may suddenly, under a new set of circumstances, or gradually, as through the process of growing older, bring into manifestation the full latent pattern of processes and manifestations inherent in that part of the central nervous system. (Korr, 1951, p. 409)

. . . there appears to be a de-emphasis of the specificity between the etiological agent on the one hand and the manifestations of the disease on the other. We see an approach to a unitary concept in which disease is conceived, not as the effect of this agent or that upon this organ or that, but rather as the reaction of the organism as a whole to noxious influences. . . . The pattern—the character of the disease—is determined by the patient, and not by the offending or invading agent; the nervous system certainly has a key role in the organization of the patterns . . . [there is an] emphasis on the similarities among diseases rather than on their differences. "There are not illnesses; there are only ill people." (Korr, 1948, p. 134)

These quotes emphasize the uniqueness of each person and suggest that there will always be a baseline of variability which cannot be resolved due to individual differences. The Cayce readings make the same point: "For what is the anatomical structure of the body? No two are alike. Do you ever find two blades of grass alike? Ever find two leaves on a tree alike? . . . So, with individual souls, with their complexities of activity" (254-114).

This is an important point with obvious implications. For example, not every spinal injury results in psychosis. Each individual possesses unique genetic loading, a particular pattern of developmental experience, and a distinct psychological style. These, among numerous other factors, influence the potential manifestation of somatic dysfunction.

Finally, readers who become familiar with the osteopathic literature will find descriptions of concepts such as the "secondary lesion" (or "reflex lesion," "sympathetic lesion," etc.) which are frequently noted in the Cayce readings. These descriptions may serve as a conceptual dictionary—an extremely helpful tool for those wishing to understand the Cayce perspective and apply it in a research format.

Electrotherapy

Bodily electrical systems were vaguely described in the readings and may represent a potentially productive area of study (e.g., direct current systems, "vibrational" energy systems, etc.). The work of Robert Becker (1985, 1990) is a prime example of research into the electrical systems in the body and deserves further consideration. The current appellation for vibrational phenomenon is "subtle energy." This field appears to be gaining research momentum (see discussion of electrotherapy in Chapter Five).

The alleged therapeutic effectiveness of the Wet Cell Battery should be high on the list of research priorities. It was often recommended in the readings, and any research findings could have immediate and dramatic clinical implications. Inasmuch as the Battery produces a measurable electrical current, it might serve as a "bridge" between subtle energy research and more traditional systems. The use of various substances in conjunction with electrotherapy is another important area with great potential. Gold was frequently recommended in this respect and was said to stimulate glandular secretions necessary for the regeneration of deteriorated nerve tissue. A study comparing plasma glandular secretions in a chronic population receiving gold chloride electrotherapy with a comparable control group could be helpful in assessing the potential of this form of therapy.

Genetic Factors

The readings are congruent with the current literature regarding the importance of heredity in schizophrenia. However, heredity was not viewed simply as a unitary process. Rather, it was differentiated into "hereditary innate" (strong genetic factor likely to manifest regardless of environment) and "hereditary tendencies" (an expression conveying a diathesis/stress emphasis; see case [5690] for an example of "hereditary tendencies"). Although the readings were generally vague about the specifics of heredity, in at least one case, the readings did provide some detailed information about the nature of the genetic factors involved. The case was Mr. [282] (see Chapter Three, Group II—Dementia Tendencies). Interestingly, the information was given in response to questions from Mrs. [457], [282]'s sister.

Mrs. [457] had been having physical problems and was very anxious and concerned that she might be approaching a nervous breakdown. Apparently, mental illness was known to have been present in the family of [457] and [282]. Specifically, an aunt was cited as suffering from major mental illness [diagnosis not provided]. In an early physical reading for [282] (prodromal), a warning was given concerning glandular dysfunction. The readings recommended the use of the Wet Cell Battery with vibratory gold. Excerpts from two readings provided for Mrs. [457] will be quoted. Readers are encouraged to draw their own conclusions about the role of heredity in this case.

457-4   F. 31   2/9/39
Q. Can I inherit or pass on to my children the mental and physical disease of my aunt?

A. POSSIBLE; but very, VERY improbable—if there is kept a normal balance of the elements in the blood supply for replenishing all nerve energies of the system; which CAN be, may be tested by an analysis of the bloodstream for those hormones of the perfect coagulation and perfect balance between red blood and white blood supply.

Q. Can childbirth cause it?

A. Not in this body.

Q. Can I be in any way affected by it?

A. Only as the mental self dwells upon same and thus create a field, an attitude for such reactions as to cause a disturbance.

Q. Could overwork or any overstrain bring about this mental snap?

A. Only as such would bring deterioration to that supply as indicated, that must be kept in balance.

Q. Is it true that this mental weakness has been in the family for generations and comes up at intervals?

A. Where there is the lack of sufficient of the negative and positive plasm about each blood center, such is a weakness. Not necessarily family hereditary, then, but a natural consequence of not proper physical and mental preparations for offspring BY the contacting or contracting parties.

457-5   F. 31   2/24/39
One of the sexes is not more subject than the other. And the injection of new blood will soon change the whole situation— or in ONE generation, though it may skip and enter the next.

The condition is, as indicated there, the number of positive units about the center of the atomic force as related to procreation; and this—as is used in body-building when there is the age or the certain environs as to cause or produce a deteriorating or lack of activities in the procreation of the atoms for its re-creation—brings about a lack of those elements as we have indicated.

Hence the active forces that create those in body—structure of the natures which add to the nerve plasm, or the grey matter in same, would be the corrective measures; as may be had by the vibratory influence of Gold or Silver—dependent upon that found to be lacking in the blood plasm. It would not be necessary that ANY have more than one such test, IF there is then ADDED, through such a vibratory means or manner, those hormones that would bring a normal balance for the cycle of procreative forces.

Ready for questions.

Q. Should the blood test be made by any or all members of my family?

A. Only if there is the desire for procreation.

Q. Should tests be made at definite intervals?

A. As we have indicated, only once is necessary IF those proportions of the influences necessary are added to bring a normal balance.

Q. Could my brother [452] affect his wife or his children in any way? [he was thinking of getting married]

A. Should not—if there are the precautions, or if there are the activities such as to bring that balance necessary in the whole system. There's NO affectation!

Q. Is my brother [282]'s case anything similar? Has he inherited anything, or has he a similar blood condition?

A. Read what has been given respecting this in times past! The warnings were given—they were NOT heeded!

Q. What precautions should be taken in the case of [282]'s children?

A. These should not be affected. No precaution necessary here.

Q. In the women of the family, would menstrual troubles or childbirth cause it to develop?

A. Not necessarily.

Q. Was my aunt's mental case due to physical condition?

A. To this deterioration as has been indicated.

Q. Has [282] inherited anything from her, or has he a similar blood condition?

A. Read that which has been given as to the warnings here—this is much better than to approach from the mental attitude of this body, [457].

Q. Any further advice to this body?

A. Do not dwell upon such. Be sure there is at all times sufficient vitamin B in the diet, as well as with the blood test if found deficient in the procreative plasm then add same through the vibratory forces of Gold [i.e., Wet Cell Battery with chloride of gold].

These excerpts are consistent with other readings which maintain that a heredity glandular deficiency is involved in some cases of schizophrenia (a hormonal secretion designated "procreative plasm"). Apparently, this deficiency can be measured by analysis of a blood sample. The readings seem to portray a diathesis/stress model in which the hereditary factor could be affected by mental stress (e.g., worry) or environmental factors. As was typical in such cases, vibratory metals (usually gold) was suggested to remedy the deficiency.

The caution about vitamin B maintenance is interesting because vitamin deficiencies have been linked to the pathogenesis of schizophrenia. In particular, vitamin B_3 has been utilized by practitioners of orthomolecular psychiatry. Readers interested in pursuing this perspective are directed to Hoffer's (1987) discussion of the subject.

Gender Differences

Gender differences in the manifestation of schizophrenia may be associated with spinal injuries. Traditionally, young males have been exposed to increased vulnerability to spinal injury due to higher levels of dangerous physical activity (e.g., contact sports such as football). Such childhood injuries may predispose some males to an earlier onset of symptoms than females who may be at increased risk during childbearing years. This is not being proposed as the only agent, or even a major agent, producing gender differences in schizophrenia, but merely as one of several possible factors which are prominent in the Cayce readings and may be relevant to schizophrenia research.

Summary

This chapter has discussed a number of research implications which are inherent in the Cayce readings. They may be summarized thusly:

1. Applied research of the therapeutic model should receive preferential status because it offers the most direct means of helping persons suffering from schizophrenia.
2. Variability is a major obstacle in current research and must be reduced significantly if consistent progress is to be made. Heterogeneity and nonspecificity are the two major sources of variability.

Suggestions have been provided to address these problems. Based upon descriptions of pathophysiological processes provided in the readings, a tentative approach to subgrouping has been proposed. Nonspecifity of certain schizophrenic phenomena (such as positive symptoms) provides the opportunity to understand the underlying systems producing these phenomena. The apparent of overlap of subgroups of epilepsy and bipolar with schizophrenia is an example of how nonspecificity can be utilized. The readings address many other diseases and syndromes which share nonspecificity with schizophrenia (e.g., unipolar depression, anxiety disorders, dementias, alcoholism, multiple sclerosis, etc.) and a comparative study of nonspecificity in these areas may be useful.

3. From the perspective of the Cayce readings, basic research in schizophrenia would profit from a partnership with manual medicine. Whereas most current research focuses on the biochemistry of the brain, the readings consistently characterize brain involvement in schizophrenia as an effect produced by somatic dysfunctions of various natures. Practitioners of manual medicine could provide the expertise required to do assessments which may be useful for subgrouping. Furthermore, the research literature of osteopathy (especially the work of Irvin Korr) contain important clues to the proposed relationship between somatic dysfunction and brain pathology. The ANS anomalies in schizophrenia represent a prime example of how this literature could contribute to the understanding of schizophrenia.

4. The readings maintain that glandular dysfunction plays a significant role in the etiology of schizophrenia. If such is the case, identification of the glands and secretions involved could provide a breakthrough in understanding the degenerative processes producing certain schizophrenic symptoms.

5. Clues to hereditary factors are sparse in the Cayce readings; however, some excerpts are provided with the hope that they may stimulate alternative perspectives in this area.

6. The various forms of electrotherapy recommended by the readings (especially the Wet Cell Battery with chloride of gold) may be useful interventions in cases of chronic schizophrenia and are therefore deserving of empirical research.

8

Summary and Conclusion

◆

THE PSYCHIC READINGS of Edgar Cayce represent an opportunity and a challenge for individuals interested in alleviating the suffering caused by major mental illness. Although this book focuses on schizophrenia, the readings also address other major disorders including anxiety, depression, personality disorders, and dementia.

The Cayce approach to treating schizophrenia can be summarized as follows:

    1. The diagnostic label of schizophrenia refers to a group of related illnesses with varied etiologies and outcome.

    2. There is a strong somatic component to this disorder which must be addressed in treatment.

    3. The symptoms of schizophrenia result from dysfunction within the brain but etiological patterns usually involve systemic dysfunction.

    4. Within the physical body, multiple systems are usually involved in the schizophrenic process, primarily the central and auto-

nomic nervous systems and the endocrine system.

5. In cases where the disorder progresses to a chronic condition, the prognosis is less favorable. This condition involves brain degeneration and is a difficult process to reverse. Early diagnosis and treatment greatly improve the prognosis.

6. Genetic factors often play a significant role in the development of schizophrenia. Genetic factors are not simplistic entities, but vary in influence from being "innate" (very likely to manifest regardless of other factors) to being only "tendencies" (i.e., inherited vulnerability as proposed in the diathesis/stress model).

7. Pregnancy and birth complications (PBCs) play a significant role in the etiology of schizophrenia.

8. Spinal injury and other forms of somatic dysfunction are important etiological factors in the production of psychotic symptoms.

9. Stress is often an important etiological factor in the production of schizophrenic symptoms.

10. The human body contains interfaces with spiritual and mental dimensions of reality. These interfaces ("centers") exist within the glandular and nervous systems. Chemical imbalances or injury to these systems can disrupt these centers producing the psychotic symptoms associated with schizophrenia.

11. The treatment of schizophrenia requires a holistic perspective which typically involves spiritual, mental, and physical interventions. These therapies include osteopathic or chiropractic treatments, massage, electrotherapy, diet, companionship, therapeutic milieu, hypnotic suggestion, exercise, and pharmacology.

12. Cayce's holistic perspective involves spiritual and metaphysical constructs such as karma and spirit possession. These transpersonal aspects were not cited in every case, and thus may be most appropriately viewed as complications of the pathological process rather than specific to schizophrenia.

Therapeutic Model

In keeping with the holistic philosophy of the Edgar Cayce readings, a therapeutic model has been proposed which addresses the dimensions of body, mind, and spirit. In the simplest possible conceptualization, this approach can be represented as:

1. Establish a *therapeutic milieu* with an emphasis on *spiritual*

qualities such as patience, gentleness, altruistic service, etc., while simultaneously providing opportunities for growth and development. Outdoor activities in the sunshine and fresh air are also emphasized. Companion therapy is sometimes necessary to implement and maintain a therapeutic milieu.

2. Provide *somatic interventions* which address the fundamental *physical* dimension of this disorder. Manual medicine, electrotherapy including vibratory metals, diet, exercise, and appropriate pharmacology play a crucial role in the *physical* treatment of schizophrenia.

3. Utilize *suggestive therapeutics* to rebuild and redirect the *mental* processes of the client. Various cognitive and behavioral techniques are employed in conjunction with naturalistic hypnosis so as to apply the principle, "*mind* is the builder."

Although the specific treatment plan may vary from individual to individual, the therapeutic principles as discussed in Chapter Four apply in all cases. While the discussion of therapeutic techniques in Chapter Five is not exhaustive, it does provide an introduction to these modalities while suggesting other available sources of information. A therapeutic model has been provided in Chapter Six which proposes two possible applications (private practitioner and institutional format) of the Cayce approach while encouraging alternative usage of the material.

Research Implications

The therapeutic model presented in Chapter Six should be subjected to empirical validation, and this eventuality is discussed in Chapter Seven. Variability resulting from heterogeneity and nonspecificity represents a formidable obstacle to schizophrenia research. The Cayce readings have important implications for abating variability. The various pathophysiological patterns noted in the readings provide a basis for recognizing subgroups in this disorder. Nonspecificity resulting from overlap of schizophrenia with other disorders such as bipolar and epilepsy provides an opportunity to understand the relationship between symptoms and the systemic interactions which produce them.

The Cayce readings recommend numerous techniques and devices which should be researched. Electrotherapy utilizing the Wet Cell Battery is a possible area of research. When this appliance was used with chloride of gold, the readings maintained that the glandular system could secrete substances capable of regenerating the nervous system of persons suffering from chronic schizophrenia. Manual medicine is another therapeutic modality which can be researched to determine its potential contribution to the treatment of schizophrenia. The research literature of osteopathy may also provide important insights into the meaning of ANS and endocrine abnormalities in schizophrenia.

Pitfalls and Potentials

A major weakness of the Cayce approach to treating schizophrenia is the lack of direct validation of the model. Although Cayce gave numerous readings for persons suffering from schizophrenia, only a few individuals applied the suggested treatments in a consistent manner. This lack of compliance is understandable given the limited resources available at the state mental hospitals of that era and the unique source of the information (psychic diagnosticians are not likely to receive much greater acceptance today).

When the suggestions were consistently followed, however, positive results were usually obtained. The extensive documentation of osteopathic and chiropractic successes using comparable models is intended to provide some clinical cross-validation of Cayce's approach. The only way to fully remedy the problem of insufficient direct validation is to replicate the treatments suggested by Cayce in a contemporary setting. With this in mind, Chapter Six proposed a therapeutic model which addressed these issues and provided a means of empirical validation.

One must seriously consider the ramifications of applying this model because the effort required for its application is obviously great. There are three reasons for considering the Cayce material: (1) it provides a comprehensive perspective on the etiology and developmental course of schizophrenia, (2) the descriptions and suggestions contained in the readings are congruent with the prevailing scientific literature, and (3) most importantly, it offers the potential for an extremely effective therapeutic model. Points 1 and 3 are interrelated because an understanding of the etiology and course of schizophrenia offers the possibility of "cure by removal of cause." These realizations underlie the thesis of this book—namely, that the psychic readings of Edgar Cayce provide a plausible perspective on the etiology and treatment of schizophrenia and are deserving of serious consideration by progressive mental health professionals.

Some Alternative Applications

Edgar Cayce often cautioned against forming a cult or idolizing his work. He consistently encouraged persons to work within and through existing institutions in a spirit of cooperation for the benefit of humanity. It is with this spirit that the Cayce perspective on schizophrenia has been presented. There will undoubtedly be many who are interested in this approach but may have various objections. The possibility that "psychic" information could be legitimate and useful may be viewed as unfeasible by many mental health professionals due to the materialistic assumptions inherent in the current scientific paradigm. Or perhaps the Judeo-Christian language and orientation of the readings will be an obstacle for others with a different religious or philosophical bias. It is not the intent of this book to convert anyone to the Cayce perspective in any regard. Rather, the purpose is to stimulate readers to consider therapeutic alternatives. It doesn't really matter what one calls the model, so long as it is helpful to those devastated by chronic mental illness.

Most of the information in the Cayce readings can be found elsewhere in reputable sources. The citations in this book can be used as stepping-stones for those persons interested in this approach but who are unable to identify with the source of the material for whatever reasons. For these individuals, some alternative applications are provided in Chapter Six. Briefly, these alternatives can be regarded as stress management programs or manual therapy models (as derived from the osteopathic and chiropractic literature). The intentional resemblance of the proposed therapeutic model (institutional format) in Chapter Six to many community mental health programs provides an open door for various alternative applications.

Conclusion

The Cayce approach to the treatment of schizophrenia is worthy of consideration by mental health professionals. It presents a comprehensive perspective with considerable clinical and research potential. Its application may provide help to many who suffer from this disorder and are not receiving benefit from prevailing programs. However, it is not being promoted as a therapeutic panacea. Although Edgar Cayce stated that many individuals suffering from this disorder could be returned to a "normal or near to normal" condition, he was also careful to explain that treatment would require patience and persistence and a response by the body involved. It is with this attitude of cautious optimism that the Cayce perspective is presented for consideration.

Appendix A

Tables, Figures, and Documents

◆

TABLE 3.1
Projected Response to Treatment
Group I: Dementia

Case #	Prognosis	Time Frame
173	normal condition	3 to 6 months
271	nearer normal reactions	not given
3315	near to hopeless	not given
3441	nearer normal condition	"it will take time"
3997	near normal	in the "third cycle" (2 to 9 years?)
4097	perfect balance	6 to 8 months
5344	departure of soul (hopeless case)	
5405	near to normal	not given
5690	violent reactions	in 3-5 months he would be safe with self and others
	normal development	later on

TABLE 3.2
Projected Response to Treatment
Group II: Dementia Tendencies

Case #	Prognosis	Time Frame
282	near to normalcy	not given
386	near to normal condition	2 to 3 months
2022	better conditions	not given
2200	near normal	3 to 6 months
2614	not given	not given
2744	near normalcy	not given
3662	near to normal	not given
4059	"greater periods of rationality, activities greatly improved"	several months
4186	normal condition	"2 moons"
4333	full equilibrium	3 to 4 months
4600	"normal forces for this body"	not given
5228	not given	not given
5715	normal, if body responds	not given

TABLE 3.3
Treatment Plan
Case # 173

THERAPEUTIC MILIEU
provide treatment with care and strict attention to suggestions

PHYSICAL THERAPY
chiropractic or osteopathic adjustments

MEDICINE
soda and gold solution taken internally
ingredients: 15 ounces of distilled water
                  15 ounces of chloride of gold
                  20 grains bicarbonate of soda
dosage: medicine to be taken twice each day; first day 3 drops, in-
        crease one drop each day until 10 drops, stop for two days;
        repeat cycle
administration: to be taken in a half a glass of water
                  50% carbonated and 50% insipid (flat) water

ELECTROTHERAPY
Radio-Active Appliance (Impedance Device) with gold
solution: 15 grains of gold
           10 ounces of pure water

TABLE 3.4
Treatment Plan
Case # 271

THERAPEUTIC MILIEU
change environment
    clean atmosphere, plenty of sunshine, outdoor activity,
    "environ that is as of a growth," individual attention
constant companion (companion therapy)
spiritual emphasis:
    patience, lovingkindness, grace, mercy, persistence

ELECTROTHERAPY
Wet Cell Battery with chloride of gold
connections: 1st day—small anode to 4th dorsal plexus, larger
                anode to umbilical center plexus over lacteals; 2nd
                day—small anode over 9th dorsal plexus and larger
                anode over umbilical plexus
    cycle: alternate pattern of connections for three to five weeks
    period of treatment: at least 20 to 30 minutes each day
Radio-Active Appliance (Impedance Device)
    connections: opposite extremities
    cycle: daily treatment for 7 to 10 days during rest period from
            Wet Cell Battery

PHYSICAL THERAPY
massage
    gentle but thorough along whole cerebrospinal system; given
    by companion

SUGGESTIVE THERAPEUTICS
during massage
    "make gentle suggestions that quiet, rest, peace, happiness,
    joy, developments in every manner that are constructive
    physically and mentally through its rest period"

DIET
well-balanced (keep away from meats)

ACTIVITY
exercises
"specific, and as much as possible both of a physical and mental nature, that are constructive—or that are building in their activity, in the open"

BIBLIOTHERAPY AND VIDEOTHERAPY
constructive reading materials and movies ("no gangland or underworld")

BEHAVIORAL THERAPY
behavorial modeling by companion
establish daily routine

TABLE 5.1

Lesion Frequency in Schizophrenia (Dunn, 1950)

Survey of 1000 cases of schizophrenia made by a member of the staff of Still-Hildreth Osteopathic Sanatorium in 1933

Lesion	Frequency
Cervical 1	37.6 %
Cervical 2	66.0 %
Cervical 3	41.2 %
Cervical 4	6.7 %
Cervical 5	1.7 %
Cervical 6	1.0 %
Cervical 7	1.2 %
Dorsal 1	18.2 %
Dorsal 2	25.3 %
Dorsal 3	32.0 %
Dorsal 4	54.5 %
Dorsal 5	74.6 %
Dorsal 6	67.6 %
Dorsal 7	41.3 %
Dorsal 8	18.7 %
Dorsal 9	7.2 %
Dorsal 10	21.4 %
Dorsal 11	30.5 %
Dorsal 12	36.2 %
Lumbar 1	12.3 %
Lumbar 2	3.2 %
Lumbar 3	1.0 %
Lumbar 4	7 %
Lumbar 5	2.7 %

TABLE 5.2
Frequency of Somatic Dysfunction in Schizophrenia Based on the
Edgar Cayce Readings
Group I: Dementia

Case #	Dysfunction	Location
173	subluxations	2nd coccyx, 5th lumbar & 12th dorsal
3441	subluxations	coccyx, lumbar, 10th dorsal & 11th dorsal
	"pressure"	organs of pelvis
3997	subluxations	1st cervical & 2nd cervical
4097	lesion	1st cervical
5405	injury	lower lumbar axis

TABLE 5.3
Frequency of Somatic Dysfunction in Schizophrenia Based on the
Edgar Cayce Readings
Group II: Dementia Tendencies

Case #	Dysfunction	Location
2022	subluxations	coccyx, 9th dorsal, 1st cervical & 2nd cervical
2200	lesions	coccyx, lower lumbar, lower dorsal & whole of cervical
	"pressure"	sacral
2744	"pressures"	pelvic region, coccyx, sacral (sacral-ileum axis), lumbar & upper portion of spine
3662	"pressures"	coccyx, lower lumbar & sacral areas
4059	(specific dysfunctions were not mentioned but massage treatments were to focus on 4th lumbar, coccyx, 9th dorsal, upper dorsals, and cervicals)	
4186	"physical defects"	3rd lumbar
4333	lesions	lower lumbar & sacral
5228	"dissociation or short circuit"	lumbar axis & sacral
5715	"pressures"	lumbar & sacral

TABLE 5.4
Frequency of Somatic Dysfunction in Schizophrenia Based on the
Edgar Cayce Readings
Group III: Schizophrenic Psychosis

Case #	Dysfunction	Location
1428	"pressures"	coccyx, lumbar & dorsal
1572	"pressures"	lumbar & lower dorsal
1789	"pressures"	coccyx & lumbar
2465	lesion	lacteal duct
2712	lesions	sympathetic ganglia
2721	"pressures"	coccyx, lumbar & 9th dorsal
3087	subluxations	coccyx, sacral & lumbar
3163	"pressures"	coccyx
3181	"pressures"	coccyx & lumbar
3223	"pressures"	coccyx, lumbar & 3rd cervical
3421	subluxation	coccyx
3440	"pressures"	sacral, 3rd cervical, 6th, 7th & 9th dorsal
3475	adhesion	pelvic organs
3589	"pressures"	1st, 2nd & 3rd cervical, coccyx
3641	"pressures"	coccyx, 4th lumbar, 3rd & 9th dorsal, 1st, 2nd & 3rd cervical
3996	"pressures"	pelvic organs
4002	adhesions	pelvic organs
	(unspecified)	sacral, lumbar & lower dorsal
4004	subluxations	lumbar & lower dorsal
4100	(unspecified)	1st, 2nd & 3rd cervical
4285	"pressures"	sacral, lumbar, dorsal & cervicals
4342	"pressures"	coccyx, sacral, lumbar & "generatory organs"
5014	"pressures"	coccyx & sacral
5274	"pressures"	coccyx

TABLE 5.5 Prevalence of Electrotherapy in the Treatment of Schizophrenia Based on the Edgar Cayce Readings

Case	Type of Electrotherapy

Group I: Dementia

Case	Type of Electrotherapy
173	Radio-Active Appliance with gold plus gold taken internally
271	Wet Cell with gold plus Radio-Active (plain)
3315	Violet Ray (possession)
3997	no electrotherapy suggested
4097	magnetic healing
5344	no electrotherapy suggested (hopeless case)
5405	Wet Cell with gold and silver (alternated)
5690	Wet Cell with gold, or gold taken orally and ultraviolet ray used while gold is in system

Group II: Dementia Tendencies

Case	Type of Electrotherapy
282	Wet Cell with gold or magnetic healing
386	Wet Cell with gold
2022	Wet Cell with gold
2200	Radio-Active Appliance
2614	Wet Cell with gold
2744	"vibratory gold," appliance not stipulated
3662	Wet Cell with gold
4059	Wet Cell with gold
4186	no electrotherapy suggested
4333	no electrotherapy suggested
4600	radium appliance
5228	Wet Cell with gold
5715	Wet Cell with gold

Group III: Schizophrenic Psychosis

Case	Type of Electrotherapy
300	magnetic healing
1310	Wet Cell with gold plus gold taken orally
1428	Wet Cell Appliance
1513	Wet Cell with gold
1572	Violet Ray (possession)

TABLE 5.5 (cont'd)
Prevalence of Electrotherapy in the Treatment of Schizophrenia
Based on the Edgar Cayce Readings

Case	Type of Electrotherapy
1789	Wet Cell with gold
1969	Violet Ray (possession)
2197	no electrotherapy suggested (surgical case)
2465	dry cell battery with gold
2712	Wet Cell with gold
2721	Wet Cell with gold
2967	Wet Cell with gold
3075	Violet Ray (possession)
3087	dry cell with gold
3158	Wet Cell with gold & Violet Ray (possession)
3163	Wet Cell with gold
3181	Wet Cell with gold
3223	Wet Cell with gold
3421	Radio-Active Appliance ("kundalini crisis")
3440	Radio-Active Appliance (nervousness, insomnia)
3475	no electrotherapy suggested
3589	no electrotherapy suggested (surgical case)
3633	no electrotherapy suggested (life reading)
3641	Wet Cell (used as Radio-Active Appliance)
3996	gold taken orally (no electrotherapy)
4002	"short-wave electrical shocks"
4004	"short-wave electrical therapy"
4100	Wet Cell with gold
4179	no electrotherapy suggested (surgical case)
4285	no electrotherapy suggested (surgical case)
4342	"alpine rays" (sunlamp)
5014	Wet Cell (used as Radio-Active Appliance)
5274	Wet Cell (used as Radio-Active Appliance)

Totals of Groups I, II & III

Wet Cell with gold 20
Violet Ray 5
Wet Cell (plain) 4

TABLE 5.5 (cont'd)
Prevalence of Electrotherapy in the Treatment of Schizophrenia
Based on the Edgar Cayce Readings

Totals of Groups I, II & III

Radio-Active Appliance (plain) 3
magnetic healing 3
dry cell with gold 2
"short-wave therapy" 2
Wet Cell with gold and silver alternated 1
Radio-Active with gold 1
alpine rays 1
radium appliance 1
ultraviolet with gold 1

TABLE 7.1 Possible Subgroups of Schizophrenia Based upon Pathophysiological Processes Cited in the Cayce Readings

Dementia Praecox Subtypes	Etiology	Symptoms	Course	Response to Medication	Biology
Glandular Deficiency					
"Hereditary Innate"	heavy genetic loading	negative or deficit symptoms	early onset, chronic course	poor	glandular deficiency, brain degeneration
"Hereditary Tendencies"	moderate or light loading + stressor (e.g., spinal lesion)	predominately negative	variable	variable	glandular deficiency, brain degeneration
Toxemia					
"Brain Toxemia"	somatic dysfunction	positive and negative	progressive	relieves positive symptoms	dysfunctional blood flow to brain, eventual degeneration
"Systemic Toxemia"	somatic dysfunction	positive and negative	progressive	relieves positive symptoms	dysfunctional emunctory system
"Pineal" Dysfunction					
"Pineal Pressure"	somatic dysfunction (e.g., spinal injury)	affective features	variable, good prognosis	fair, may respond to lithium	glandular dysfunction
"Pineal Activation"	somatic dysfunction, lower spine or reproductive tract	positive with transpersonal features	variable	good	"lyden" center affects pineal

FIGURE 3.1

ETIOLOGICAL FACTORS
Group 1: Dementia/Chronic Schizophrenia

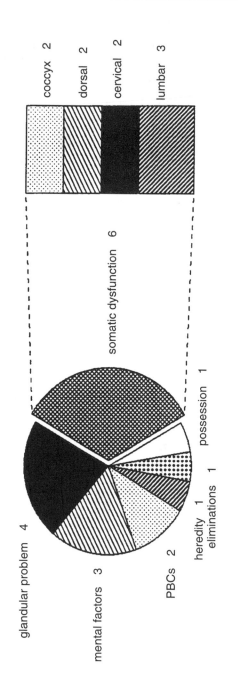

coccyx 2
dorsal 2
cervical 2
lumbar 3

somatic dysfunction 6

glandular problem 4

mental factors 3

PBCs 2

heredity 1
eliminations 1
possession 1

Factor Frequency

Location & Frequency

FIGURE 3.2

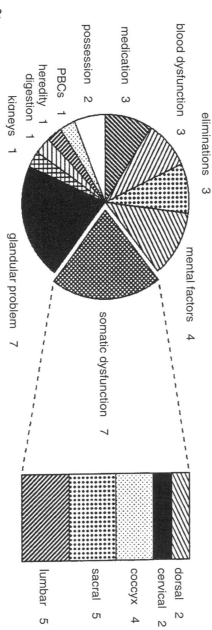

ETIOLOGICAL FACTORS
Group 2: Dementia Tendencies

Factor Frequency

Location & Frequency

FIGURE 3.3

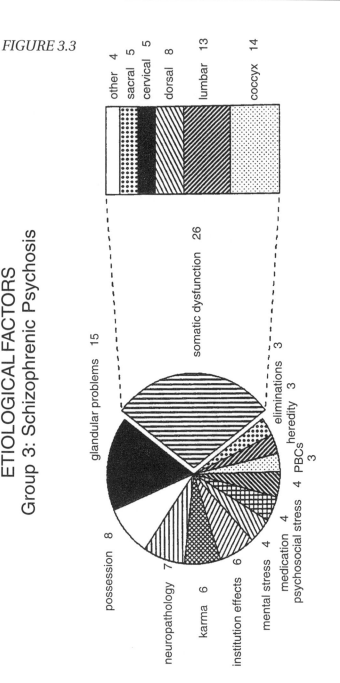

ETIOLOGICAL FACTORS
Group 3: Schizophrenic Psychosis

other 4
sacral 5
cervical 5
dorsal 8
lumbar 13
coccyx 14

glandular problems 15

somatic dysfunction 26

eliminations 3
heredity 3
PBCs 3

possession 8

neuropathology 7

karma 6

institution effects 6

mental stress 4
medication 4
psychosocial stress 4

Factor Frequency

Location & Frequency

FIGURE 3.4

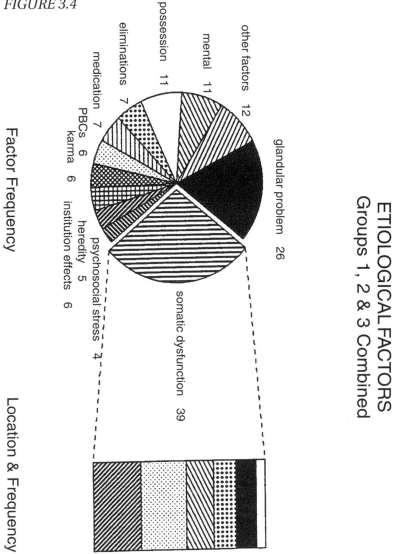

ETIOLOGICAL FACTORS
Groups 1, 2 & 3 Combined

Factor Frequency

glandular problem 26

other factors 12

mental 11

possession 11

eliminations 7

medication 7

PBCs 6

karma 6

institution effects 6

heredity 5

psychosocial stress 4

somatic dysfunction 39

Location & Frequency

other 4
cervical 9
sacral 10
dorsal 12
coccyx 20
lumbar 21

DOCUMENT 5.1
Text of Letter from Edgar Cayce to A. G. Hildreth

May 16, 1935

Dr. A. G. Hildreth
Still-Hildreth Sanatorium
Macon, Missouri

Dear Dr. Hildreth:

I appreciate your letter of the 8th more than I can tell you; I appreciate your giving me the background for your interest in a work of this nature. While the time was short that I spent with Dr. Still on his visit some years ago in Kentucky, the most of it was spent in talking over many things that had happened in the experience of each. Of course, you can realize that during the thirty-five years that I have been doing this work I have come in contact with physicians of almost every school. A great many have shown interest. More have said taboo. And quite a number have, after years, come back and said, "We have found it worthwhile." That the information in the readings has more often and more consistently suggested osteopathy than any other one character of treatment, of course, is one of the things that has caused many of the medical profession to question same. Why it has done this I do not know, but we have quite a number of osteopaths throughout the country who are very well acquainted with the results individuals have obtained, even when applying medicine and other local applications in connection with osteopathy. Osteopaths seem more open-minded and willing to cooperate with any school of treatment which may help the individual. Just as our friend Dr. Frank Dobbins of New York City said some weeks ago, "When I have forty-eight cases that come with the readings, and I follow the treatments suggested—even though some of them are not exactly as I have been trained to give them, and I see all forty-eight patients get the results as promised in the readings, then I have to believe something." Or as Dr. Gravett of Dayton, Ohio, said some years ago, "When I see seventy-five cases osteopathically correctly diagnosed through the readings, I know there's something to it."

Dr. Hildreth, I do hope that sometime we may have the opportunity to each view personally the other's field of activity. I would indeed deem it a privilege to be able to go through your institution. And if you are ever this way again, I do want you to stop in and see the amount of data we have on hand, and the reports we have had from people all over the country who have gotten results by carrying out their readings—most of whom we have never met personally . . . We have had quite a number of cases of dementia praecox, but never one thoroughly tested yet with the treatment suggested through the readings; because the ones we have had have been so closely allied with the medical profession that no cooperation could be obtained in following any other mode of treatment suggested. In a few cases we have seen people removed from insane institutions by some sympathetic physician administering some simple remedy outlined in the readings, but these have been very few—and have been scattered through the entire thirty-five years of experience with this work. So, it is indeed a wonderful thing that such an institution as yours exists. I'm sure Dr. A. T. Still was happy, is happy, to know that such an institution exists—for the good it has done and may do for suffering humanity . . .

DOCUMENT 5.2
Letter from A. G. Hildreth to Edgar Cayce

STILL-HILDRETH OSTEOPATHIC SANATORIUM
MACON, MISSOURI

Office of Superintendent
A. G. HILDRETH, D.O.

May 24, 1935

Dr. Edgar Cayce
Association for Research & Enlightenment
Virginia Beach, Virginia

Dear Doctor Cayce:

Your highly appreciated letter and literature came. I have read with very much interest all you had to say. The facts are, Mr. Cayce, I have been raised in an atmosphere similar to that which you found in Dr. Still and as to belief and liberality relative to the type of work you are doing my mother and father were spiritualists for a great many years before I was born before there was much known about that phenomenon and they were steadfast in their attitude, even through all criticism and ridicule heaped upon their belief.

I am very sure you are doing a splendid work, one that is of vast benefit to a great many people.

Note what you say about Dr. Still's joy over the work at this institution. He always stated when the time came our profession could own buildings of our own and surround those people with the right kind of an atmosphere there was a great number of the mentally sick that could be cured osteopathically and this institution here was in line with his thought and his desire and his sons contacted this property before I did and they selected me, or said they would consider it if I would agree to take charge of it.This was a source of great pleasure to Dr. Still and while its establishment came so late in his life that he was never able to visit us at Macon, only thirty-two miles from Kirksville, yet he was vitally interested and frequently sent for me to talk over our work here and always expressed his delight over the fact we had this institution here where we could offer our services to humanity along the line of his discovery. There is no question in our minds not only that he enjoyed this institution while alive but he is equally interested in it now and happy over the results we are able to produce.

I note what you say about *dementia praecox* and relative to Miss [. . .]'s brother. We will be very glad if we can serve them. There is no way to know other than by trial what can be accomplished for him, but a trial is certainly worthwhile. We are deeply grateful to you for your attitude. We are grateful we can offer to those poor individuals whose lives if they must live to the end insane, which is worse than death, a chance to get well. Don't misunderstand me, I appreciate fully your good words and your interest in our type of work but over and above my own benefit and my profession's comes first the glory of helping some body get well who has been pronounced incurable.

I presume you are well acquainted with conditions relative to dementia praecox, or rather the fact there is no treatment for it so far as the old system is concerned; hence, if we can establish, as we are, a percentage of cures great enough to interest the reading public perhaps the time will come when the whole world can recognize that insanity may be cured through osteopathic treatment or some similar method.

As to the attitude of the old school men relative to our work and yours, it does not bother me any because I know it is based on prejudice. It is too bad the whole medical world could not extend their right hand to any and all avenues that offer more and better results in the cure of dementia praecox and in the cure of disease.

Like yourself I would be happy if I could meet you and have a long talk and visit and I assure you should we travel east anytime again we will try and make that opportunity. We would be happy to have you visit Macon, see and know for yourself of our work and our results. It is very fine of you to take the time you do in writing me such interesting letters. By the way, I am well acquainted with Dr. Gravett of Dayton and consider him one of my

DOCUMENT 5.2
Letter from A. G. Hildreth to Edgar Cayce (cont'd)

real friends. The facts are I know a great many osteopaths throughout the length and breadth of the land and only hope I can return at least in part to you in a way that will help you personally for the good things you say and do for our profession.

With good wishes, I am,

Sincerely yours,

A. G. Hildreth D.O.

A. G. Hildreth, D.O.

Appendix B

The Pineal

◆

THIS AND SUBSEQUENT appendices will address various topics relevant to the treatment of schizophrenia by providing a general discussion of each subject which is followed by a selection of excerpts from the readings. In this initial appendix addressing the pineal, the discussion section will be approached from three perspectives: a brief literature review, Edgar Cayce's view of the pineal, and a look at some contemporary perspectives on the clinical significance of a form of pineal dysfunction designated as "kundalini crisis."

Literature Review

For centuries the pineal gland has been associated with paranormal phenomena and insanity. Eastern philosophies have tended to view the pineal as an important "chakra" or energy vortex, which, if activated, opened the individual to psychic experiences and cosmic vision (Judith, 1987). Contemporaneous Western philosophies also attached mystical significance to the pineal:

The ancient Greeks considered the pineal as the seat of the soul, a concept extended by Descartes, who philosophically suggested that this unpaired cerebral structure would serve as an ideal point from which the soul could exercise its somatic functions. Descartes thus attributed to the pineal a prominent function in uniting the immortal soul with the body. Being influenced by this thesis, many 17th and 18th century physicians associated the pineal causally with "madness," a link that has been uncannily prophetic for the present day. (Miles & Philbrick, 1988, pp. 409-410)

The reference to "unpaired cerebral structure" is an example of one of the many anatomical peculiarities of the pineal gland. The brain exhibits a high degree of bilateral symmetry, a characteristic not shared by the pineal because it is not generally regarded as having left and right divisions. The pineal is a small, cone-shaped gland attached to the posterior ceiling of the third ventricle of the brain, suspended in cerebrospinal fluid. Its location in the center of the brain, combined with its unique proclivity to calcify, make it a valuable landmark for neuroradiologists.

Recognition of the pineal as an active endocrine gland is a recent advancement because the highly sensitive bioassays required to detect pineal secretions are relatively new. Melatonin is the most easily detected of the pineal productions and has therefore received the most attention in current research. Thus, the frequent references to melatonin throughout this review is a reflection not only of its primary biochemical status among pineal secretions but also of its accessibility.

There are numerous anatomical and physiological idiosyncrasies associated with the pineal. "Relative to total body weight the pineal is small (50-150 mg in man; 1 mg in the rat), but its blood flow is second only to the kidney" (Arendt, 1988, pp. 205-206). Morphologically, the pineal has been considered as a homologue of the "third eye" in certain lizards (*Gray's Anatomy*, 1977). The photosensitivity of pineal in humans derives from nerve impulses from the retina and may have a basis in the structure of the gland.

Furthermore, it is interesting to note that some of the pigmented cells were arranged in a rosette-like structure reminiscent of developing retinal structures. When one considers these findings along with the electron microscopic observation . . . it is reasonable to conclude that human pineal glands exhibit transient cellular features reminiscent of developing photoreceptor cells as shown in other mammals. (Min, 1987, p. 728)

The pineal has been labeled a "photoneuroendocrine transducer" due to its photoperiodic influences on reproductive cycles, coat color, coat growth, and seasonal variations in behaviors of many mammals (Arendt, 1988). "Many other seasonal variations both physiological and pathological exist in humans and it will be of interest to consider their possible relationship to daylength and other seasonal synchronizers" (Arendt, 1988, p. 210). Ralph (1984) has reviewed the role of the pineal in thermoregulation and emphasized the "adaptive" nature of the gland.

The key word to understanding the pineal organ probably is "adaptation." That is, one can argue, with substantial justification, that the pineal organ participates in preparation for future conditions . . . While the literature relating pineal organs to thermoregulation is not nearly as large as that dealing with reproduction, or rhythmycity, it is substantial and compelling. (Ralph, 1984, p. 193)

Pineal involvement in cycles of growth and development during the life span has long been recognized. Pineal tumors have been associated with both precocious and delayed puberty in humans (Kitay & Altschule, 1954; Turner & Bagnara, 1971). Blindness has been linked to earlier menarche in girls and blind adults also appear to exhibit disynchronicities related to photosensitivity (Parkes, 1976; Lewy & Newsome, 1983). Melatonin secretions is known to decrease in amplitude from infancy to adulthood (Young et al., 1986) and during old age (Iguchi et al., 1982).

Pineal involvement in circadian rhythms, particularly the sleep cycle within these rhythms, has received considerable attention in recent years.

Melatonin secretion increases during sleep and decreases during waking hours (Axelrod, 1974; Arato, et al., 1985). Since light both entrains and suppresses melatonin secretion, melatonin has been called a "darkness hormone" (Arendt, 1988). Arginine vasotocin (AVT), another pineal secretion linked to sleep cycles, has been found to induce slow-wave sleep in cats (Pavel, Psatta & Goldstein,

1977) and a specific AVT antiserum markedly increases the number of REM (rapid eye movement or dream sleep) periods while decreasing REM latency (Pavel & Goldstein, 1981). However, the role of the pineal in the modulation of circadian rhythms such as sleep cycles cannot be considered as primary. Rather, it works in conjunction with other systems and has its basis in evolutionary processes.

Among the vertebrates, two areas seem to have assumed major importance in the organization of circadian systems— the pineal organ and the SCN (suprachiasmatic nucleus). The pineal organ of lower vertebrates is photosensory in nature and it may have been this, presumably ancient, function that caused the pineal organ to assume such a predominant role with circadian systems. Clearly, light is the preeminent entraining or synchronizing stimulus for circadian systems, and the pineal organ may have been involved in the perception of LD (light-dark) cycles. (Underwood, 1984, pp. 245-246)

In addition to being sensitive to variations in environmental light, the pineal appears to possess sensitivity to the earth's magnetic field and various electromagnetic influences.

There is ever-increasing evidence that the magnetic irradiation of a strength equal or approximate to that of the geomagnetic field exerts a variety of behavioral and physiological effects on the organism. Some studies focused on the pineal gland as the most feasible candidate for a mediator of magnetic irradiation on the organism. Such an approach is quite in keeping with the generally accepted concept that the pineal gland plays its physiological role through the modulation of the homeostatic and behavioral responses upon the changes in the living microambient. (Milin, Bajic & Brakus, 1988, p. 1083).

The pineal may also serve as a somatic interface with other sources of environmental energy designated as extremely low frequency (ELF) electric and magnetic-field exposure. Wilson, Stevens, and Anderson (1989) reviewed studies of ELF electromagnetic-field exposure in relation to health risks such as cancer, depression, and birth outcome (e.g. miscarriage, stillbirth). Citing work from their laboratory and elsewhere which shows that ELF field exposure alters the normal circadian rhythm of melatonin synthesis and release in the pineal gland, the authors present evidence which suggest pineal susceptibility to such sources:

> Whether directly affected or not, the pineal is a convenient locus for monitoring dyschronogenic effects of these fields. It appears ever more plausible, however, that the pineal may also play a central role in the biological response to this environmental factor. (Wilson, Stevens & Anderson, 1989, p. 1328)

The link between pineal dysfunction and suppressed immune response highlights another active area of pineal research. In particular, research has focused on melatonin and its relation to cancer. Depletion of melatonin by pinealectomy has been associated with proliferation of cancer cells (Rodin, 1963).

> Loss or reduction of oncostatic melatonin in the circulation is only one of the several possible mechanisms for increased cancer risk resulting from pineal gland dysfunction. Melatonin appears to have a stimulatory effect on immune function in the whole animal. (Wilson et al., 1989, p. 1323)

The minireview of this topic provided by Wilson et al. is a concise discussion of pineal research and is highly recommended to readers interested in the pineal/immune interface. In recognition of the role of the pineal in current cancer research, Blask (1984) has referred to the pineal as an "oncostatic gland" and an entire conference was recently devoted to this subject (Gupta et al., 1988).

Pinealectomy has been implicated in the production of convulsive states (Philo & Reiter, 1978). Furthermore, melatonin has been shown to suppress seizure activity in humans and other mammals (Fariello et al., 1977).

> Surgical removal of the pineal gland apparently produces rather uniform alterations in EEG activity and, under special circumstances (e.g., when rats are previously parathyroidectomized), severe seizures occur when the pineal gland is surgically extirpated. Several other rodent species . . . and certain strains of mice convulse after simple pinealectomy, i.e., loss of the parathyroid gland is not a prerequisite . . . The appearance of the convulsions suggests basic alterations in the biochemi-

cal and electrical activity of the CNS which are presumably due to the loss of some pineal constituent. (Reiter, 1977, p. 257)

The role of melatonin in brain excitability is an interesting example of the widespread explorations of pineal functioning, and Albertson et al. (1981) have provided an excellent review, including results of their own research. Their paper is an excellent resource for those readers interested in the relationship between the pineal and epilepsy.

The neuroendocrine functions of the pineal affect a wide variety of glandular and nervous system processes.

Although experimental results suggested many years ago that the pineal may inhibit growth of the gonads, substantial progress in this field has occurred only in the last ten years, since the pineal began to be considered as one of the central regulating mechanisms in charge of pituitary control rather than as an endocrine gland only. (Moszkowska, Kordon & Ebels, 1971, p. 241)

Evidence that the pineal gland exerts a regulatory influence on several endocrine functions is rapidly growing. (Motta, Schiaffini, Piva & Martini, 1971, p. 279)

The prevalence of sigma receptors in the pineal has been noted by Jansen, Dragunow & Faull (1990) and may be an important interface with several systems and pathologies:

The highest concentration of sigma receptors was seen in the pineal gland, an area which has not been previously studied. This is of interest as both sigma receptors and the pineal gland have recently been shown to play a role not only in the nervous system but also in the immune and endocrine systems . . . Haloperidol and some other antipsychotic drugs bind sigma receptors, as do psychotomimetic benzomorphan opiates, suggesting that the receptor may be involved in psychosis. (Jansen, Dragunow & Faull, 1990, p. 158)

Research indicates that pineal involvement in mental health may go beyond psychosis. It is very likely that the pineal plays a significant role in the manifestation of several mental illnesses.

Currently, much interest is focused on the role that melatonin may play in various psychiatric disorders, and pineal research now represents one of the active areas of current psychiatry research . . . Present ideas suggest a positive involvement of melatonin in affective disorders, possible involvement in the schizophrenic psychosis, and potential involvement of this hormone in other psychiatric categories. (Miles & Philbrick, 1988, p. 405)

Reduced nocturnal melatonin secretion has been noted in depression (Wetterberg et al., 1979, 1981 & 1984) and schizophrenia (Ferrier et al., 1982). Brown et al. (1985) found that lowered nocturnal melatonin concentrations differentiated between melancholic patients and patients suffering from major depression without melancholia. The role of the pineal in depression may be related to neurotransmitters associated with depression.

In that various theories of depression have suggested reduced serotonergic and noradrenergic function, and both of these products are involved in the synthesis of melatonin as a precursor and neurotransmitter, it would not in fact be at all surprising to find low melatonin in depression . . . It is tempting to speculate that all anti-depressants increase melatonin production. (Arendt, 1988, pp. 218-219)

Recognition that the pineal is photosensitive and plays a major role in the regulation of seasonal physiological adaptations has led to speculation that pineal dysfunction may be related to SAD (seasonal affective disorder). SAD is a recurring winter depression presenting with weight gain, hypersomnia, and carbohydrate craving (Rosenthal et al., 1984). Phototherapy has been utilized in this and other forms of depression to ameliorate depressive symptoms (Kripke & Risch, 1986).

Persons suffering from bipolar have been shown to be supersensitive to the inhibiting effect of bright light on nocturnal melatonin secretion (Lewy et al., 1981). Research by Lewy et al. (1979) suggests that during mania (particularly during the early phase of mania) bipolar patients exhibit consistently elevated levels of melatonin throughout the day and night. Because lithium has been shown to affect pineal functioning and may be linked to decreased photosensitivity, some researchers have speculated that some individuals diagnosed as bipolar may be suffering from circadian disorganization (see review by Miles & Philbrick, 1988). Structural similarities between melatonin and agents of known hallucinogenic potency (i.e., harmine, bufotenine, and psilocybin) has led to speculation about a possible connection between this pineal hormone and schizophrenia (Arendt, 1988). Psychotomimetic agents (lysergide, dimethyltryptamine, mescaline, and harmaline) induce HIOMT, a methylating enzyme, which increases melatonin production in the pineal (Klein & Rowe, 1970; Hartley & Smith, 1973). Furthermore, agents which produce symptoms closely resembling schizophrenic psychosis (i.e., cocaine, L-dopa, and amphetamine) also increase melatonin production. Research into the assimilation of LSD in monkey brains reveals a propensity for LSD concentrations in the pineal and pituitary glands, these accumulations being 7-8 times those found in the cerebral cortex (Snyder & Reivich, 1966). Winter et al. (1973) report that the pineal must be capable of functioning for hallucinogens to have behavioral effects. Although melatonin has direct biochemical effects on dopaminergic function (Wendel et al., 1974; Zisapel & Laudon, 1983; Bradbury et al., 1985) and haloperidol is highly concentrated by pineal tissue (Naylor & Olley, 1959), direct evidence of melatonin involvement in schizophrenia has not been forthcoming (see excellent review by Miles & Philbrick, 1988).

There exists a vast pineal literature which is undergoing phenomenal expansion. As the present discussion is intended to serve as an introduction to the subject, interested readers are directed to these useful reviews for further elaboration: Wilson et al., 1989; Arendt, 1988; Ebels & Balemans, 1986; Miles & Philbrick, 1988; Mullen & Silman, 1977; and Reiter, 1984.

In summary, whereas only a few decades ago the pineal was widely viewed as a vestigial entity, current research has revealed it to be an important neuroendocrine gland involved in thermoregulation, immune response, and the mediation of various cycles (i.e., circadian rhythms involving the regulation of sleep, seasonal rhythms affecting patterns of reproduction and physiological adaptations to the environment, and cycles of growth and development during the life span such as sexual maturation). In consideration of the pineal's influence on the other endocrine glands, it can be viewed as a "regulator of regulators" (Reiter, 1984, p. v). Further, pineal functioning may play an important role in mental illnesses such as schizophrenia and affective disorders. Perhaps the most controversial area of pineal research may involve the gland's functioning as a transducer of environmental energies such as electromagnetic fields. "After years of disregard the pineal has taken its place in mainstream biology and medicine. It is an organ of particular fascination in that it serves as an interface between the environment and the body" (Arendt, 1988, p. 205).

The pineal gland, viewed historically as a "sphincter to control the flow of thought," as the "seat of the soul," as a "third eye," and depicted more recently as a "neuroendocrine transducer organ," now promises to portray more complex physiological functions than originally believed and forecasts to reveal more extensive implications in pathological processes than once deemed possible . . . Future investigations should be directed toward comprehension of the functions of numerous neglected neurotransmitters and biological substances found in the pineal gland. The results of these investigations may bring forth multifunctional significance for [the] pineal gland not only in "temporal arrangement of various reproductive events" in mammals, in "rhythmical thermoregulatory process" in some ectotherms, and in "nightly pallor response" in amphibians, but also in major arenas of human suffering such as seizure disorders, sleep disorders, and behavioral abnormalities. (Ebadi, 1984, pp. 1 & 27)

Cayce's Perspective of the Pineal

The relatively frequent references to the pineal in the Cayce readings reflect the importance which the readings attached to this gland. As previously mentioned, during the early decades of this century, the pineal was widely regarded as a vestigial organ of little physiological significance. The readings acknowledged the prevailing view of medical science by describing the pineal as a "mass without apparent functioning" (294-141). However, the readings continued to insist upon the preeminent role of the pineal as a major mediator of physiospiritual processes. The research literature just cited in this Appendix suggests that contemporary views regarding the pineal are rather expansive and tend to support the readings' insistence that the pineal is much more than a dormant, vestigial organ.

To fully appreciate Cayce's perspective of the pineal, it is necessary to discuss the various ways in which the term pineal was used in the readings. Although pineal was often used to designate a discrete, glandular entity in the center of the brain (a notion consonant with contemporary views of the pineal), the readings also occasionally spoke of the pineal as if it were a system. This is more than just a problem of semantics, for in the readings the "pineal system" represents the interface of mental and spiritual dimensions within the body—it was described as the body/mind/spirit connection.

When viewed as a system, other terms were often associated with the pineal, such as the "cord of life," the "silver cord," the "Appian Way," and the "imaginative system." In this context, the pineal seemed to be regarded as a life energy system as well as a glandular entity. This perspective is congruent with certain Eastern religions and occult traditions which emphasize the paranormal aspects of pineal activity by labeling it a major "chakra," or energy center in the body (e.g., Bailey, 1932; Besant, 1959). In the Cayce readings, the energies associated with the pineal system carry several designations including: "kundalini," "kundaline," "life force," "psychic force," "aerial activity," and "creative energy."

The status of the pineal as a system is established in the readings by noting the diversity and essentiality of its functioning. The pineal system was said to function through nerve impulse (e.g., 2197-1, 4800-1), glandular secretion (e.g., 567-1, 2200-1), and vibratory energies such as the life force or kundalini energy (e.g., 281-53) while mediating numerous processes including fetal growth, sexual development and functioning, and alterations in consciousness. Two brief excerpts from the readings will be provided to portray the physiological and psychospiritual parameters of the system:

567-1   M. 25   6/1/34
. . . for the PINEAL center is engorged, especially at the 3rd and 4th LUMBAR and the 1st and 2nd cervical . . . the mental capacities as related to the imaginative system refuse to coordinate with the rest of the activity of the body . . . as we have indicated, a constitutional condition, you see, which affects the glands of the body, as related to the pineal—which runs all the way through the system and is the GOVERNING body to the coordinating of the mental and physical.

288-29   F. 27   4/16/32
In this particular body [Edgar Cayce] through which this,

then, at present is emanating, the gland with its thread known as the pineal gland is the channel along which same then operates, and with the subjugation of the consciousness—physical consciousness—there arises, as it were, a cell from the creative forces within the body to the entrance of the conscious mind, or brain, operating along, or traveling along, that of the thread or cord as when severed separates the physical, the soul, or the spiritual body.

These excerpts contain some important examples of the diverse influences attributed to the pineal system. The references to "the gland with its thread known as the pineal" and "the pineal—which runs all the way through the system and is the *governing* body to the coordinating of the mental and physical" indicate the anatomical expansiveness of this system. The "thread" or "cord" which emanates from the pineal gland may be physical (e.g., nerve tissue), nonphysical (e.g., "vibratorial" or subtle energy), or both. The readings are particularly vague on the subject. The readings compared the *activity* of the pineal to an aerial:

281-53   4/2/41
    In your radio you have what you call an aerial for communications that are without any visible connection. This is not a part of that making up the framework, yet it is necessary for certain characters of reception or for the better distribution of that which takes place in the instrument as related to communication itself.
    So in the physical body the aerial activity is the flow through the pineal, to and through all the centers. It aids the individual, or is an effective activity for the individual who may consciously attempt to attune, coordinate, or to bring about perfect accord, or to keep a balance in that attempting to be reached or attained through the process . . . Understand the processes of activity through which there are the needs of the aerial in reception. For, of course, it is a matter of vibration in the body, as well as that illustrated in the physical condition.

This evocative description of pineal activity brings to mind contemporary research into the pineal's ability to detect variations in geomagnetic and electromagnetic fields (as discussed earlier in this Appendix). Reading 2501-6 suggests a similar phenomenon relating the phase of the moon to behavioral changes—an association apparently mediated by the pineal through the sympathetic nervous system (see the excerpt section which follows).

Regardless of whatever the pineal and its "cord" may represent, the readings stated that it extended throughout the body and governed the coordination of mental, spiritual, and physical energies (311-4). Note also that the pineal provides the connections of body, mind, and spirit which was regarded as a prerequisite for the functioning of consciousness (1001-9).

The "pineal system" may be conceptualized as including the endocrine glands (262-20, 281-49, 1001-9, 1593-1). The holistic perspective of the readings was frequently reflected in a systems approach to anatomy and physiology: " . . . there is to be considered ever the whole activity; not as separating them one from another but the whole anatomical structure must be considered EVER as a whole . . . Then we find the endocrine system—not glands but system . . . " (281-38)

Certain glands within this system were noted as having an especially close affinity—the pineal/pituitary interaction was frequently cited in the readings. The interface between pineal and Leydig gland was also particularly important and deserving of close study (e.g., 263-13, 294-141, 294-142).

The pineal system's close association with the nervous systems is exemplified by its role as mediator between the "mental body" and the central nervous system (1523-17). There are frequent references to both the pineal and the sympathetic systems as the "imaginative system" and the "impulse system"—expressions intimating the role of mind, in particular the unconscious mind, in the phenomenon of imagination. The readings referred to the sympathetic nervous system as the nervous system of the unconscious mind while the CNS was identified with the conscious mind. Thus, the readings' frequent association of pineal dysfunction with incoordination between the sympathetic and central nervous systems may be related to its role as mediator of states of consciousness. In this capacity, the pineal was said to be involved in such common phenomena as imagination and sleep, paranormal experiences such as kundalini awakening and past-life recall, and pathological conditions such as psychosis and epileptic seizures.

The "life force" energy discussed in the readings was said to function in two modes: (1) a growth and development mode (a health maintenance mode) and (2) a "supercharged" mode which the readings associated with "kundalini" experiences similar to those described in the meditative literature of the Orient (281-53). In the growth and development mode, the pineal was said to begin activity within the third week after conception by organizing fetal development (294-141, 281-141). In its activity, the pineal system could be conceptualized as a morphogenetic blueprint for embryonic elaboration, particularly the formation of the brain (294-141). Just as it would later serve as the interface of physical, mental, and spiritual bodies in the newborn child, during gestation the pineal system was said to serve as a conduit for mental and spiritual impulses from the pregnant woman (281-53, 294-141).

Across the life span, the pineal system was viewed as a regulator of cycles of growth and development and was responsible for the maintenance of health. In this capacity, the life force was referred to as *élan vital* (281-24) and was related to youth and vigor. "Keep the pineal gland operating and you won't grow old—you will always be young" (294-141). The life force was said to "strengthen and maintain equilibrium in the system" (1026-1) and "sustain coordination to the organs of the body" (5162-1).

The readings recommended various forms of energy healing to reestablish a healthy state in bodies with insufficient or unbalanced energy. Magnetic healing was one such modality and could be accomplished by raising the life force (i.e., "kundalini") and passing this energy into the body of the afflicted person by "laying on of hands" (281-14). The readings described a specific technique for this intervention and provided guidelines for persons interested in utilizing it (e.g., using the hands in polarity, resting between sessions to maintain vigor, etc.—see Circulating File on magnetic healing for details; available from the A.R.E.).

This life force could be rebalanced by an apparatus called the Radio-Active Appliance (currently referred to as the Impedance Device; see Chapter Five under "Electrotherapy"). The readings stated that magnetic healing and the Radio-Active Appliance utilized the same energy, frequently referred to as "vibratory energy" or the "low form of electrical energy," which was said to be the basis of life. This energy flows through the body and is particularly accessible along the spine at seven "centers" (3428-1), apparently corresponding to the seven chakras of Eastern meditative traditions. Three of these centers were preferentially noted as being key interfaces between the physical and soul forces:

3676-1   M. 8   2/19/44
... the 3rd cervical ... the 9th dorsal, and ... the 4th lumbar
... These are the centers through which there is the activity of
the kundaline forces that act as suggestions to the spiritual
forces for distribution through the seven centers of the body.

It is no coincidence that these three centers (and specifically the
9th dorsal) were frequently specified locations for attachment of the
Wet Cell Battery utilizing "vibratory metals" (i.e., gold and silver) to
stimulate the regeneration of the nervous system in cases of dementia praecox. These key centers were also consistently pointed out to
osteopaths and chiropractors making the spinal adjustments. Cayce
even gave specific instructions for coordinating these centers using
massage and manipulation.

In the "growth and development" mode, the life force was described as a subtle influence which was generally not physically perceptible in its action or effects. In the "supercharged" mode (such as
kundalini), the life force was much more easily perceptible (occasionally painfully so) in its action and effects. In this mode, the life
force was said to vary its circulation through the body (281-53) by
arising along the spinal cord to the base of the brain. The "opening
of the lyden [Leydig] gland" was a prerequisite for this activity and
could be accomplished by a variety of meditative and pathophysiological processes. The utilization of traditional yogic techniques
such as altered breathing (2475-1) and incantations (275-43) were
noted as effective means of "awakening the kundalini."

In several cases of psychopathology noted in the readings, the
awakening of the kundalini was associated with somatic dysfunctions such as spinal injury and lesions in the reproductive system.
Throughout this book, such cases have been designated as "kundalini crisis." A further consideration of this topic from the perspective of contemporary sources will be included in the final section of
this discussion.

To fully appreciate the readings' perspective on "kundalini crisis," one must keep in mind that the *pineal system* includes a
"thread" or "cord" which extends from the pineal gland proper,
along the spinal cord to various centers in the body (281-46). Pressure upon this system can produce hallucinations and dementia
(294-141, 4333-1). It is unclear whether this pathology resulted from
the secretion of a glandular substance by the Leydig gland or as a
result of some change in the "subtle energy" balance within the pi-

neal system. The readings are not explicit about this process and these two scenarios are not mutually exclusive, nor do they preclude other interpretations of this process. The important psychopathological implication here is that the pineal system is quite vulnerable to somatic insult, particularly along the spinal column.

The psychic readings of Edgar Cayce were said to have resulted from the activation of the kundalini within the pineal system (288-29, 2475-1) resulting in cosmic consciousness (2109-2). In other words, Cayce apparently had a kundalini experience during each reading. The possibility that he could be rendered insane by a misapplication of this process was noted in the readings and cautions were provided for the maintenance of a healthy physical vehicle for a safe and optimal psychic experience.

If one accepts the plausibility of psychic productions such as the Cayce readings or other such manifestations which are common within the tradition known as the perennial philosophy, one comes to view the pineal system as the "consciousness system"—i.e., altered states of consciousness such as kundalini experiences are produced by alterations within this system. Psychosis which is produced by pineal system dysfunction (i.e., kundalini crisis) may thus be viewed as one of the alterations in consciousness mediated by this system.

Epilepsy is another major pathology involving altered states of consciousness—a phenomenon which the readings frequently associated with pineal activity. The overlap between epilepsy and schizophrenia has been discussed in Chapter Seven and will not be recapitulated here. However, several excerpts from the readings on epilepsy have been included in this Appendix to provide a context for comparing the role of the pineal in these two major pathologies.

The pineal system is involved in two other major alterations in consciousness—sleep and death. Sleep was said to be a "shadow of, that intermission in earth's experience of, that state called death" (5754-1). According to the readings, the soul temporarily disengages during sleep to "visit" other dimensions and have experiences which are remembered during the waking consciousness as dreams. "Each and every soul leaves the body as it rests in sleep." (853-8) The idea that some aspect of the self dissociates during sleep and transits between dimensions (e.g., astral travel) is not original to the Cayce readings. This is a common theme in the traditions of many cultures (Hanson, 1989). In the readings, sleep is viewed as an opportunity for the mental being to review previous experiences and plan future actions accordingly (hence the retrospective and pre-cognitive function of dreams). During sleep, connection of the physical, mental, and spiritual bodies is maintained by a "silver cord" which sounds strikingly similar to the "thread" or "cord" of the pineal system. Death involves the severance of this cord (262-20) whereas sleep may be viewed as merely a temporary "stretching" of it. The "projection" of consciousness out of the body during sleep may be related to the projection which Edgar Cayce experienced during his psychic readings. In other words, perhaps everyone has a "kundalini" experience and psychic awakening each night while he or she sleeps. The physiological alterations which occur during "dream sleep" (i.e., REM or paradoxical sleep) seem to parallel those described in the readings as occurring during kundalini arousal.

This may relate directly to schizophrenia research because for several decades clinicians and researchers have recognized the similarities between hallucinations and dreams. This apperception has led to the hypothesis that hallucinations represent dream intrusions into waking consciousness. "Schizophrenia may be characterized by a breakdown in the normal boundaries between the REM-sleep and waking states." (Wyatt, 1971, p. 46) This hypothesis was bolstered by research confirming that schizophrenics tend to exhibit distinctive sleep patterns (most significantly, decreased REM rebound after deprivation; e.g., Azumi et al., 1967). As with most areas of schizophrenia research, sleep and dream studies have suffered the effects of variability, thus the sleep anomalies in schizophrenia remain unexplained.

From a transpersonal perspective, many dreams represent a conscious experience of paranormal realities (i.e., not just epiphenomena resulting from brain activation during sleep). Dreams may reflect an altered state of consciousness where the conscious mind has access to other dimensions of reality normally unavailable during waking states (Roberts, 1974). The experience of precognition, direct communications with discarnate entities, past-life recall, etc., during dreams is thus viewed as representing a valid perspective of "reality."

Hence some persons experiencing acute psychosis with paranormal features could be viewed as suffering from a form of "kundalini crisis," or a pathological activation of the pineal system resulting in psychotic symptoms such as hallucinations. The Cayce readings indicated that such persons were close to the "borderland" and that pathological symptoms such as auditory hallucinations were "real" experiences to those individuals. This pathological aspect of pineal functioning is the focus of the final part of the discussion section and will consist of contemporary formulations of pineal activation which result in psychosis.

Current Perspectives on Kundalini

Numerous accounts of spontaneous "awakening" of the kundalini energy can be found in the modern clinical literature. Gopi Krishna believed that the awakening of the kundalini force could go awry and produce acute psychosis. His personal experience with kundalini provides valuable firsthand information about its effects:

> The condition [kundalini awakening] denotes, from the evolutionary point of view, a physiologically mature system ripe for the experience, and a highly active Kundalini pressing both on the brain and the reproductive system. But the activity of Kundalini, when the system is not properly attuned, can be abortive and, in some cases, even morbid. In the former case [when the brain is not ready], the heightened consciousness is stained with complexes, anxiety, depression, fear, and other neurotic and paranoid conditions, which alternate with elevated blissful periods, visionary experiences, or creative moods. In the latter [when the reproductive system is dysfunctional], it manifests itself in the various hideous forms of psychosis, in the horrible depression, frenzied excitement, and wild delusions of the insane. (in Kieffer, 1988, pp. 138-139)

Thus, Krishna's emphasis on the enlightening properties of kundalini is balanced by his awareness of its destructive potential when awakened prematurely. As Krishna observes, in some cases the difference between the two outcomes is difficult to assess:

> There is a close relationship between the psychotic and the mystic. In a mystic, there is a healthy flow of prana into the brain, and in the psychotic the flow is morbid. In fact, the mystic and the psychotic are two ends of the same process, and the ancient traditions class mad people as mad lovers of God, or something divine. (in Kieffer, 1988, p. 110)

Joseph Campbell expressed the same idea poetically by stating,

"The schizophrenic is drowning in the same waters in which the mystic swims with delight" (in Mintz, 1983, p. 158). Sannella (1987), a psychiatrist, also notes the dual manifestations of the kundalini experience:

> I have also witnessed this regrettable tendency among those who have stumbled onto the kundalini experience. But this says nothing about the experience itself, which is not inherently regressive. On the contrary, I view the kundalini awakening as an experience that fundamentally serves self-transcendence and mind-transcendence. (p. 20)

In 1974 Sannella co-founded the Kundalini Clinic in San Francisco, a facility dedicated to helping persons undergoing sudden kundalini arousal.

The transformative potential of spiritual awakening with psychotic features (which we have designated as kundalini crisis) has been noted by Christina and Stanislav Grof and labeled "spiritual emergency." Christina's description of her spiritual emergency and Stanislav's clinical insight into the transformative potential of these experiences provide a valuable resource in this area. Their criteria for distinguishing between spiritual emergency and psychosis provide a helpful "yardstick" for clinical assessment.

> Among favorable signs [indicating spiritual emergency] are a history of reasonable psychological, sexual, and social adjustment preceding the episode, the ability to consider the possibility that the process might originate in one's own psyche, enough trust to cooperate, and a willingness to honor the basic rules of treatment. Conversely, a lifelong history of serious psychological difficulties and of marginal sexual and social adjustment can generally be seen as suggesting caution. Similarly, a confused and poorly organized content of the experiences, presence of Bleuler's primary symptoms of schizophrenia, strong participation of manic elements, the systematic use of projection, and the presence of persecutory voices and delusions indicate that traditional approaches might be preferable. Strong destructive and self-destructive tendencies and violations of basic rules of treatment are further negative indicators. (p. 256)

Christina Grof founded the Spiritual Emergence Network (SEN) in 1980 to provide educational information and a referral service for people experiencing transformational crises. It is currently located at the Institute of Transpersonal Psychology (250 Oak Grove Ave., Menlo Park, CA 94025; 415/327-2776).

Mariel Strauss (1985) provides a practical source of information about kundalini awakening in all its aspects. *Recovering from the New Age: Therapies for Kundalini Crisis* documents the symptoms of kundalini arousal and suggests therapies to minimize its distress. Strauss describes "kundalini crisis" from her personal experience, while providing a scholarly review of the kundalini literature. Her familiarity with the Cayce philosophy and frequent citations from the readings serve as valuable stepping-stones between the various sources and perspectives in this literature. Her recognition of the pervasiveness of kundalini manifestations, both clinically in psychosis and subclinically in "dis-ease," accurately portrays the readings' perspective of this phenomenon:

> We must remember that Cayce found degrees of kundalini imbalance in many individuals, not just in those with the syndrome of extreme symptoms we have delineated [i.e., kundalini crisis]. His cases ranged from those who were simply nervous and fatigued . . . to those who had been confined to hospitals or their homes for many years, sometimes since early childhood. Therefore, his remedies dealt less with large alterations in diet and more with the other aids . . . such as spinal adjustment and massage, mental regroupment, and treatments with the electrical appliances he designed. (p. 45)

Another excellent source of information regarding kundalini is John White's *Kundalini: Evolution and Enlightenment.* White's expertise as an editor is evident in this thorough discussion of the kundalini phenomenon.

Summary

In summary, the pineal is an important endocrine gland which is probably involved in a wide spectrum of developmental and health maintenance processes including major mental illnesses such as schizophrenia. Its association with paranormal processes is documented in traditional and current sources and is congruent with the

Cayce readings on the subject. Cayce viewed the pineal as the focal point of a system utilizing subtle energies (e.g., kundalini) capable of pathological disruption. Because such disturbances may present with paranormal features, clinicians are advised to become more familiar with the operation of this system and all of its transpersonal manifestations. From the Cayce perspective, the most significant aspect of pineal functioning is its role as the interface of mental and spiritual facets of the self with the physical body. This role has been acknowledged historically, and restated succinctly by Mullen:

> The human pineal is now under intensive investigation by various groups throughout the world. In the next few years we can confidently expect the physiological and pathological roles of this mysterious gland to be elucidated. The pineal which for Descartes was the seat of the mind and the immortal soul may yet turn out to be of interest for biological psychiatry. The pineal has been called a neuroendocrine transducer but it could one day be more accurately termed a psychosomatic transducer standing as a mediator on the boundary between soma and psyche. (Mullen et al., 1978, p. 370)

Excerpts from the Cayce Readings

22-1 M. [age unknown] 12/23/24 [epilepsy]
. . . for we have incoordination through the system, in the nerve supply especially, and this disturbs the mental equilibrium, and the locomotion is affected by ganglions in the body at times. These we find affect directly the pineal nerve and gland. Hence the whole system throughout the cerebrospinal system becomes involved in the conditions.

179-1 F. 13 10/19/26 [epilepsy]
In the first condition, we find there are some prenatal [karmic?] conditions to be considered, and other conditions as were produced by physical conditions as were seen in the body at the time of birth. These were those conditions, for the pressure as produced in the presentation brought to certain cervicals that nonalignment which produces a pressure, not so much on the cerebrospinal cord as on that of the gland situated at the base of the brain. This, then, is the cause of the character of repression and the variation in their severity, and the apparent cause of that as brings about the cycle of the vibration for, as we see, the pineal gland is affected.

254-68   9/7/33
Q. What caused the extraordinary physical reaction with Edgar Cayce at the close of the reading [254-67] this morning, at the beginning of the suggestion?
A. As was seen, through the seeking of irrelevant questions there was antagonism manifested. This made for a contraction of those channels through which the activity of the psychic forces operates in the material body; as we have outlined, along the pineal, the lyden and the cord—or silver cord. The natural reactions are for sudden contraction when changing suddenly from the mental-spiritual to material.

262-20   6/5/32
In the psychic forces, or spiritual forces (which are psychic forces), there has ever then been a vehicle, or portion of the anatomical forces of the body, through which the expressions come to individual activity, and these may find various forms of manifestations, or MOVEMENTS of—as has been given, that finds its seat in the creative energies and forces of the body. In the body we find that which connects the pineal, the pituitary, the lyden, may be truly called the silver cord, or the golden cup that may be filled with a closer walk with that which is the creative essence in physical, mental and spiritual life; for the destruction wholly of either will make for the disintegration of the soul from its house of clay.

263-13   F. 29   12/16/40
Let it be understood as to how each phase of consciousness or experience affects the other; that is, the associations or connections between the spiritual and the mental body, the spiritual and the physical body, and between the mental and the physical and mental and spiritual . . .
Then, there are centers, areas, conditions in which there evidently must be that contact between the physical, the mental and the spiritual.
The spiritual contact is through the glandular forces of creative energies; not encased only within the [Leydig] lyden gland of reproduction, for this is ever—so long as life exists—in contact with the brain cells through which there is the constant reaction through the pineal.
Hence we find these become subject not only to the intent and purpose of the individual entity or soul upon entrance, but are con-

stantly under the influences of all the centers of the mind and the body through which the impulses pass in finding a means or manner of expression in the mental or brain itself . . .

Thus we find the connection, the association of the spiritual being with the mental self, at those centers from which the reflexes react to all of the organs, all of the emotions, all of the activities of a physical body.

275-43   F. 22   4/1/35

These [incantations] as they make for the raising of that from within of the Creative Forces, as it arises along that which is set within the inner man as that cord of life that once severed may separate, does separate, that balance between the mind, the body, the soul . . .

281-13   11/19/32

. . . it [kundalini/life force] rises from the glands known in the body as the lyden, or to the lyden [Leydig] and through the reproductive forces themselves, which are the very essence of Life itself with an individual—see? for these functionings never reach that position or place that they do not continue to secrete that which makes for virility to an individual physical body. Now we are speaking of conditions from without and from within!

The spirit and the soul is within its encasement, or its temple within the body of the individual—see? With the arousing then of this image, it [kundalini] rises along that which is known as the Appian Way, or the pineal center, to the base of the BRAIN, that it may be disseminated to those centers that give activity to the whole of the mental and physical being. It rises then to the hidden eye in the center of the brain system, or is felt in the forefront of the head, or in the place just above the real face—or bridge of nose, see? . . . for ye are raising in meditation actual creation taking place within the inner self!

281-14   12/14/32

Q. Please explain the sensations during meditation of vibration running up through the body and ending in a sort of fullness in the head.

A. The various portions, as given, represent the activities that are being set, either when considered from the purely scientific or from the metaphysical standpoint, as an active force emanating from the Life itself within. Then, these become all-embracing; hence the better understanding should be gained, whether used to disseminate and bring healing or for the raising of the forces in self. When one is able to so raise within themselves such vibrations . . . then the body of that individual becomes a magnet that may (if properly used) bring healing to others with the laying on of hands. This is the manner in which such a healing becomes effective by the laying on of hands.

281-24   6/29/35

As we have indicated, the body-physical is an atomic structure subject to the laws of its environment, its heredity, its soul development.

The activity of healing, then, is to create or make a balance in the necessary units of the influence or force that is set in motion as the body in the material form, through the motivative force of spiritual activity, sets in motion.

It is seen that each atom, each corpuscle, has within same the whole of the universe—with its own structure.

As for the physical body, this is made up of the elements of the various natures that keep same in its motion necessary for sustaining its equilibrium; as begun from its (the individual body's) first cause.

If in the atomic forces there becomes an overbalancing, an injury, a happening, an accident, there are certain atomic forces destroyed or others increased; that to the physical body become either such as to add to or take from the *élan vital* that makes for the motivative forces through that particular or individual activity . . .

There is the physical body, there is the mental body, there is the soul body. They are One, as the Trinity; yet these may find a manner of expression that is individual unto themselves. The body itself finds its own level in its own development. The mind, through anger, may make the body do that which is contrary to the better influences of same; it may make for a change in its environ, its surrounding, contrary to the laws of environment or hereditary forces that are a portion of the *élan vital* of each manifested body, with the spirit or the soul of the individual.

Then, through pressure upon some portion of the anatomical structure that would make for the disengaging of the natural flow of the mental body through the physical in its relationships to the soul influence, one may be dispossessed of the mind; thus ye say rightly he is "out of his mind."

Or, where there are certain types or characters of disease found in various portions of the body, there is the lack of the necessary *vital* for the resuscitating of the energies that carry on through brain structural forces of a given body. Thus disintegration is produced, and ye call it dementia praecox—by the very smoothing of the indentations necessary for the rotary influence or vital force of the spirit within same to find expression. Thus derangements come.

Such, then, become possessed as of hearing voices, because of their closeness to the borderland. Many of these are termed deranged when they may have more of a closeness to the universal than one who may be standing nearby and commenting; yet they are awry when it comes to being normally balanced or healthy for their activity in a material world.

281-27   6/11/36

Q. Please explain just what took place the night I heard what sounded like a large top spinning—felt a strong vibration sweep through my body and when I spoke saw a bluish spark close to the top of my head and it felt like electricity.

A. As hath been indicated for the group, for members of same, there is that line, that connection, that point of contact in the body-physical to the spiritual forces as manifest through same. There are the centers of the body through which contacts are made, or are physically active . . . [which] finds expression in emotions of varied centers, varied characters. Thus the experience is that of the broader contact. Thus there are the vibrations of the electrical energies of the body, for Life itself is electrical—it manifests itself in its contacts in a physical being in much the same manner. Thus the experience in self of the emotions—physical being contacted by emotions—spiritual manifesting in the body.

281-41   6/15/39

. . . but as ye find your bodies made up of the physical, mental and spiritual, it is the attuning of the mental body and the physical body to its spiritual source . . .

But there are physical contacts which the anatomist finds not, or those who would look for imaginations or the minds. Yet it is found that within the body there are channels, there are ducts, there are glands . . . In many individuals such become dormant. Many have become atrophied. Why? Nonusage, nonactivity! . . . For as has been indicated, there are physical contacts in thy own body with thy own soul, thy own mind. Does anyone have to indicate to you that if you touch a needle there is pain felt? Ye are told that such an awareness is an activity of consciousness that passes along the nervous system to and from the brain. Then, just the same there are contacts with that which is eternal within thy physical body. For there is the bowl that must one day be broken, the cord that must one day be severed from thine own physical body—and to be absent from the body is to be present with God.

281-46   9/25/40
The cord that is eventually known or classified as the pineal is the first movement that takes place of a physical nature through the act of conception; determining eventually—as we shall see—not only the physical stature of the individual entity but the MENTAL capacity also, and the spiritual attributes.

281-47   10/2/40
That gland [pineal?] a nucleus extending in the shape or form of a moving atom, gathers from its surroundings physical nourishment; and from the mind of the body it takes its PHYSICAL characteristics, or the moulding as it were of its features as related to the external expression of same . . .
It is centered first, then about that known as the cranial center; next the ninth dorsal or that which is the motivative force to other portions through the umbilical cord, that begins then in the third week to give material manifestations in physical development.
Then the centers of the heart, liver and kidney areas begin their expression.
Thus we have first the pineal, the aerial, the adrenals, the thymus—or the pump gland of the heart itself . . .
The seeking here is for that area, that center, in which the system makes its relative relationships or associations with spiritual, mental and physical being.
These areas indicated, that have come through growth into being in relation to the mental, spiritual and physical attitude of the mother, are constantly dependent upon that one from which the body draws its PHYSICAL sustenance; but purpose, desire and hope are through the mental. Thus these centers are opposite the umbilical cord, or those areas through which ALL messages of desire, or of the mental nature, pass; not only to the brain in its reflexes but along the cords to the pineal—that has been and is the extenuation of its first cause.

281-48   10/23/40

In that which has been given there is an attempt to show the necessary coordination of the mental with the physical and spiritual; or, to be exact, the coordinating of the mental with the spiritual that so alters the characteristics, the purposes, the hopes of the individual entity materialized and manifested. That entity is, however, altered by choices made under its own impulse . . . We find the preparations of the parents, mentally and physically, was such that there was an elongation of activity in the endocrine system of the pineal; so that the stature of the entity then was of a different type, a different nature, and the mental and spiritual so balanced and coordinated that through the experience of the entity there was a physical and mental development equaled and surpassed by few.

281-51   1/15/41

. . . the pineal, through which the brain forces make manifest . . .

281-53   4/2/41

Q. Are the following statements true or false? Comment on each as I read it: The life force rises directly from the Leydig gland through the Gonads, thence to Pineal, and then to the other centers.

A. This is correct; though, to be sure, as it rises and is distributed through the other centers it returns to the solar plexus area for its impulse through the system.

For the moment, let's consider the variation here in this life force—or as respecting this life force. The question is asked not in relation to the life alone as manifested in the human body, but as to the process through which coordination is attained or gained in and through meditation, see?

Hence physically, as we have indicated, there is first the nucleus—or the union of the first activities; and then the pineal as the long thread activity to the center of the brain, see? Then from there, as development progresses, there are those activities through reflexes to the growth or the developing of the body.

Interpret that variation, then, as being indicated here. One life force is the body-growth, as just described. The other is the impulse that arises, from the life center, in meditation.

Q. As the life force passes through the glands it illuminates them.

A. In meditation, yes. In the life growth, yes and no; it illuminates them to their activity in life growth.

Q. The Leydig gland is the same as that we have called the lyden, and is located in the gonads.

A. It is in and above, or the activity passes through the gonads. Lyden is the meaning—or the seal, see? while Leydig is the name of the individual who indicated this was the activity. You can call it either of these that you want to.

Q. The life force crosses the solar plexus each time it passes to another center.

A. In growth, yes. In meditation, yes and no; if there remains the balance of attunement, yes.

When we are considering these various phases, the questions should be prepared so that they would not crisscross, or so that there would not be a confusion or a misinterpretation as to what is meant.

You see, what takes place in the developing body, or in life growth (which we have used as the demonstration, or have illustrated), may be different from that which takes place as one attempts to meditate and to distribute the life force in order to aid another—or to control the influence as in healing, or to attain to an attunement in self for a deeper or better understanding. These questions or statements are such that they will be confusing to some; but if they are asked properly there will not be confusion.

Q. The solar plexus is the aerial gland.

A. No. By the term aerial we mean that impulse or activity that flows in an upward, lifting, raising or rising movement. It is an activity in itself, you see; not as a gland but as an activity UPON glands as it flows in, through, from or to the various centers of activity in the system itself. It is a function. Let's illustrate—possibly this will give an interpretation such that you may understand:

In your radio you have what you call an aerial for communications that are without any visible connection. This is not a part of that making up the framework, yet it is necessary for certain characters of reception or for the better distribution of that which takes place in the instrument as related to communication itself.

So in the physical body the aerial activity is the flow through the pineal, to and through all the centers. It aids the individual, or is an effective activity for the individual who may consciously attempt to attune, coordinate, or to bring about perfect accord, or to keep a balance in that attempting to be reached or attained through the process.

As the process begins in the physical body, it is along the pineal; or it is the same movement that is the controlling or attuning influence from the mother with the developing forces of the body through the period of gestation. That is the manner, or the process, or the way in which the impressions are made. So, if there is beauty about the body of the mother through such periods, there are those influences to bring about accord. It may be indicated in contour of face. It may be indicated in the process of change in the activity of the thyroid as related to all the forces—even to the color of hair or eyes, or the skin's activity; the nails, or more toes than should be—or less, or such activities. Or, the influences existent through such processes might make for a lacking of something in the body itself, pathologically; by the attempt to create a normal balance without the necessary influences being available.

All of this is what we have referred to as the aerial activity, see? ... Understand the processes of activity through which there are the needs of the aerial in reception. For, of course, it is a matter of vibration in the body, as well as that illustrated in the physical condition. Thus there are activities about a body that is supplying the needs physically and mentally for a developing body, that become a part of the process, see?

281-57   8/27/41

Where is the dwelling place of the soul in the physical body? What is the connection or center through which the mind and soul function, that makes one individual a devil and another a saint? ...

Ye have gained that the first movement of same physically reaches out and becomes the brain, through which the pineal in its activity brings its physical development; and that it is related to the mind of the body and the environs of the body supplying physical activities to that developing physical entity.

288-29   F. 27   4/16/32

There must be in the physical or material world a channel through which psychic or spiritual forces may manifest. It must become concrete, or definite, with some channel, some manner of manifestation. The anatomical condition of the human body lends itself to such an experience, then, through some portion of the physical organism of a body . . .

In this particular body [Edgar Cayce] through which this, then, at present is emanating, the gland with its thread known as the pineal gland is the channel along which same then operates, and with the subjugation of the consciousness—physical consciousness—there arises, as it were, a cell from the creative forces within the body to the entrance of the conscious mind, or brain, operating along, or traveling along, that of the thread or cord as when severed separates the physical, the soul, or the spiritual body. This uses, then, the senses of the body in an introspective manner, and they are not apparent in functioning in a physical normal manner as when awake. All faculties of the body become more alert. As to the loss of consciousness, how great is the ability of the development of the psychic sources to completely cut off consciousness from the physical or anatomical brain and still retain—in the shell—those abilities of functioning through that such an entity may have experienced in its passage through physical experience.

294-140   M. 55   4/22/32

Suggestion by Mrs. Cayce: You will have before you the information [in 288-29] given through this channel on April 16, 1932, concerning the psychic development of the entity known as Edgar Cayce, present in this room. You will give further information which may be correlated with the data already on hand to aid those studying this work to better understand this channel and sources of information. You will answer questions.

Mr. Cayce: Yes, we have the information as given as respecting manifestation of psychic forces through these channels . . .

The glands of reproduction in a body gives up something that creation may be reached, or tuned into, when such an one—a psychic—attunes self to the infinite . . .

In the body as given, there are channels through which all forces do manifest. To some there are the voices heard. To others there is the vision seen. To others there is the impression, or feeling of the presence of those sources from which information may radiate; and then there are those channels that are submerged or awakened during such periods.

The lyden [Leydig], or "closed gland," is the keeper—as it were—of the door, that would loose and let either passion or the miracle be loosed to enable those seeking to find the Open Door, or the Way to find expression in the attributes of the imaginative forces in their manifestation in the sensory forces of a body . . .

294-141   M. 55   4/23/32

First, this shows that there is innate in each physical individual that channel through which the psychic or the spiritual forces, that are manifest in material world, may function. They are known as glands, and affect the organs of the system . . .

Q. Please discuss in detail the functions of the pineal gland.

A. If this is discussed from the anatomical viewpoint, in the fetus as is begun in first of gestation, we find this may be termed as the Builder. As is seen, the location of same is in the beginning in that of the center or the nucleus about which all of the matter takes its first form, and becomes the brain as is guiding or directing the building of the body as its development in the womb takes place. As it then reaches from the umbilical cord to the brain, there is builded that as is centered about same by the physical attributes of that pro-generated from those bringing such an action into being. When there has reached that stage when there is the separation of same, the cord then being broken, this forms then its own basis in the lower portion of the brain, or cerebellum, and through the medulla oblongata to the central portion of the cerebrospinal cord itself is held intact, and with the removal of same, or pressure on same, the various forms of hallucinations are evident, whether in the developing stage or when it has reached the elderly or older years in an experience. Its functioning, then, is as that, of that, which makes for—or known as—the impulse or imaginative body. Hence one that may be called demented by others, who has hallucinations from a pressure in some portions, may be visioning that which to him is as real (though others may call him crazy) as to those who are supposed to have an even balance of their senses; which [such visioning?] has been formed by the circulation, or the activity of the gland—as it is called—in its incipiency, until it becomes—or is—as a mass without apparent functioning. If the imaginative body, or the trained body (as is called in a material world) is, trained constantly away FROM the activities of same, it—in natural consequence of things in physical being—draws, as it were, within self. Hence senility sets in. Keep the pineal gland operating and you won't grow old— you will always be young!

In this activity, then, as is seen, there is within the genital organs the activity through that as may be called the lyden gland [Leydig], which has within itself that closed door, or open door, as makes for activity through that to the base of the brain, or the PINEAL gland— as is at the base of the brain itself—which opens up for its activities and associations to those other portions of the brain; that sends out its sensations either through the sensory organism or the sympathetic organism, or the purely physical organism . . .

294-142   M. 55   4/23/32
Q. What other glands in the body, if any, besides the Leydigian, pineal, and glands of reproduction, are directly connected with psychic development?
A. These three are the ducts, or glands. In some developments these have reached a stage where they do not function as ducts or glands, but are rather dormant; yet much passes through same, especially for the various stages of a psychical sojourn or development. These, as we find—the genitive organism is as the motor, and the Leydig as a sealed or open door . . . Hence these may literally be termed, that the pineal and the Leydig are the SEAT of the soul of an entity.
Ye have gained that the first movement of same physically reaches out and becomes the brain, through which the pineal in its activity brings its physical development; and that it is related to the mind of the body and the environs of the body supplying physical activities to that developing physical entity.

311-4   M. 28   4/11/31
Q. How can I overcome the nerve strain I'm under at times?
A. By closing the eyes and meditating from within, so that there arises—through that of the nerve system—that necessary elements that makes along the PINEAL (Don't forget that this runs from the toes to the crown of the head!), that will quiet the whole nerve forces . . .

504-3   F. 53   2/12/34
[Certain life experiences produce] . . . tiny shivers in the body itself, as they move along those of the pineal that make for the awakening that is in the real heart and SOUL of the entity. For, its psychic forces—from its developments through many sojourns—have made for one that is VERY sensitive . . .

543-17   F. 23   3/15/32   [epilepsy]
There will be found that the various portions of the organs as involved—that make for pressures upon the nerve system, which act through those of the pineal direct to the organs of gentation in system—will react in the various ways, as the various stages of activity or impulse are created in the system. Hence these would be followed rather closely by the one USING such applications, and see that

there is created—as near as possible—those of positive, coordinating forces in the system.

663-1   F. 4   9/18/34   [epilepsy]
 ... for the tendency for the contraction is to produce in the brush end of the spine—or from the 4th lumbar to the lower end of the spine—contraction of the muscular forces there; for here we contact during the periods of development especially the activity of the pineal reaction to the brain centers, which makes for the differentiation of the actions of the imaginative forces in the body.

693-1   M. 11   10/13/34   [epilepsy]
 Again we find the same in the caecum and the lower portion of the lacteal duct centers ... Their activity to the system is to produce along the course of the pineal center to the duct in the lower portion of the brain center itself where through the medulla oblongata there enters the coordinations between sympathetic impulses and the cerebrospinal system, and through the duct or gland of the lyden [Leydig] that makes for the GOVERNING of impulse in reaction to the torso or body from the brain centers themselves.

1001-9   M. 23   9/23/30   [epilepsy]
 Q. What is it that brings on or incites said attacks?
 A. The attempt of the physical body—through the forces in the imaginative body—to coordinate through that condition existent in the lyden [Leydig] gland, or in the base of the brain itself. Hence the contraction, and the lack of coordination in such conditions.
 Q. From what part of the body do the attacks originate? and why does body lose consciousness during attack?
 A. From the solar plexus to that of the lyden [Leydigian] gland, or through the pineal. The lyden [Leydig] is IN the pineal, see?
 Q. Why does body lose consciousness?
 A. That's just what we have been giving! It is the imaginative forces and the cerebrospinal forces, or the nerve supply through the cerebrospinal system cuts off—through the lyden [Leydig?] forces—which is sealed gland, see? they lie within those of the pineal themselves, see? When these become of such an activity, through conditions as excite in the system—as thrown out from those of the genitive forces, acting through those of the solar plexus, and the attempt to coordinate—they push in so much it pushes out consciousness.

1026-1 F. Adult 10/21/35

The vibrations from the Chloride of Gold solution would add to the vitality for blood and nerve building, aiding more specifically the activities through the lyden gland, through the activities of the glands in the system's reproductive activities that make for an expression in the system through the emotions of the body; making for an activity to the glands that strengthen or maintain the equilibrium in the system—that is, as to the pineal's reaction.

1387-2 F. 40 6/12/39

Q. Have headaches any connection with psychic development?

A. Rather is it the effect of the OPENING centers that are disturbed. Leave off psychic development, or the attempt to RAISE the vital forces, until there has been more of a purifying of the bloodstream.

1468-5 F. 48 8/5/38

As is understood by the body, there is the physical, the mental, the spiritual. All are one, but with their attributes have their activity through the one or the individual entity or body.

The spiritual arises from the centers in the lyden . . . glandular forces that are as hidden energies, or the very nature of the creative or reproductive forces. There are the abilities of each center, each gland, each atom to reproduce itself within the body—which is the very nature of glandular reaction.

1523-15 F. 33 4/28/42

Q. Please explain the physical reaction which took place in the movies the afternoon of Friday the 24th, which started with a hot flush, then a sensation of pin pricks that moved up the spine covering the head and terminating in the feeling of a band being tightened around my head, leaving me with a dull headache.

A. This was an emotion arising from the periods and the flow of emotion from the kundaline center, or the lyden [Leydig—Leydigian] gland, to the ones in the center and frontal portion of the head. This was partly a psychic experience, but kept as a physical reaction by the resistances of the body.

This is nothing to be fearful of, but keep the emotions better balanced.

1523-17   F. 35   12/29/43
   Q. Why has the heartbeat been so rapid, especially just after retiring?
   A. This is the system attempting to adjust itself to the variations in tempo of the physical and the mental body. This is just as described. The impulses arising from centers along the spine from deep meditation, deep imagination or deep thinking, radiate to various portions of the body. With the congestion which has arisen from toxic poisons resulting from cold, it makes everything work fast. You had just as well ask why does it make the liver work faster, the kidneys work faster, the toes work faster! It doesn't the tongue, or the eyes, or the smell, or any of the sensory organs—for these become dull or slow. It's the central nervous system, attuning to the mental system!
   Here you may have a very good demonstration of a physical body and a mental body. Tune them together!

1593-1   F. 68   5/20/38
   In the mental reactions as related to body-building, these have become so disturbed as to bring a distortion through the activity of the coordinating forces or centers along the cerebrospinal system from which awarenesses may be gained by the rising of the spiritual forces through the glandular forces along the pineal to the brain forces themselves.

1703-2   F. 51   12/12/38
   Q. What can be done to clear up the congestion in the fluid inside the spine, called by some the kundalini: Will yogi breaths aid?
   A. As we find, rather the influences of the massage that will alleviate the pressures on those centers along the spine from which impulses are received to the superficial circulation from the deeper cerebrospinal impulses, could bring the better assimilated forces in the glandular activity.
   The yogi breathing have their place, but when a condition has reached the place where there is the lack of the forces that PRODUCE same, then supply them by the release in the system of those centers from which impulse may be had.

1749-1   F. 48   11/16/38
   ... there has been the inclination for the body, through activities of the mental self in its anxiety, to raise or open the centers of the

body through meditation and activity when the physical forces were not in the condition for such.

This produced upon the nerve system, especially the sympathetic, what might be called a contaminated stream of negative reaction; causing or producing a nervous breakdown.

1861-11 M. 35 1/30/42
Q. What are the reactions of the kundaline forces—physically, mentally, spiritually?
A. We might write five or six books upon this! Just which one is desired to be known? There are twelve centers acted upon, each in a different manner, and from the varying sources from which these vibrations are raised in and through these centers—and for what purposes? How many characteristics and desires does the body have? Figure those and multiply it by about fifteen, and you'll have just how much variation there may be in such activities in the body! How many dispositions have you seen in the body? These are all activities of the kundaline forces acting upon some reactory force in the centers of the body.

1916-4 F. 19 8/9/29 [epilepsy]
. . . the pineal gland, with its correlation of the cerebrospinal and sympathetic system, do not coordinate.

1994-1 M. 14 9/6/39 [epilepsy]
As we find, through the lacteal duct center, this is affecting the activities of the glands in the pineal as well as the genital system . . .

2109-2 F. 51 2/22/40
As indicated—how oft has remaining quiet aided thee in seeing and feeling and experiencing the full cosmic consciousness! Yes!
This is found, as has been the experience, by the opening of those channels within the physical body through which the energies of the Infinite are attuned to the centers through which physical consciousness, mental activity, is attained—or in deep meditation.

2153-4 F. 12 8/31/40 [epilepsy]
There are NO brain lesions, but there is that which at times hinders the coordination between the impulses of the body and the normal physical reactions—or that break between the cerebrospinal and the sympathetic or vegetative nerve system, that coordi-

nates from the lacteal duct through the adrenals and their reaction to the pineal; causing the spasmodic reaction in the medulla oblongata, or that balance at the base of the brain.

2197-1   F. Adult   3/12/24

The nerve systems in the physical we find that depression first caused in the lyden [Leydig] gland that pressed, or indentations made on the perineurial and the pineal nerve center connected with the lyden [Leydig] gland. This then gives the hallucinations in the vibration to the brain center or through the cerebellum oblongata, you see. In the impression as this receives, there comes those conditions of melancholia, of self-destructive forces, of aberrations, of depression as received and hallucinations to all the functioning of the sensory organism, through which these nerve connections find manifestations with the pineal nerve in its course through the system.

2200-1   M. Adult   1/20/31

In times back we find there was an accident to the body that produced a lesion in the coccyx . . . While lesions have resulted from same in the lower lumbar, in the lower dorsal, and with the combined conditions that have been applied, we find SYMPATHETIC lesions in the whole of the cervical region. This produces, through these pressures, those spasmodic conditions to the reaction between the sympathetic and the cerebrospinal system—which has been termed a MENTAL disorder. The reaction is not mental, but a physical—that acts to, or on, the mental so that the reflexes that come through the sympathetic system are those that prevent a normal impulse from their reaction, causing that pressure, that condition in the lower end of brain proper that makes for the tendency of the body to move, to react in a wondering manner, to make as for responses of those forces in self of first condemnation in self, then as of that as to REMOVE those conditions from self. These come through, then, as repressions in first the sympathetic nerve system, from the lower lumbar plexus to the sacrals and coccyx, then to those activities in the glands themselves that secrete for the functioning through the pineal, and making for an engorgement and an inactivity or an ungoverning of the supply of impulse, as well as blood supply to the brain itself proper. Not dementia praecox, nor even softening of tissue. Unless these conditions are changed in the impulses TO the nerve system this deterioration must eventually set in.

2329-2   F. 41   9/17/40
In the nervous system—here we find PHYSICALLY, or pathologically, some effects of the raising of the kundalini, or the imaginative
system, to the reactions along the centers of the cerebrospinal system, without their SOURCES being GRATIFIED . . .
These as we find are much of the sources of the nervous tensions.
Not that these—the raising of such forces—should not be accomplished in a body; but their sources, their reactions must of necessity find expression.
For this body we find that these may find the greater expression
in just aiding, helping, someone not so fortunate as self—in the
mental, the spiritual and the physical balance.

2402-1   F. 56   11/16/40
As to the activities through the centers, here—for the moment,
let's indicate the SOURCES of this disturbance, that arises along the
cerebrospinal system when at times the body OPENS—and has
opened—the centers for the raising of the spiritual forces and pow-
ers through the body . . .
The soul body manifesting in the physical, as we have heretofore
indicated, finds expression in what we call today the GLANDULAR
systems of the body . . .
Then, when under stress there has been raised—from the lyden
gland (internal), through the activities of sex as well as the gland
forces internally—that which has brought this engorgement—
which in the natural consequence or sources of activity has formed
a lesion in the lower portion of the 9th dorsal center, which reflects
both upward and downward to organs of the physical system . . .
The mind then moving much faster than the abilities or the impulses, becomes at times confused; and forgetting becomes a part,
and superactivity becomes another part of this reflex action.

2465-1   F. 28   3/17/41
There has been a lesion in the lacteal duct and that as coordinating with the organs of the pelvis.
Hence at times such a state is produced as to almost become an
obsession, but possession in same.
The reaction to the pineal becomes so severe as to short circuit
the nerve impulse; carrying or producing a fluttering or an engorgement in static waves to the base of the brain.
Thus periods are caused when there is lack of self-control.

2475-1   M. 44   3/27/41

Yes, we have the body, the enquiring mind, [2475]; and those conditions, those experiences of the body in the use of Yoga exercise in breathing . . .

These exercises are excellent, yet it is necessary that special preparation be made—or that a perfect understanding be had by the body as to what takes place when such exercises are used.

For, BREATH is the basis of the living organism's activity. Thus, such exercises may be beneficial or detrimental in their effect upon a body . . .

There is the body-physical—with all its attributes for the functioning of the body in a three-dimensional or a manifested earth plane.

Also there is the body-mental—which is that directing influence of the physical, the mental and the spiritual emotions and manifestations of the body; or the way, the manner in which conduct is related to self, to individuals, as well as to things, conditions and circumstances. While the mind may not be seen by the physical senses, it can be sensed by others; that is, others may sense the conclusions that have been drawn by the body-mind of an individual, by the manner in which such an individual conducts himself in relationship to things, conditions or people.

Then there is the body-spiritual, or soul-body—that eternal something that is invisible. It is only visible to that consciousness in which the individual entity in patience becomes aware of its relationship to the mental and the physical being.

All of these then are one—in an entity; just as it is considered, realized or acknowledged that the body, mind and soul are one . . .

Then in the physical body there ARE those influences, then, through which each of these phases of an entity may or does become an active influence.

There may be brought about an awareness of this by the exercising of the mind, through the manner of directing the breathing.

For, in the body there is that center in which the soul is expressive, creative in its nature—the Leydig center.

By this breathing, this may be made to expand—as it moves along the path that is taken in its first inception, at conception, and opens the seven centers of the body that radiate or are active upon the organisms of the body . . .

As this life-force is expanded, it moves first from the Leydig center through the adrenals, in what may be termed an upward trend, to the pineal and to the centers in control of the emotions—or reflexes through the nerve forces of the body.

Thus an entity puts itself, through such an activity, into association or in conjunction with all it has EVER been or may be. For, it loosens the physical consciousness to the universal consciousness. To allow self in a universal state to be controlled, or to be dominated, may become harmful.

But to know, to feel, to comprehend as to WHO or as to WHAT is the directing influence when the self-consciousness has been released and the real ego allowed to rise to expression, is to be in that state of the universal consciousness—which is indicated in this body here, Edgar Cayce, through which there is given this interpretation for [2475] . . .

Q. Is there at present any danger to any particular body-function, such as sex; or to general health?

A. As we have indicated, without preparation, desires of EVERY nature may become so accentuated as to destroy—or to overexercise as to bring detrimental forces; unless the desire and purpose is acknowledged and set IN the influence of self as to its direction—when loosened by the kundaline activities through the body.

2501-6   F. 20   3/24/30

That physical conditions exist that are accentuated by influences in the entity's experience is apparent, as does also the [Moon] influence most (This would be very interesting to the physician in charge to watch the changes in the moon and watch the effect it has upon the body). Now, when we have the new moon we will find that for the first two days, as it were, following same, a WILD, HILARIOUS reaction of the stronger; as the WANE begins, then we will find the changes will come about, as will of a bettered condition. These are merely INFLUENCES, NOT those that may not be overcome by the activities as may be changed in a physical organism; for with pressure in the lumbar and sacral region, as has been first indicated, there is that activity to those forces as operate to and through the pineal gland to the upper portion of the body, which corresponds to those forces as are spoken of, even in that of the [Book of] Revelation. Be very good for the doctor here to read [The] Revelation and understand it! especially in reference to this body! These forces as applied to this are the activities as are seen in the sympathetic nerve system, and ADVANCE in their activities as the force of same impel through the sympathetic and the cerebrospinal plexus from the 9th dorsal to the brain itself—at top, see? Hence in the changes as are being brought about in the system through the activity of the change, there is seen less pressure is on the solar plexus center. Hence there is less INCOORDINATION THROUGH the pineal FROM the effect of the sympathetic system.

2684-1 F. 43 2/13/42

Q. What causes and what should be done for sensitivity to sounds?

A. This arises from the raising of the kundaline influence in the body to those areas from which the auditory forces receive their impulse. And these, as it were, have been congested there.

Hence, as we have indicated, the necessity of relaxation to those nerves AND the centers and ganglia along the area from the upper dorsal throughout the cervical area.

3082-1 M. 25 7/3/43 [epilepsy]

. . . the body has these convulsions . . . as well as the reflexes in brain, to the activity of glands relating to the pineal.

3156-1 M. 8 8/14/43 [epilepsy]

As we find, there are conditions that disturb the physical, the mental, and the soul entity. This we find is a prenatal condition; and must be met by the body as well as by those responsible for the body . . .

We find that there is a lesion in the lacteal duct area affecting the activities of the pineal gland; causing those periods of incoordination at the 1st and 2nd cervical, causing spasmodic reaction to the mental body or those losses of hold on self, or the control of the rational body-mind.

3421-1 F. 39 12/27/43

We find that there has been the opening of the lyden (Leydig?) gland, so that the kundaline forces move along the spine to the various centers that open with this attitude, or with these activities of the mental and spiritual forces of the body—much in the same manner as might be illustrated in the foetus that forms from conception. These naturally take form. Here these take form, for they have not in their inception been put to a definite use.

The psychological reaction is much like that as may be illustrated in one gaining much knowledge without making practical application of it. It then forms its own concepts.

Now we combine these two and we have that indicated here as a possession of the body; gnawing, as it were, on all of the seven centers of the body, causing the inability for rest or even a concerted activity—unless the body finds itself needed for someone else. Then the body finds, as this occurs, the disturbance is retarded or fades—in the abilities of the body to exercise itself in help for others.

3428-1 M. 60   11/21/43
And here we find some of those conditions of which many bodies should be warned—the opening of centers in the body-spiritual without correctly directing same, which may oft lead to wrecking of the body-physical and sometimes mental.

Q. Is the focal center of the disease in the brain or some other part of the body?

A. As indicated, it is in those centers—the seven centers of the body—where sympathetic and cerebrospinal coordinate the more; 1st, 2nd and 3rd cervical; 1st and 2nd dorsal; 5th and 6th dorsal; 9th dorsal; 11th and 12th dorsal; and through the lumbar and sacral areas. These are the sources. This is not an infection—it is the lack of coordination between the impulses of the mental self and the central nerve and blood supply . . .

Q. Does sexual expression or repression cause this condition, or have any effect on same?

A. This was a part of the beginnings of it; for when the lyden (Leydig) glands are opened, which are in the gonads—or the centers through which the expression of generation begins, they act directly upon the centers through the body. Unless these find expression they disintegrate, or through thy association cause disassociation in impulse and the central or body-nerves.

3481-1 F. 46   12/23/43   [Theosophist, vegetarian]
Individuals can become too zealous or too active without consideration of the physical, mental and spiritual. True, all influences are first spiritual; but the mind is the builder and the body is the result. Spiritualizing the body without the mind being wholly spiritualized may bring such results as we find indicated here, so as to raise even the kundaline forces in the body without their giving full expression.

The lack of elements is causing such disturbances in this body [vegetarian diet] . . . These, then, are the sources of disturbances

here: etherealizing mentally and the lack of materializing physically in body-forces; from excesses of diets that do not supply the full or complete needs of a body physically active in the vibrations that surround this body . . .
Q. Are the pituitary, pineal, thyroid and adrenal glands working?
A. Overworking! . . .
Q. What is the condition of the female organs?
A. All of these suffer under the disturbances, and the raising of the kundaline forces is causing activities here that are not in keeping with best conditions.

3481-3	F. 47	8/24/44
Q. What is the condition of the Kundalini now, which was mentioned in my first reading?
A. This depends upon how and in what manner the body attempts to raise same during its meditation. This doesn't change, for it is the seat, or the source of life-giving forces in the body. The effect upon the body depends upon the use to which an individual entity puts same. Thus the warning, as was indicated, as to how and for what, such influences are raised within the body itself.

3498-1	F. 43	11/12/43
Then, through deep meditation, even leaving the body almost in same, find there the answer—through the raising of the kundaline forces in the body itself, from the cells within the Leydig gland, so as to carry energies through the body.

3676-1	M. 8	2/19/44
. . . the 3rd cervical . . . the 9th dorsal . . . the 4th lumbar . . . These are the three centers through which there is activity of the kundaline forces that act as suggestions to the spiritual forces for distribution through the seven centers of the body.

3790-1	F. 23	7/22/26	[epilepsy]
These all must be considered, taken into consideration when those conditions are applied to the body for the correction of physical defects that are of the nature of a prenatal affection [infection?] in the glands that have to do with the equilibrium of the body—pineal gland—that runs through the body, from the base of the brain.

3997-1   M. 19   5/11/28
Q. What is the lyden [Leydig] gland and where is it located?
A. Lyden meaning sealed; that gland from which gestation takes place when a body is created through coition, or inception, through conception of two bodies meeting in creating a body. Located in and above the gland called genital glands, see? In the male, above the glands corresponding to testes. In the female, that above gland responding to testes in the male. Here in this particular case, near the size of a wren's egg. Nominally should be about the size of a small pea.

4002-1   F. 28   3/28/44
We find that there are adhesions in the organs of the pelvis causing definite reactions to the pineal gland. These as they react to and through the reflexes of brain cause those periods when there are the exaggerated repressions, and there enters all of those experiences through which the entity in transition has passed [past-life memories] . . .
Q. What brought on the mental breakdown?
A. As just indicated the adhesions in the pelvic organs, as directly connected or associated with the lyden (Leydig) and the pineal glands.

4087-1   M. 6   4/15/44
For as we find this entity has more than once been among those who were gifted with what is sometimes called second sight, or the superactivity of the third eye. Whenever there is the opening, then, of the lyden (Leydig) center and the kundaline forces from along the pineal, we find that there are visions of things to come, of things that are happening.

4333-1   F. Adult   5/17/27
The pressure, then, on account of the fall of the body in the sixth (6th) year that injured the spinal center near the lower lumbar and the sacral, produces a pressure in the overtaxed condition that produces reflexes in the pineal gland. Then we have these occurrences of the hallucinations, or the inability for the body to function normal.

4342-1   F. Adult   8/21/26
. . . the gray, the white tissue itself . . . when these become unbal-

anced, or distorted, the reaction in the brain, and hence the activities to those incentives of the physical forces in body become distorted also, and to another mind becomes unbalanced. In this body, the pressure as produced at birth was in the presenting of the body itself, in that known as breech birth, and the pressure was produced in the last lumbar, and the 2nd portion or structure portion of the sacral, and the sacral then producing a pressure to those of the generatory system brought about that enlargement in those centers about these organs in pelvis, that direct connect with the base of the brain in this gland situated there [pineal]. The thread of same, which traverses the system from brain to the end of the cerebrospinal cord proper.

5014-1   M. 11   4/8/44

These conditions began with the period of presentation. For this was a breech or foot, breech and foot presentation. This brought about pressures in the coccyx and sacral areas that have prevented the normal reactions through the pineal. Not that portion having to do with growth but the exterior portions or to the left side, where there are connections in the lumbar axis, 9th dorsal, the brachial center and the upper cervical center.

5028-1   F. 31   4/13/44

For the entity takes most every experience by intuition. Easily may the entity, by entering deep meditation raise the kundaline [kundalini] forces in body to the third eye as to become a seeress; so that it may see the future and the past. But the law of such is that, unless these are used for constructive and never for selfish motives or purposes, they will bring more harm than good.

5162-1   M. 41   4/19/44

We would not make or take the exercises as to raise the kundaline forces in the body without leaving that kind of an experience that is of a nature to coordinate the activities of such exercises through the organs and centers of the body. Not that these are not good, but it is not very good to give a child a razor, not very good to use a razor to sharpen pencils and try to shave with same. So it is in the activities of those who disregard the means to an end of bringing coordination to organs of the body.

5274-1   F. 39   5/17/44

There are pressures in the coccyx end of the spine from an injury received thirty-seven years ago . . .

Q. What causes the hallucinations and the persisting in wearing a cardboard or metal pad above her right eye?

A. These are the reactions from former appearances of the same entity in the earth.

Q. Why does she imagine she is being abandoned and tortured by people who dislike her?

A. This, again, is the impression from other appearances in the earth.

5286-1   F. 29   6/29/44

As for the physical forces, the weakness in the nerve tensions through the body has come from periods when there has been opening of centers of the body without direction to the use of the energies that have been and are created in and through the kundaline forces as they act along the spine . . .

This may be better done when there are better coordinations between sympathetic and cerebrospinal systems. Don't overtax the imaginative body to the detriment of the physical being . . .

As has been just indicated, there is progress made but at times to the detriment of the nervous forces. We would, then, correct the physical being and the mental and spiritual forces may manifest the better.

5399-2   F. 28   8/26/44

Q. Have I ever caught glimpses of past lives, or are these things more dreams and fancy?

A. The entity has caught glimpses of past lives when it has gone out of itself or has allowed the energies of the kundaline force to pass along the centers of the body. Beware unless you are well balanced in your purposes . . .

Appendix C

Dementia Praecox
———————◆———————

DEMENTIA PRAECOX WAS the diagnostic category in vogue during most of Edgar Cayce's life. Therefore it was used by him in cases where actual organic deterioration of the brain was present.

The earliest recognition of dementia praecox was by Willis, the English anatomist, in 1672. Sydenham described a similar condition in 1772. From 1862 to 1869, Kahlbaum described hebephrenia and catatonia. In 1896, Kraepelin classified dementia praecox into the three types, hebephrenia, catatonia, and paranoia, and did a great amount of detailed research, so to him we are indebted for much of our present-day knowledge. (Still, 1933, p. 382)

The term dementia praecox became untenable when further clinical observation revealed that it was semantically inaccurate. Dementia was considered to be a permanent condition of mental deterioration. Since a small but consistent percentage of individuals carrying this diagnosis recovered without any serious mental impairment, the term dementia was unacceptable. Similarly, praecox was used to broadly signify adolescence. Since occasional cases were noted as developing as late as the fourth decade of life, praecox failed to convey the variability of occurrence across the life span. "Kraepelin's concept of dementia praecox as a disease entity was largely displaced by Eugene Bleuler's concept of schizophrenia, a concept which denoted a psychological process capable of all degrees of gradation rather than a disease entity with an inevitable outcome" (Bockoven, 1963, p. 95). Schizophrenia, as conceived of by Bleuler (1911), indicated a split in the personality of the afflicted person and this diagnostic label has remained in use to the present day. Bleuler also insisted that schizophrenia represented a group of related syndromes and not a single disease.

The relationship between Kraepelin's dementia praecox and Crow's Type II schizophrenia has been noted in Chapter One. This connection correlates closely with Cayce's descriptions of dementia praecox and the classification recognized by the early osteopathic physicians treating this disorder. The important commonality among all these perspectives is the recognition of progressive brain deterioration resulting in poor outcome.

It is particularly interesting to note the congruency between the osteopathic concept of dementia praecox and Cayce's perspective. Compare the following quotation from the osteopathic literature with the rather graphic descriptions found in the reading excerpts presented later in this Appendix and with the etiologies in the case study summaries found in Chapter Three.

> Lesions predispose the body to infections and maintain them in a chronic state, with absorption of bacterial poisons. Lesions disturb the ductless glands, whose secretions may thus become toxic. A starved and poisoned brain cannot function well. So the mind breaks down under a strain that normally would not affect it. (Hildreth, 1929, p. 519)

Irvin Korr is more explicit in his physiological description of the effects of somatic dysfunction on brain functioning:

> We know of course that the sympathetic innervation extends to the blood vessels supplying the brain and the central nervous system and can exert a profound influence on blood

flow to these tissues. Ordinarily this is a negligible role because brain circulation is regulated largely through arterial blood pressure, but it is well established that under certain conditions, when the sympathetics are stimulated in a given area, for example the superior cervical ganglion, there is strong contractile activity in the vessels to the brain to the degree that cerebral ischemia may be produced . . . Beyond this neurovascular control is the fact that sympathetic innervation has a profound influence on cerebral function itself, even the highest intellective functions. The results in experimental animals have demonstrated, for example, that various interventions in the superior cervical ganglia can either impede or accelerate the rate of learning or forgetting of conditioned reflexes and profoundly modify brain-wave patterns. So we see that the sympathetics have influences which are not ascribable merely to regulation of smooth-muscle or secretory activity. (Korr, 1970, pp. 32-33)

Regardless of the pathophysiology involved, the osteopathic literature and the Cayce readings are in agreement that somatic dysfunction is directly linked to abnormal brain functioning in certain cases of chronic schizophrenia (i.e., dementia praecox).

Developmental Course of Dementia Praecox

Since dementia praecox was regarded as a degenerative process resulting in brain damage, the osteopathic and psychiatric view was generally that once actual organic deterioration was present, the patient could never fully recover. The Cayce readings differ on this point. Cayce recognized the seriousness of the condition. However, in some cases the readings maintained that significant improvement was possible and that frequently the individual could be brought to a *"normal or near to normal"* condition with persistent and consistent application of the suggestions provided in the readings. The use of electrotherapy (primarily the Wet Cell Battery and gold solution) was crucial in these cases. Cayce stated that gold would stimulate glandular secretions necessary for producing normal neurotransmission and tissue regeneration. "This [osteopathic adjustment] will remove strain, yet would not enliven tissue in itself. We begin, then giving *internally,* and through a vibratory force [Wet Cell Battery], those forms of soda and gold, internally, that rejuvenates the whole system, as to repropagation of nerve energy. Stimulating same, see?" (173-1)

Cayce's perspective closely follows the traditional osteopathic dictum of "cure by removal of causes" based upon the body's inherent tendency toward maintaining health. It also accounts for the small but consistent number of cases, who after years of chronic illness, spontaneously improve or are entirely cured. In these cases, perhaps something has happened to allow the body's systems to become coordinated and produce regeneration at an anatomical level.

It is important to recognize that Cayce did not state that all cases of dementia praecox could be cured. To the contrary, in cases where the condition was advanced, he emphasized the difficulty in reversing the process. He also noted that the possibility of possession increased as the brain deteriorated and that possession vastly complicated the recovery process (see reading excerpts from cases [2614] and [3315]). In several cases, the process of degeneration had proceeded to the point where there was a dissociation of the spiritual from the physical and all hope for recovery was lost (e.g. [586], [3315], [5344]).

The readings are congruent with the osteopathic literature of that era in which early intervention was cited as a crucial ingredient for a successful intervention. A. G. Hildreth, using records maintained at the Still-Hildreth Sanatorium, emphasized the importance of early diagnosis and intervention with the following statistics (1938, p. 275):

RESULTS IN 840 CASES of DEMENTIA PRAECOX

Admitted within first 6 months of illness
263 patients. Recovered 179, or 68 percent.

Duration of illness 6 months to 1 year
163 patients. Recovered 78, or 48 percent.

Duration of illness 1 to 2 years
129 patients. Recovered 37, or 29 percent.

Duration of illness over 2 years
285 patients. Recovered 57, or 20 percent.

When all cases of dementia praecox were considered as a group, a cure rate of 38 percent was reported. The dramatically improved prognosis produced by early intervention led Hildreth to proclaim, "It is our firm belief that if patients could be given osteopathic treatment at the onset of the condition in dementia praecox, the percentage of cures would be much greater: nearer one hundred percent than thirty-eight." (1924, p. 8) Cayce also emphasized early intervention in cases of dementia praecox: "Had this been taken from six to seven years ago, easily might this have been corrected" (4432-1). The current psychiatric literature likewise suggests that early intervention is associated with improved prognosis (e.g., Wyatt et al., 1988).

It is also interesting to note that many of the cases of dementia praecox diagnosed by Cayce involved mental distress and worry. One cannot be sure whether the mental distress caused the physical condition or vice versa (perhaps a reciprocal interaction existed). Cayce does state that mental distress can cause degeneration in the nervous system (e.g., 1452-1). Jensen et al. (1982) studied survivors of torture and found ventricular enlargement and symptoms of premature dementia. Survivors of concentration camps of World War II presented similar patterns (Thygesen, Hermann, & Willinger, 1970; Eitinger & Strom, 1973). It is highly likely that any combination of persistent mental or physical distress could lead to brain pathology. Perhaps ventricular enlargement and brain degeneration result from a variety of etiological factors such as genetic predisposition, mental distress, spinal injury, etc. As this is one of the "hottest" areas of current research, one can expect major discoveries ahead in this field.

In summary, the concept of dementia praecox as elucidated by Kraepelin and utilized in the Cayce readings represents a diagnostic category of chronic psychosis with brain degeneration and poor prognosis. The nearest current equivalent of this term is Crow's Type II schizophrenia. Because schizophrenia is diagnosed by the presence of symptoms, the term as it is presently used includes individuals who may have no organic damage but do manifest the symptoms considered pathognomonic to this disorder. In the Cayce readings, such persons in the prodromal stages of psychosis (or even experiencing an acute episode) would not be diagnosed as dementia praecox although the tendency toward this process might be noted. More often, Cayce would simply state the etiological factors involved and the status of the various physiological systems, and note the presence of symptoms such as hallucinations, delusions, social withdrawal, etc.

Perhaps the most significant effect associated with dementia praecox in the Cayce readings was the characteristic dissociation of body, mind, and spirit. This tendency for separation or detachment of the aspects of the self (which together make up a whole person) lies at the heart of the degenerative process. In the early stages of the illness, the readings would frequently use the term "incoordination" to describe the precarious relationship among the physical, mental, and spiritual. In these cases the readings would often note that the physical body was good and the mental body was good, but that they were not coordinating with each other (this incoordination was often associated with incoordination of the CNS and ANS). In chronic cases where the degeneration was irreversible, dissociation or severance was often noted.

A group of excerpts on dementia praecox conclude this Appendix. These selections were extracted with the hope that such a collection will facilitate the use of this resource by researchers and other interested parties.

Excerpts from the Cayce Readings

271-1   M. 34   2/13/33

In a general manner the condition may be termed dementia praecox (as some have diagnosed it) . . . softening of cell cord and brain tissue.

271-7   M. 34   5/29/33

[There is] deterioration in the white matter of the brain impulse . . .

281-24   6/29/35

There is the physical body, there is the mental body, there is the soul body. They are One, as the Trinity; yet these may find a manner of expression that is individual unto themselves. The body itself finds its own level in its own development. The mind, through anger, may make the body do that which is contrary to the better influences of same; it may make for a change in its environ, its surrounding, contrary to the laws of environment or hereditary forces that are a portion of the *élan vital* of each manifested body, with the spirit or the soul of the individual.

Then, through pressure upon some portion of the anatomical

structure that would make for the disengaging of the natural flow of the mental body through the physical in its relationships to the soul influence, one may be dispossessed of the mind; thus ye say rightly he is "out of his mind."

Or, where there are certain types or characters of disease found in various portions of the body, there is the lack of the necessary *vital* for the resuscitating of the energies that carry on through brain structural forces of a given body. Thus disintegration is produced, and ye call it dementia praecox—by the very smoothing of the indentations necessary for the rotary influence or vital force of the spirit within same to find expression. Thus derangements come.

Such, then, become possessed as of hearing voices, because of their closeness to the borderland. Many of these are termed deranged when they may have more of a closeness to the universal than one who may be standing nearby and commenting; yet they are awry when it comes to being normally balanced or healthy for their activity in a material world.

386-1   F. 20   8/9/33
This, then, is the difference between an unbalanced condition in a mental reaction and that of dementia—which destroys the reaction in the plasm of the nerve as fixed from the blood supply itself; though, unless there are some material changes, this may become the condition that will ensue.

2022-1   F. Adult   10/9/39
. . . conditions are rather serious. And if there is the continuation of the bromides, this may cause such a softening of the nerve tissue as to produce dementia praecox.

2200-1   M. Adult   1/20/31
This produces, through these pressures, those spasmodic conditions to the reaction between the sympathetic and the cerebrospinal system—which has been termed a mental disorder. The reaction is not mental, but a physical—that acts to, or on the mental—so that the reflexes that come through the sympathetic system are those that prevent a normal impulse from their reaction, causing that pressure, that condition in the lower end of the brain proper that makes for the tendency of the body to move, to react in a wondering manner, to make as for responses of those forces in self of first condemnation in self, then as of that as to remove those conditions

from self. These come through, then, as repressions in first the sympathetic nerve system, from the lower lumbar plexus to the sacrals and coccyx, then to those activities in the glands themselves that secrete for the functioning through the pineal, and making for an engorgement and an inactivity or an ungoverning of the supply of impulse, as well as blood supply to the brain itself proper. Not dementia praecox, nor even softening of tissue. Unless these conditions are changed in the impulses to the nerve system this deterioration must eventually set in.

2614-1   F. 37   11/7/41
These are the result of chemical and glandular reactions in the body; producing a deteriorating reaction in nerve impulses.

Thus the mental aberrations that appear, the hallucination as to lack of desire for associations and activities, faultfinding in self and in environs, as well as those about the body.

If these are allowed to progress they may bring a very detrimental condition—either that of possession or such a deteriorating as to become dementia praecox in its nature.

3315   F. 40   10/27/43
The conditions here, as we find, have been so aggravated by animosities, and by hates, that we have a deterioration in the nerve force along the spinal system; so that this is dementia—and now possession, such that this may appear near to hopeless in this experience.

Through the application of the low electrical forces as shocks to the body, with patience, care, persistence, there may be aid . . .

Q. What was the original cause, or what brought about this condition?

A. Changes in the glandular system, and then aggravated by animosities and hate.

3441-1   F. 33   11/24/43
As we find, there are disturbances, and there are tendencies towards the destruction of the reflexes to brain centers. These are produced from pressures that are associated and connected with organs of pelvis.

Hence there should be those corrections made and pressures removed where those subluxations exist in the coccyx, the lumbar also in the 10th and 11th dorsal areas, so that better connections will be established . . .

Sure, dementia praecox is indicated, but it is from pressure—that will respond. It will take time, but be patient, be persistent.

3997-1 M. 19 5/11/28

Dementia in the act that the repressions are as magnified, and will eventually—without correction—bring the softening of cell tissue in brain itself. Hence we find there are periods when the body is not controlled by any reaction in self... unless corrections are made [osteopathically]... we may expect a continued reaction; though at times bettered, then the general breaking down of the gray portion of nerve tissue, nerve cell matter, in the body.

4097-1 M. Adult 9/16/22

In the nerve center of head itself, the seat of the emotions and expressions [limbic system?] as received or transmitted through the sensory system, we find the action of the brain itself to be that of dementia praecox—that is, the softening of the tissue used to present the reaction of impressions to the centers as distributed from the action of the sensory system in itself, action of the body itself. That is, impressions as received to this body act refractorily on the centers giving off the impressions received to this body, so that we have only a partial action of the brain to give the proper incentive to the movements of the other forces in the body; or the impossible forces present themselves through the action of other portions of the body. So that the expressions from this mind become of a demented force in the actions; yet to the mind itself it is rational. In its impressions to others it expresses the irrational.

This, we find, has been produced by the breaking of cell force itself in the blood supply, as we have given here, to the brain force itself. Though this may be removed by the stimulus of nerve tissue and sensations, by the use of forces within the system to remove the condition as shown or expressed in the brain action itself; by applying to the centers that give the supply of blood to the brain and that remove from the circulation the used forces as given off by the flow of blood through the brain, that can absorb from the system those impurities that have been left and caused the hallucinations of the body at the present time . . .

Q. What produced these conditions, Mr. Cayce?

A. Extreme nervous tension that overtaxed the system, as received through the sensory forces, until the cells broke here at the 1st cervical.

5167-1 M. 30   1944

As we find, there are serious disturbances here. These are apparently a series of what might be called accidents, but are there accidents? These have caused fractures to the structural portion of the head or cranium, and with those healings there has been brought the formation of lesions and of pressures across from the left side toward the right, and then from the upper portion. My! What a mess! These have been allowed to remain so long that other than what is being administered in the present would not be of special help, unless there was a series of operations. For these have begun to cause deterioration of brain flexes themselves, or dementia praecox . . .

Q. Is the brain itself injured or is there a brain tumor?

A. It is a tumor. As has been indicated, the seams cause pressure in the casement and these run crosswise, as well as downward. Hence all of the reflexes are abnormal. This is the reason why most diagnoses are: dementia praecox. It isn't true dementia, but a gradual wasting of gray matter. X-ray should indicate it. These have been made, but fluids form, you see, and these do not show in X-rays. Flouroscope would be the better manner of examination, or infrared X-rays, or shadowgraph.

Q. Are there any glandular defects or malfunctioning of glands underlying this condition?

A. No glandular disturbance.

5228-1 M. 31   6/2/44

Yes, as we find, here are those conditions which if neglected will lead to such poor reflexes from brain to activities of the inferior muscles of the locomotories as to bring about dementia praecox, or such softening of reflexes as for there to be little effect of the gray matter impulse indicated in thought, or activity, either voluntary or involuntary.

Such violent reactions have existed until they brought that dissociation or short circuit in the areas between the cerebrospinal and sympathetic nervous systems, both in those areas in lumbar axis and in the brachial centers, here, or a violent nervous breakdown by overtaxing and more from worry about those things which were "not too good to think about."

5344-1 F. 35   7/15/44

There has already been departure of the soul, which only waits by here. We have the physical being but the control of same only needs the care, the attention, the greater love which may be shown in and under the circumstances, which will give the best conditions for this body. For already there are those weakenings so of the centers of the cerebrospinal system that no physical help, as we find, may be administered, only the mental or soul help as will be a part of the mental or superconscious self.

The condition has come from pressures which caused dementia praecox.

5405-1 M. 22 8/22/44

In the present environs, and under the existent shadows, very little may be accomplished, for those individuals in authority take little interest in even possibilities, where there have been, and are evidences of this nature or character of dementia praecox which indicates the inability of the body to respond to suggestive forces, as indicated, or the reaction of reflexes from brain to the organs of sensory forces in their activity to the physical being . . . There is no obsession—there is no possession, but a weakness, as in the first periods of stress in study, and in an activity that brought a pressure upon the sympathetic nervous system which broke the connection with the reflexes in central portion of the brain, as to cause lapses, or loss of memory—inability to recall what had been . . .

Q. Do I understand that overstudy and strain was the cause of his condition?

A. Overstudy and strain, and, as indicated, an injury in the lower portion of the lumbar axis, where the Gold is to be applied; and the massages should be daily, following the use of the Appliance [Wet Cell Battery].

5690-1 M. 27 3/6/31

There are physical defects in the cerebrospinal nerve system. There are also the lacking of elements in the physical forces, as produced by conditions—some a lacking of elements in the physical forces, as produced by conditions—some a tendency in innate influences; not as wholly hereditary innate, as much as hereditary tendencies [genetic vulnerability?]. Then, with the physical defects, these in their combination bring about that as has been called dementia praecox. This an inability of coordination between sympathetic, cerebrospinal, and the general physical body . . .

5715-1   M. Adult   6/17/30

. . . there are distresses caused in the coordination of the sympathetic and cerebrospinal nerve system, produced by pressure in the lumbar and sacral region, which prevents that proper reaction as should come with the activities of the pineal gland and the lyden [Leydig] gland, through the medulla oblongata to the brain . . . the application of those properties as will bring for the replenishing of the white tissue in the nerve cells themselves—these, we find, would be aiding and bringing the nearer normal reaction, will these be taken in time, before the pressure produces the softening of the brain tissue itself; until there is dementia in its reaction.

5715-2   M. Adult   8/4/30

In the physical forces of the body we do not find the response in the coordination in the cerebrospinal and brain forces, nor in the activity of the white and gray nerve matter, nor in the proper distribution of active forces as may be termed discernment, and this must mean—unless changes are made—the softening of the tissue itself, or the beginning of dementia praecox, as it is termed.

Appendix D

Karma
———◆———

KARMA IS AN ancient concept which refers to the law of cause and effect.

> The word karma itself means "action," but implies action and reaction. All actions have consequences, some immediately, some delayed, others in future incarnations. Thus we bear responsibility for all our actions and cannot escape the consequences, although bad actions may be expiated by good actions. (Shepard, 1984, p. 714)

The Cayce readings present a panoramic view of the human condition which parallels the Eastern religions (particularly Hinduism, Buddhism, and Taoism). From this perspective humans are regarded as immortal beings evolving toward unity with the divine source of being. This view includes reincarnation and the ability of each individual to choose certain key probabilities concerning a particular lifetime. Naturally, genetics plays an important role because heredity provides a relatively stable and predictable means of having the necessary life experiences to encounter one's personal karma.

In many cases where readings were given for persons inflicted with serious congenital disorders, Cayce would comment that it was a karmic condition. In clinical terms, this meant that it would be a particularly difficult condition to heal and that the spiritual aspects of the experience would play a crucial role in achieving a constructive result. In such cases, Cayce would often comment, "The entity is meeting self," and caution the person to use the experience as a stepping-stone rather that a stumbling block. From a theoretical perspective, karma provides a link among key concepts such as choice, responsibility, and the continuity of consciousness.

Karmic conditions often involved the glandular system, which Cayce viewed as the spiritual connection within the physical body. Several of the individuals diagnosed by Cayce as suffering from karmically linked dementia praecox apparently had glandular problems. In these cases, karma was often a family affair where the care of the afflicted person was a karmic responsibility of the parents or guardians. Spiritual suggestions were prominent in these readings.

Excerpts from the Cayce Readings
263-13 M. 29 12/16/40
As has been indicated through these channels respecting that which takes place at the moment of conception, as to ideals and purposes of those who through physical and mental emotions bring into being a channel through which there may be the expression of a soul-entity—each soul choosing such a body at the time of its birth into material activity has its physical being controlled much by the environs of the individuals responsible for the physical entrance. Yet, the soul choosing such a body for a manifestation becomes responsible for that temple of the living God, when it has developed in body, in mind, so as to be controlled with intents, purposes and desires of the individual entity or soul. So in this body, in this physical condition that exists here with this body, [263], we find it subject to those attributes of a physical being it has chosen for the mental and soul expression of self.

440-5 M. 23 12/20/33
Well that karma be understood, and how it is to be met. For, in various thought—whether considered philosophy or religion, or

whether from the more scientific manner of cause and effect—karma is all of these and more. Rather it may be likened unto a piece of food, whether fish or bread, taken into the system; it is assimilated by the organs of digestion, and then those elements that are gathered from same are made into the forces that flow through the body, giving the strength and vitality to an inanimate object, or being, or body. So, in experiences of a soul, in a body, in an experience in the earth. Its thoughts make for that upon which the soul feeds, as do the activities that are carried on from the thought of the period make for the ability of retaining or maintaining the active force or active principle of the thought through the experience. Then, the soul reentering into a body under a different environ either makes for the expending of that it has made through the experience in the sojourn in a form that is called in some religions as destiny of the soul, in another philosophy that which has been builded must be met in some way or manner, or in the more scientific manner that a certain cause produces a certain effect. Hence we see that karma is all of these and more . . .

852-12   F. 18   11/15/35

Environs and hereditary influences are much deeper than that which is ordinarily conceded in the psychology of the present day.

For the environs and the hereditary influences are spiritual as well as physical, and are physical because of the spiritual application of the abilities of the entity in relationship to spiritual development.

For the purpose of each soul's experience in the earth is to become one with the Creative Forces that manifest in human experience, if [the soul] will apply [this] in its relationships to its fellow man.

Hence what one is today is because of what one (the individual soul) has done about that the soul knows of the Creative Force or God in its experience, in whatever environ or consciousness it—the soul—may manifest.

2359-1   F. 41   8/23/40

In giving the interpretations of the records that are written upon the skein of time and space, these are the forces and influences that each soul builds in its passing through time and space. Thus they become a part of that which the entity must meet in all phases of its activity . . .

These then are the lines that create what some call karma. Hence meeting them is the law. For, what ye sow, so shall ye reap. But as has been interpreted by the entity in much of its study, its analysis of the atonement, or at-onement with Creative Forces—being the law, one meets or overcomes. But such overcoming must be a continuous practice in the daily experiences with others . . .

Q. What are my obligations to my husband?

A. These have been as problems ye have worked out together before. It was this companion who forced thee to be in that relationship during those periods of his journeys in other lands—which has brought to thee the opportunity for the meeting of same in the present.

2575-2   M. 19   4/19/43   [karmic condition]

. . . [healing] will require time, patience and persistence, AND an expectance on the part of mental attitude of the body itself. If there are the conclusions that the treatment won't do any good (because the relief doesn't happen in the moment), then don't try it! Keep on with the condition and you'll meet it in the "law" way!

2779-1   M. 11   7/7/42

Before this, then, the entity was in the land of the present nativity, but during the early periods when there were those disturbances wrought by the activity of the minister of a church—as of one Marshall Whittaker. The entity then was the minister, or the associate minister, who caused the uprising and the condemnation of children who say, who hear, who experienced the voices of those in the interbetween. And because of the entity's condemning there was brought a hardship into the experience of the entity, especially the adopting of that rule of "ducking" others.

Q. What made me revert to the habit of bed wetting after having stopped?

A. Read what we have just given! This is not merely a physical condition, but it reverts to the disturbance the entity brought to others because of their beliefs, faiths or activities.

2828-4   M. 41   1/10/44

Remember the sources, as we have indicated are the meeting of one's own self; thus are karmic.

3063-1　M. 56　6/26/43
. . . the entity was among the descendents of Esau . . . the name was Jared. The entity took advantage of a group. Hence expect a group to take advantage of thee! For what ye measure, it must be, it will be measured to thee. For ye must pay every whit that ye measure to others. And this applies in the future as well as in the past. Do you wonder that your life is in such a mess!

3249-1　M. 46　9/29/43
Karmic conditions, of course, are cause and effect.

3313-1　F. 58　10/26/43　[Cancer]
Karma is cause oft of hereditary conditions so called. Then indeed does the soul inherit that it has builded in its experience with his fellow man in material relationships.
Q. What is the cause of my condition and what treatment is recommended?
A. The basic cause is karmic.

3395-2　F. 63　1/15/44
Q. Is the ill health which I have been experiencing the past years the result of mistakes of a past life or is it due to something amiss in this present life?
A. Both. For there is the law of material, there is the law of the mental, there is the law of the spiritual. That brought into materiality is first conceived in spirit. Hence as we have indicated, all illness is sin; not necessarily of the moment, as man counts time, but as a part of the whole experience. For God has not purposed or willed that any soul should perish, but purgeth everyone by illness, by prosperity, by hardships, by those things needed, in order to meet self . . .

3468-3　M. 73　8/25/44
In these if the body will accept it there is the meeting of self—or karmic conditions.

3504-1　M. 29　12/12/43
Sources of these are prenatal conditions as well as karmic. These, of course, may be rejected by many. Yet those who reject same do not supply better reasons, do they?

3684-1 M. 56 2/21/44

Yes. As we find, there are disturbances with this body—physical, mental, spiritual. For while a very material-minded individual might say that "bad luck" had come to the body, we find that nothing happens by chance. For each soul is as precious in the sight of the Creative Forces or God as another—just as a mother doesn't have her love changed for another, no matter how many children there may be—unless she's a foolish mother. For God is not a respecter of persons. And when an individual as this, through conditions brought about physically, has sudden collapses by the breaking of cells as to cause paralysis to portions of the body, while it is pathological, it is also psychological, it is partly karma. Then, if there will be a release of the physical conditions that are at present useless, there must be a change of attitude towards spiritual and mental things. For mind is the builder. There have been periods when the mind has been hindered, as might be expressed, or "touched." Yet these are not wholly through experiences of the entity in the present. Just because there has been the breaking of cellular force in the brain so that reflexes are not possible in the body at present, does not indicate that these need necessarily to remain so. For the body renews itself, every atom, in seven years. How have ye lived for the last seven? . . . the manner in which ye treat thy neighbor is the manner in which ye are treating thy Maker. And be not deceived, God is not mocked; whatsoever a man soweth that must he also reap. Then, kick not against the pricks, because ye are meeting thine own self.

5044-1 M. 9 5/5/44

In interpreting the physical and mental disturbances here, the sources and basis for these are in the karmic conditions of this body. To those responsible for this body: Rather than feeling it is a calamity, know that it is an opportunity to meet not only those things in self, but to help this individual entity or soul in search for its oneness with the Creative Forces, or God.

Appendix E

Possession

◆

POSSESSION IS A difficult subject to discuss in relation to mental illness due to the atrocities which have been inflicted upon the insane over the centuries in the name of religion. Nevertheless, the Cayce readings explicitly acknowledge the reality of possession in certain cases of insanity. Therefore it is important to understand the precise meaning of possession in the readings.

The readings affirm the continuity of consciousness and state that souls do not proceed immediately after death to some eternal resting place (be it heaven, hell, or whatever). Instead, the process of evolution toward unity with the Creator continues on various "planes" or dimensions of reality other than the earth. Unfortunately, some individuals have such strong attachments to the earth experience that they are unable to detach from this dimension at death. Instead, they may exist in a realm which Cayce describes as the "borderland." Such discarnate souls seeking expression in a physical manner, may find it through persons whose spiritual centers are open to cosmic influences. This opening may result from cases of insanity (i.e., dementia praecox), alcoholism, epilepsy, and various other organic disorders or from misdirected attempts at spiritual evolvement (e.g., certain occult practices, obtaining "higher knowledge" without applying it, etc.).

Keep in mind that the readings referred to "definite points" within the body which serve as connections between body, mind, and spirit (i.e., the *pineal system*, Appendix B). These interfaces could be adversely affected by somatic dysfunction, biochemical imbalances, and so forth. Severe weakening of these centers could thus leave the body open to outside influences seeking expression in the earth plane.

In certain cases cited in Chapter Three, possession was indicated because the individuals had lost control themselves and had little, if any, ego strength or sense of personal identity due to the degenerative effects of dementia praecox. In cases where dementia praecox was not indicated, the experience was more of obsession (e.g., [5221]) due to the opening of the spiritual centers of the body to outside influences.

It is also important to note that Cayce's use of the word possession in the readings does not suggest demonic possession. The intrusive entities were always earthbound spirits seeking expression in the earth plane. The readings' portrayal of life after death can be best be described as a "continuity of consciousness." In other words, patterns of thought and action are carried over into the discarnate state. Interpersonal patterns of "possession" developed during one's earthly life would thus be maintained by earthbound discarnates (e.g., a marriage partner who dominates a spouse, a parent who lives vicariously through an offspring, an employer who controls employees, etc.). With this in mind, one can appreciate the readings' frequent use of the term *influence* (e.g., "discarnate influence" or "outside influence," etc.) to describe the manifestation of possession.

Possession is not necessarily always a negative experience. Throughout history people of all cultures have sought possession by benevolent spirits and have engaged in rituals and ceremonies for that purpose (e.g., the Holy Spirit in Christianity).

Mediumship is a form of trance possession whereby individuals willingly allow discarnate entities to use their bodies for communication. In this form, possession does not necessarily interfere with an individual's course of life or produce pathological dissociation, and is time limited so that the individual can resume normal con-

scious daily living. The prime consideration in this type of possession is the conscious voluntary involvement of the person being
possessed. The popularity of spiritualism in the nineteenth century
and the current interest in channeling are examples of trance possession.

Electrotherapy and hypnotherapy were two of the most common
forms of therapy for the treatment of possession in the Cayce readings. Specifically, Cayce stated that electricity would drive out the
discarnate influences. Wickland (1924) was an early twentieth-century M.D. who used electrotherapy in conjunction with other techniques (including hypnosis) to encourage the earthbound entities
to detach from their hosts and proceed forward in the evolutionary
process of soul growth.

The Unquiet Dead (Fiore, 1987) is an informative and readable
introduction to this subject. Fiore is a clinical psychologist who uses
hypnosis to perform "depossession therapy." Her view of possession
in relation to schizophrenia is similar to that presented in the Cayce
readings: "I do *not* feel that all schizophrenics are psychotic *because*
of the possibility of possession. I do feel that—in addition to their
mental illness—they are undoubtedly possessed. The possession is
an extra burden for them" (p. 163).

Numerous clinicians are currently involved in various applications of depossession therapy. Baldwin's (1989) work with "spirit
releasement therapy" echoes many of the themes developed by
Fiore and attempts to provide a research format for exploring this
subject. His work is scholarly and highly recommended to readers
seeking further information.

Naegeli-Osjord (1989) is a Swiss medical doctor who provides
assessment criteria for the distinguishing possession from schizophrenia. The range of criteria includes interpersonal contact, presence
of phobias, auditory phenomenon, sudden changes in personality,
and mediality (mediumistic). His discussion of auditory hallucinations will serve as an introduction to his diagnostic procedure.

In the theory of established psychiatry, hallucinations—
voices—are, for the most part, considered to be primary symptoms of schizophrenia. In my opinion, this is wrong. We have
to consider that "voices" which another person cannot hear
are real sensations, but only heard by the individual in the
subtle interaction of the anatomic auditory center of the brain.
This may be caused by either a very intense personal feeling,

or by a being of the ethereal dimensions, a "suffering soul" or a demon. But the existence of an ethereal body is not considered. In my opinion, it is an absolute proof of possession or harassment when these "voices" constantly repeat the same words, for example, "kill yourself" or "you are a fool," for a long time, without stopping. (pp. 471-472)

There is abundant literature in this area and it is not necessary to wade through it because possession is not the primary focus of this book. Rather, this Appendix is intended to provide a context from which to consider Cayce's occasional reference to it in cases of dementia praecox.

Because Cayce's use of the term possession in the readings was not satanic, but more a matter of influence and obsession, the manifestation of this state was closely allied to the symptoms of the mental disorder. In other words, one would not expect a person receiving a psychic reading from Cayce which indicated possession to be exhibiting symptoms and behaviors which are graphically portrayed in innumerable movies about satanic possession (i.e., no rotating heads and vomit). Rather, one might observe a lack of control, periods of unconsciousness, obsessive thought patterns, etc.

The written correspondence associated with the readings where possession was involved provides vivid and personal accounts of the experience of possession in this context. There are three Circulating Files and a research bulletin on possession which are available through the A.R.E. James Windsor has written a brief paper entitled *Commentary on Possession* which provides an excellent overview of possession as noted in the readings. A concise quotation from this work will be provided, and interested readers are encouraged to review this insightful paper in its entirety.

Possession was not a major theme of the Cayce readings. It was mentioned several times, almost as an aside, in cases where the primary concern was either physical or mental health. Possession was presented as a consequence of other problems such as insanity, epilepsy, and alcoholism, rather than a cause. The disease, and resulting weakness, opened the person to the possibility of possession. (Windsor, 1989, p. 2)

Clinicians (e.g., Fiore, Baldwin, Naegeli-Osjord, etc.) have provided assessment criteria for differential diagnosis for those interested in pursuing the relationship between possession and mental illness in a clinical setting. Oesterreich's (1966) *Possession: Demonical and Other Among Primitive Races, in Antiquity, the Middle Ages, and Modern Times* is a comprehensive treatment of the subject from an historical perspective while Rogo's (1987) *The Infinite Boundary* focuses on twentieth-century clinicians who have investigated the relationship between mental illness and possession. Admittedly, this Appendix is an abridgment of this controversial subject and will only serve as an introduction. Although William James was perhaps a little hard on the medical profession, his view of this subject is still timely:

> I am not as positive as you are in the belief that the obsessing agency is really demonic individuals. I am perfectly willing to adopt that theory if the facts lend themselves best to it: for who can trace limits to the hierarchies of personal existence in the world? But the lower stages of mere automatism shade off so continuously into the highest supernormal manifestations, through the intermediary ones of imitative hysteria and "suggestibility," that I feel as if no general theory as yet would cover all the facts. So that the most I shall plead for before the neurologists is the recognition of demon possession as a regular "morbid-entity" whose commonest homologue today is the "spirit-control" observed in test-mediumship, and which tends to become the more benignant and less alarmingly, the less pessimistically it is regarded . . . I am convinced that we stand with all these things at the threshold of a long inquiry, of which the end appears as yet to no one, least of all to myself . . . The first thing is to start the medical profession out of its idiotically conceited ignorance of all such matters—matters which have everywhere and at all times played a vital part in human history. (in Murphy & Ballou, 1960, p. 261)

Excerpts from the Cayce Readings
281-6   5/12/32

Q. What has caused the severe attacks during the past week?
A. The return of those influences and forces seeking a home.
Q. Why should those entities return to this body after our prayer?
A. They are as material as individuals, why doesn't an entity return home? They are seeking a home, the same as individuals, personalities!

281-24   6/29/35

Q. In certain types of insanity, is there an etheric body involved? If so, how?

A. Possession.

Let's for the moment use examples that may show what has oft been expressed from here:

There is the physical body, there is the mental body, there is the soul body. They are One, as the Trinity; yet these may find a manner of expression that is individual unto themselves. The body itself finds its own level in its own development. The mind, through anger, may make the body do that which is contrary to the better influences of same; it may make for a change in its environ, its surrounding, contrary to the laws of environment or hereditary forces that are a portion of the *élan vital* of each manifested body, with the spirit or the soul of the individual.

Then, through pressure upon some portion of the anatomical structure that would make for the disengaging of the natural flow of the mental body through the physical in its relationships to the soul influence, one may be dispossessed of the mind; thus ye say rightly he is "out of his mind."

Or, where there are certain types or characters of disease found in various portions of the body, there is the lack of the necessary *vital* for the resuscitating of the energies that carry on through brain structural forces of a given body. Thus disintegration is produced, and ye call it dementia praecox—by the very smoothing of the indentations necessary for the rotary influence or vital force of the spirit within same to find expression. Thus derangements come.

Such, then, become possessed as of hearing voices, because of their closeness to the borderland. Many of these are termed deranged when they may have more of a closeness to the universal than one who may be standing nearby and commenting; yet they are awry when it comes to being normally balanced or healthy for their activity in a material world.

436-3   M. 28   11/11/33

Q. Are there entities, because of a psychic opening, feeding on or sucking my vitality?

A. Entities that would seek to find expression through that left open ... yet the harmony even of the spheres may be the experience of the entity with the aid in self builded to such an extent as to gain from the meditation healing influences from the higher sources, and give out to those who would as vultures feed upon the body—that they may find for themselves that guiding influence in their present environ and sphere of experience.

638-1   F. 72   8/21/34
Mr. Cayce: Yes, we have the body here, [638]. [In undertone, after long pause: "We have possession here."] Now, as we find, from the physical or material standpoint we have conditions that disturb the better physical functioning of this body. These have to do with the coordinations between the sympathetic and cerebrospinal responses to the activities in the physical forces of the body . . . we have . . . corresponding cold spots on various portions of the body . . .
Q. What causes the illusions?
A. Incoordination between the sympathetic and cerebrospinal nerve system, from those areas or ganglia as indicated. We must create for the physical forces of the body that which will make coordinations in these areas.

900-20   M. 29   1/15/25
For the subconscious, as given, is the storehouse of every act, thought, or deed . . . Hence the condition as is seen about such entity having passed into the spirit plane; it seeks the gratification of such through the low-minded individuals in an earth plane.

1183-3   F. 56   1/22/38
Q. What causes him to lose control of himself?
A. Possession!
Q. Is there any way I can help him?
A. Kindness, gentleness and prayer. These offer the channels through which the greater help may come at this time . . .
Q. Regarding my husband, what is meant by "possession"?
A. Means possession!
Q. Does that mean by other entities, while under the influence of liquor?
A. By others while under the influence that causes those reactions and makes for the antagonism, and the very change of the activities.
For this body [the husband], if there could be a sufficient period of refraining from the use of alcoholic stimulants and the diathermy electrical treatments used these would drive these conditions out!
But do not use same with the effects of alcohol in the system—it would be detrimental!

But such information for the physical condition of the body had best be approached from the individual, to be sure.

Q. Is he crazy, or mentally deranged?

A. If possession isn't crazy, what is it?

1553-6   F. 71   8/19/38

Q. Is it possible that this body is possessed by an unclean or evil spirit which causes peculiar crying and expression of rage at times?

A. As has been indicated, there is the inclination for the inner self to GATHER the influences of same. Not a case of complete possession, but ENTERTAINING of such influences at times. Hence the electrical forces will aid, with the suggestions, in eliminating these IMPRESSIONS—or POSSESSIONS of the mental attitudes.

1553-17   F. 72   10/30/39

This can only be met through the suggestions—for, as has been indicated, these periods come and go; and, as has been outlined heretofore, it is a lack of the coordinating between the cerebrospinal and sympathetic impulses or reflexes.

Q. Is there POSSESSION in this body?

A. No—not in the present. As has been indicated, there have been periods; but these have passed.

1572-1   F. 50   4/18/38

Hence pressures are indicated in the lumbar and the lower dorsal area . . . As has been given, this is the incoordination between the cerebrospinal and the sympathetic nervous system. And as the glandular system is affected as related to the genitive system, and especially affecting directly the center above the puba, there is produced—with the toxic forces in the system—this burning, and the EFFECT of POSSESSION!

1789-1   F. 32   1/13/39

The beauty of this soul, its abilities as a creative influence in the lives of those who may bring it back as it were from the very borderland, is worth all the effort, all the love, all the kindness one may give.

Such is so near possession that there needs to be great care taken.

1969-1   M. 38   7/28/39

In the present environs (this is not meant to be as a disputation), it is not thoroughly understood. For here we have a condition that is as much POSSESSION as a weakening of the nerve forces in the system; and the general nerve breakdown will NOT be eliminated by the administering of drugs nor by the mere activity of suppression.

2067-3   F. 52   9/30/40
Q. When my vitality is low and I get discouraged, is it still possible for undesirable discarnate beings to obsess me and make a statement unbeknown to me, as I believe they did in 1938 in [1387]'s office?
A. May obsess anyone that opens self to listen to same!

2465-1   F. 28   3/17/41
There has been a lesion in the lacteal duct and that as coordinating with the organs of the pelvis.
Hence at times such a state is produced as to almost become obsession, but possession in same.
The reaction to the pineal becomes so severe as to short circuit the nerve impulse; carrying or producing a fluttering or an engorgement in static waves to the base of the brain.
Thus periods are caused when there is lack of self-control.

2544-1   F. 50   7/25/41
Now we find, there are disturbing conditions. These are the result of external injuries to the body. [thrown up in air in an automobile accident]
And the pressures that exist especially in the coccyx area of the spine cause a deflection of nerve energies and impulses; producing hallucinations to the mental reaction.
But from external injuries the nerves in the coccyx end of the spine have been jammed, as well as the reaction upon the nerves in the lumbar axis and the brachial and cervical.
In the reaction to the nerves, as the pressures upon the coccyx end and the brush end of the cerebrospinal, congested areas have formed there.
Periods come when there is self-condemnation, self-realization of the reaction; and at times the feeling or expression of POSSESSION.

2614-1   F. 37   11/7/41
These are the result of chemical and glandular reactions in the

body; producing a deteriorating reaction in nerve impulses.

Thus the mental aberrations that appear, the hallucination as to lack of desire for associations and activities, faultfinding in self and in environs, as well as those about the body.

If these are allowed to progress they may bring a very detrimental condition—either that of possession or such a deteriorating as to become dementia praecox in its nature.

2863-2   F. 45   7/21/43

When the adjustments or manipulations are given, now about once a week, follow same with the ultraviolet light—this to be the Mercury Light, and project the green glass between it and the body; this to be applied mainly to the spinal system.

Q. What material conditions are upsetting to the body, and what adjustments need to be made to prevent this?

A. These have just been outlined. As the centers are opened, that is why we are giving the electrical treatments in the two forms—one external to act upon the structural portion, the other to the centers that will prevent any form of possession or impression from the psychic forces outside the body.

2865-1   F. 31   12/7/42

As we find, there are physical or pathological, as well as mental-psychological, disturbances. These, while they do not work together, are caused or produced by retentions in the mind—or that which is partially, or at times possession.

The body-mind lost control of itself through overtaxing of the body-mind, combined with a type of fever that was part of the experience when the body so taxed itself; reducing the body-forces to such an extent that in many centers along the spinal column there came to be less and less ability for the centers to coordinate between sympathetic and cerebrospinal nervous systems.

First there was caused absentmindedness, the tendencies towards a little temperature, the driving of self too much, and then the hallucinations, and then debilitation in the impulses to be carried back and forth through the ganglia.

3075-1   M. 24   7/2/43

As we find, the conditions that disturb this body are as much of a psychological nature as of a pathological nature.

Pathologically, these would have to do with conditions which existed during the period of gestation.

Psychologically, these have to do with the karma of this body, and those responsible for the physical body.

Hence we have here conditions that at times approach near to that of possession of the mind by external influences, or that very close to the spiritual possession by disincarnate forces.

To be sure, these interpretations would not be accepted by some as an explanation. And yet there will come those days when many will understand and interpret properly . . .

Owing to those conditions which existed in the manner in which coordination is established in the physical reactions between impressions received through sensory system and the reactions upon the reflexes of brain, we find these at times become very much disassociated . . .

At such times possession near takes place.

With the capsule of the inner brain itself, these cause the distortions, the associations with not the normal reflexes but with the impressions received in the suggestive forces.

3315-1   F. 40   10/27/43

The conditions here, as we find, have been so aggravated by animosities, and by hates, that we have a deterioration in the nerve force along the spinal system; so that this dementia—and now possession, such that this may appear near to hopeless in this experience.

Ready for questions.

Q. What was the original cause, or what brought about this condition?

A. Changes in the glandular system, and then aggravated by animosities and hate.

3410-1   F. 20   12/19/43

As we find, there are disturbing conditions. Part of these are pathological, part are psychopathic. There has been the opening of the lyden [Leydig] gland and thus a disturbance through glandular system. Possession at times is the result.

3421-1   F. 39   12/27/43

. . . there has been the opening of the lyden [Leydig] gland, so that the kundaline forces move along the spine to the various centers that open . . . with these activities of the reaction is much like that as may be illustrated in one gaining much knowledge without making practical application of it . . . Now we combine these two and we have that indicated here as possession of the body; gnawing, as it were, on all the seven centers of the body, causing the inability for rest or even a concerted activity—unless the body finds, as this occurs, the disturbance is retarded or fades—in the abilities of the body to exercise itself in [giving] help for others.

5221-1   F. 53   6/9/44
. . . the body is a supersensitive individual entity who has allowed itself through study, through opening the [gland] centers of the body, to become possessed with reflexes and activities outside of itself . . .

Q. How did I happen to pick this up?

A. . . . the body in its study opened the [gland] centers and allowed self to become sensitive to outside influences.

Q. What is it exactly that assails me?

A. Outside influences. Discarnate entities.

References

Albertson, T. E., Peterson, S. L., Stark, L. G., Lakin, M. L. & Winters, W. D. (1981). The anticonvulsant properties of melatonin on kindled seizures in rats. *Neuropharmacology, 20,* 61-66.

Albus, M., Ackenheil, R. & Muller, F. (1982). Situational reactivity of autonomic functions in schizophrenic patients. *Psychiatry Research, 6,* 361-370.

Albus, M., Engel, R. R., Muller, F., Zander, K. J., & Ackenheil, M. (1982). Experimental stress situations and the state of autonomic arousal in schizophrenic and depressive patients. *International Pharmacopsychiatrica, 17,* 129-135.

Alpert, M. & Friedhoff, A. J. (1980). An un-dopamine hypothesis of schizophrenia. *Schizophrenia Bulletin, 6*(3), 187-390.

American Psychiatric Association. (1987). *Diagnostic and statistic manual of mental disorders (3rd ed. revised).* Washington, DC: Author.

Andreasen, N. C. (1982). Negative vs. positive schizophrenia: Definition and validation. *Archives of General Psychiatry, 39,* 789-794.

Andreasen, N. C. (1985). Positive vs. negative schizophrenia: A critical review. *Schizophrenia Bulletin, 11*(3), 380-389.

Andreasen, N. C. (1987). The diagnosis of schizophrenia. *Schizophrenia Bulletin, 13*(1), 9-47.

Anthony, W. A. & Liberman, R. P. (1986). The practice of psychiatric rehabilitation: Historical, conceptual, and research base. *Schizophrenia Bulletin, 12*(4), 542-559.

Arato, M., Grof, E., Laszlo, I. & Brown, G. M. (1985). Reproducibility of the overnight melatonin secretion pattern in healthy men. In G. M. Brown & S. D. Wainwright (eds.), *Advances in the biosciences: The pineal gland; Endocrine aspects* (pp. 277-282). Oxford: Pergamon Press.

Arendt, J. (1988). Melatonin. *Clinical Endocrinology, 29,* 205-229.

Axelrod, J. (1974). The pineal gland: A neurochemical transducer. *Science, 184,* 1341-1348.

Azumi, K., Takahashi, S., Takahashi, K., Maruyama, N. & Kikuti, S. (1967). The effects of dream deprivation on chronic schizophrenics and normal adults: A comparative study. *Folia Psychiatric et Neurologica Japonica, 21,* 205-225.

Bailey, A. A. (1932). *From intellect to intuition.* New York: Lucis Publishing Co.

Baldwin, W. J. (1989). Clinical parapsychology: A new perspective on spirit possession. In K. P. Freeman, M. L. Albertson & D. S. Ward (eds.), *Proceedings of the Second International Conference on Paranormal Research* (pp. 443-466). Fort Collins, CO: Rocky Mountain Research Institute.

Ballanger, J. C. (1988). The use of anticonvulsants in manic-depressive illness. *Journal of Clinical Psychiatry, 49*(11), suppl., 21-24.

Bandura, A. (1977). *Social learning theory.* Englewood Cliffs, NJ: Prentice-Hall.

Bartko, G., Maylath, E. & Herczeg, I. (1987). Comparative study of schizophrenic patients relapsed on and off medication. *Psychiatry Research, 22,* 221-227.

Beard, J. H., Propst, R. N. & Malamud, T. J. (1982). The Fountain House model of psychiatric rehabilitation. *Psychosocial Rehabilitation Journal, 5,* 47-59.

Becker, B. O. (1990). *Cross currents.* Los Angeles: Jeremy P. Tarcher, Inc.

Becker, B. O. & Seldon, B. (1985). *The body electric.* New York: William Morrow and Company, Inc.

Bellak, L. & Strauss, S. (1979). Overview: The heuristic need for subgroups of the schizophrenic syndrome. *Schizophrenia Bulletin, 5*(3), 441-442.

Bernstein, A. S. (1987). Orienting response research in schizophrenia: Where we have come and where we might go. *Schizophrenia Bulletin, 13*(4), 623-636.

Besant, A. (1959). *A study in consciousness.* Wheaton, IL: The Theosophical Press.

Bierman, J. M., Siegel, E., French, F. E. & Simonian, K. (1965). Analysis of the outcome of all pregnancies in a community. *American Journal of Obstetrics and Gynecology, 91,* 37-45.

Bigelow, L. B. (1974). Effects of aqueous pineal extract in chronic schizophrenia. *Biological Psychiatry, 8*(1), 5-15.

Blask, D. E. (1984). The pineal gland: An oncostatic gland? In R. J. Reiter (ed.). *The pineal gland* (253-284). New York: Raven Press.

Bleuler, E. (1911). *Dementia praecox or the group of schizophrenias.* Translated by J. Zinkin (1950). New York: International Universities Press.

Bockoven, J. S. (1963). *Moral treatment in American psychiatry.* New York: Springer Publishing.

Bolduc, H. L. (1985). *Self-hypnosis: creating your own destiny.* Virginia Beach, VA: A.R.E. Press.

Bolton, B. (1969). *Edgar Cayce speaks.* New York: Avon Books.

Boyd, J. H., Pulver, A. E. & Stewart, W. (1986). Season of birth: Schizophrenia and bipolar disorder. *Schizophrenia Bulletin, 12*(2), 173-186.

Bradbury, A. J., Kelly, M. E. & Smith, J. A. (1985). Melatonin action in the midbrain can regulate forebrain dopamine function both behaviorally and biochemically. In G. M. Brown & S. D. Wainwright (eds.). *Advances in the biosciences: The pineal gland: Endocrine aspects* (pp. 327-332). New York: Pergamon Press.

Bradbury, T. N. & Miller, G. A. (1985). Season of birth in schizophrenia: A review of evidence, methodology, and etiology. *Psychological Bulletin, 98,* 569-594.

Bradley, B. W. & McCanne, T. R. (1981). Autonomic responses to stress: The effects of progressive relaxation, the relaxation response, and expectancy of relief. *Biofeedback and Self-Regulation, 6*(2), 235-251.

Brantingham, J. W. (1986). Still and Palmer: The impact of the first osteopath and the first chiropractor. *Chiropractic History, 6,* 19-22.

Bro, H. H. (1990). *A Seer Out of Season.* New York: Penguin Books.

Brockington, I. F., Cernik, K. F., Schofield, E. M., Downing, A. R., Francis, A. F. & Keelan, C. (1981). Puerperal psychosis. *Archives of General Psychiatry, 38,* 829-833.

Brown, G. W. & Birley, J. L. T. (1968). Crises and life changes and the onset of schizophrenia. *Journal of Health and Social Behavior, 9,* 203-214.

Brown, G. W., Monck, E. M., Carstairs, G. M. & King, J. K. (1962). Infuence of family life on the course of schizophrenic illness. *British Journal of Preventive and Social Medicine, 16,* 55-68.

Brown, R. P., Kocsis, J. H., Caroff, S., Amsterdam, J., Winokur, A., Stokes, P. E. & Frazier, A. (1985). Differences in nocturnal melatonin secretion between melancholic depressed patients and control subjects. *American Journal of Psychiatry, 182,* 811-816.

Brown, W. A. & Herz, L. R. (1989). Response to neuroleptic drugs as a device for classifying schizophrenia. *Schizophrenia Bulletin, 15*(1), 123-128.

Callan, J. P. (1979). Holistic health or holistic hoax? *Journal of the American Medical Association, 241*(11), 1156.

Calvert, R. (1989). Massage and chiropractic: A healing partnership. *The Digest of Chiropractic Economics,* 37-40.

Cancro, R. (1979). Genetic evidence for the existence of subgroups of the schizophrenic syndrome. *Schizophrenia Bulletin, 5*(3), 453-459.

Cannady, D. (1982). Chronics and cleaning ladies. *Psychosocial Rehabilitation Journal, 5*, 13-16.

Caplin, R. B. (1969). *Psychiatry and the community in nineteenth-century America.* New York: Basic Books, Inc.

Carpenter, W. T. & Heinrichs, D. W. (1981). Treatment-relevant subtypes of schizophrenia. *The Journal of Nervous and Mental Disease, 169*(2), 113-119.

Carpenter, W. T., Heinrichs, D. W. & Alphs, L. D. (1985). Treatment of negative symptoms. *Schizophrenia Bulletin, 11*(3), 440-450.

Carpenter, Jr., W. T., & Stephens, J. H. (1979). An attempted integration of information relevant to schizophrenic subtypes. *Schizophrenia Bulletin, 5*(3), 490-506.

Cayce, C. T. (1978, January). *Concerning a physical basis for mental illness.* Paper presented at the Medical Symposium, A.R.E. Clinic, Phoenix, Arizona. Available as Child Development Series, No. 9, A.R.E., Virginia Beach, VA.

Cayce, J. G. (1973). *Osteopathy: Comparative concepts—A. T. Still and Edgar Cayce.* Virginia Beach, VA: Edgar Cayce Foundation.

Chouinard, G. (1988). The use of benzodiazepines in the treatment of manic-depressive illness. *Journal of Clinical Psychiatry, 49*(11), 15-19.

Cott, A. (1971). Controlled fasting treatment of schizophrenia in the U.S.S.R. *Schizophrenia,* 2-10.

Cottingham, J. T. (1985). *Healing through touch.* Boulder, CO: Rolf Institute.

Crow, T. J. (1980). Molecular pathology of schizophrenia: More than one disease process? *British Medical Journal, 280,* 66-68.

Crow, T. J. (1985). The two-syndrome concept: Origins and current status. *Schizophrenia Bulletin, 11*(3), 471-484.

Csernansky, J. G., Holman, C. A. & Hollister, L. E. (1983). Variability and the dopamine hypothesis of schizophrenia. *Schizophrenia Bulletin, 9*(3), 325-328.

Cyriax, J. (1977). Deep massage. *Physiotherapy, 63*(2), 60-61.

Cyriax, J. (1980). Clinical applications of massage. In J. B. Rogoff (ed.), *Manipulations, traction and massage* (pp.152-169). Baltimore: Williams & Wilkins.

Dawson, M. E. & Neuchterlein, K. H. (1984). Psychophysiological dysfunctions in the developmental course of schizophrenic disorders. *Schizophrenia Bulletin, 10*(2), 204-230.

DeBenedette, V. (1988). Getting fit for life: Can exercise reduce stress? *The Physician and Sportsmedicine, 16*(6), 185-186, 191-200.

Dennerstein, L., Judd, F. & Davies, B. (1983). Psychosis and the menstrual cycle. *The Medical Journal of Australia,* May, 524-526.

Depue, R. A. & Fowles, D. C. (1973). Electrodermal activity as an index of arousal in schizophrenics. *Psychological Bulletin, 79,* 233-238.

Dorian, B. & Garfinkel, P. E. (1987). Stress, immunity and illness—a review. *Psychological Medicine, 17,* 393-407.

Duggan, J. & Duggan, S. (1989). *Massage, hydrotherapy & healing oils.* Inner Vision Publishing Company: Virginia Beach: VA.

Dunn, F. E. (1950). Osteopathic concepts in psychiatry. *Journal of the American Osteopathic Association,* March, 354-357.

Ebadi, M. (1984). Regulation of the synthesis of melatonin and its significance to neuroendocrinology. In R. J. Reiter (ed.), *The pineal gland* (1-38). New York: Raven Press.

Ebels, I. & Balemans, G. M. (1986). Physiological aspects of pineal functions in mammals. *Physiological Reviews, 66*(3), 581-605.

Edgar Cayce Foundation (1971). *Basic diet.* Virginia Beach, VA: A.R.E. Press.

Eisner, V., Brazie, J. V., Pratt, M. W. & Hexter, A. C. (1979). The risk of low birthweight. *American Journal of Public Health, 69,* 887-893.

Eitinger, L. & Strom, A. *Mortality and morbidity after stress.* New York: Humanities Press.

Erb, J. L., Kadane, J. B. & Tourney, G. (1981). Discrimination between schizophrenic and control subjects by means of plasma dehydroepiandrosterone measurements. *Journal of Clinical Endocrinology and Metabolism, 52,* 181.

Falloon, I. R. (1986). Family stress and schizophrenia. *Psychiatric clinics of North America, 9*(1), 165-182.

Fariello, R., Bubenik, G., Brown, G. & Grota, L. (1977). Epileptogenic action of intraventricularly injected antimelatonin activity. *Neurology, 27,* 567-570.

Ferrier, I. N., Arendt, J., Johnstone, E. C. & Crow, T. J. (1982). Reduced nocturnal secretion of melatonin in chronic schizophrenia: Relationship to body weight. *Clinical Endocrinology, 17,* 181-187.

Figueiredo, E., Conclaves, P. & Mota Cardoso, R. (1980). Massages and schizophrenia. *Revue de Medecine Psychosomatique et de Psychologie Medicale, 22*(3), 313-321.

Fink, M., Shaw, R., Gross, G. E. & Coleman, F. S. (1958). Comparative study of chlorpromazine and insulin coma in therapy of psychosis. *Journal of the American Medical Association, 166*(15), 1846-1850.

Fiore, E. (1987). *The unquiet dead.* New York: Doubleday & Co.

Fitch, L. & LaRoche, R. (1984). Earth House: An alternative for persons suffering from the schizophrenias. *Journal of Orthomolecular Psychiatry, 14*(2), 136-142.

Flor-Henry, P. (1975). Psychiatric surgery. *Canadian Psychiatric Association Journal, 20,* 157-167.

Floyd, M. (1984). The employment problems of people disabled by schizophrenia. *Occupational Medicine, 34*(3), 93-95.

Frederick, J. & Adelstein, P. (1978). Factors associated with low birth weight of infants delivered at term. *British Journal of Obstetrics and Gynecology, 85,* 1-7.

Gallagher, B. J., III, McFalls, J. A., Jr. & Jones, B. J. (1983). Racial factors in birth seasonality among schizophrenics: A preliminary analysis. *Journal of Abnormal Psychology, 92,* 524-527.

Garver, D. L., Reich, T., Isenberg, K. E. & Cloniger, C. R. (1989). Schizophrenia and the question of genetic heterogeneity. *Schizophrenia Bulletin, 15*(3), 421-430.

Garza-Trevino, E. S., Volkow, N. D., Cancro, R. & Contreras, S. (1990). Neurobiology of Schizophrenic Syndromes. *Hospital and Community Psychiatry, 41*(9), 971-980.

Gaziano, E. P., Freeman, D. W. & Allen T. E. (1981). Antenatal prediction of women at increased risk for infants with low birth weight. *American Journal of Obstetrics and Gynecology, 140,* 99-107.

Gerber, R. (1988). *Vibrational medicine.* Santa Fe, NM: Bear and Co.

Gerdine, L. V. H. (1919). Mental diseases. *The Western Osteopath, 13*(8), 5-6.

Gilligan, S. (1987). *Therapeutic Trances.* New York: Brunner/Mazel, Inc.

Gitlin, M. J. & Pasnau, R. O. (1989). Psychiatric syndromes linked to reproductive function in women: A review of current knowledge. *American Journal of Psychiatry, 146,* 1413-1422.

Glueck, B. C. & Stroebel, C. F. (1975). Biofeedback and meditation in the treatment of psychiatric illnesses. *Comprehensive Psychiatry, 16*(4), 303-321.

Goldberg, S. C. (1985). Negative and deficit symptoms in schizophrenia do respond to neuroleptics. *Schizophrenia Bulletin, 11*(3), 453-456.

Goldstein, J. M. & Kreisman, D. (1988). Gender, family environment, and schizophrenia. *Psychological Medicine, 18,* 861-872.

Goldstein, J. M., Santangelo, S. L., Simpson, J. C. & Tsuang, M. T. (1990). The role of gender in identifying subtypes of schizophrenia: A latent class analytic approach. *Schizophrenia Bulletin, 16*(2), 263-275.

Goldstein, J. M. & Tsuang, M. T. (1990). Gender and schizophrenia: An introduction and synthesis of findings. *Schizophrenia Bulletin, 16*(2), 179-183.

Goldstein, M. J. (1987). Psychosocial issues. *Schizophrenia Bulletin, 13*(1), 157-169.

Grady, H. (1988). *Study of the impedance device.* Phoenix, AZ: Fetzer Energy Medicine Research Institute & A.R.E. Medical Clinic.

Grau, B. W. (1986). Measurement of negative symptoms—past issues: Comments and responses. *Schizophrenia Bulletin, 12*(1), 7-8.

Gray, H. (1977). *Gray's Anatomy.* New York: Bounty Books.

Green, M. F. & Nuechterlein, K. H. (1988). Neuroleptic effects on electrodermal responsivity to soft tones and loud noise in schizophrenia. *Psychiatry Research, 24,* 79-86.

Greist, J. H., Klein, M. H., Eischens, R. R., Faris, J., Gurman, A. S. & Morgan, W. P. (1979). Running as treatment for depression. *Comprehensive Psychiatry, 20*(1), 41-54.

Grof, C. & Grof, S. (1990). *The stormy search for the self.* Los Angeles: Jeremy P. Tarcher, Inc.

Gruen, R. & Baron, M. (1984). Stressful life events and schizophrenia. *Neuropsychobiology, 12,* 206-208.

Gruzelier, J., Connolly, J., Eves, F., Hirsch, S. Z., Weller, M. & Yorkston, N. (1981). Effect of propanolol and phenothiazines on electrodermal orienting and habituation in schizophrenia. *Psychological Medicine, 11,* 93-108.

Gruzelier, J. & Venables, P. H. (1972). Skin conductance orienting activity in a heterogeneous sample of schizophrenia. *Journal of Nervous and Mental Disease, 155,* 277-287.

Gruzelier, J. & Venables, P. H. (1973). Skin conductance responses to tones with and without attentional significance in schizophrenic and nonschizophrenic psychiatric patients. *Neuropsycholigia, 11,* 221-230.

Gunderson, J. G. (1980). A reevaluation of milieu therapy for nonchronic schizophrenic patients. *Schizophrenic Bulletin, 6*(1), 64-69.

Gupta, Das, T. K. & Terz, J. (1967). Influence of pineal gland on the growth and spread of melanoma in the hamster. *Cancer Research, 27,* 1306.

Gur, R. E. & Gur, R. C. (1990). Gender differences in regional cerebral blood flow. *Schizophrenia Bulletin, 16*(2), 247-254.

Hanson, R. C. (1989). A preliminary investigation of out-of-body experience from a comparative, dialectical perspective. In K. P. Freeman, M. L. Albertson & D. S. Ward (eds.), *Proceedings of the Second International Conference on Paranormal Research* (pp. 235-253). Fort Collins, CO: Rocky Mountain Research Institute.

Hardin, J. G. (1989). Rheumatoid arthritis therapy: The slow-acting agents. *Hospital Practice,* 163-173.

Harris, A. E. (1988). Physical disease and schizophrenia. *Schizophrenia Bulletin, 14*(1), 85-96.

Harris, M. J. & Jeste, D. V. (1988). Late-onset schizophrenia: An overview. *Schizophrenia Bulletin, 14*(1), 39-55.

Hartley, R. & Smith, J. A. (1973). The activation of pineal hydroxyindole, O-methyltransferase by psychotomimmetic drugs. *Journal of Pharmacology, 25,* 751-752.

Havens, R. (1985). *The wisdom of Milton Erickson.* New York: Irvington Publishers.

Heimann, H. (1985). Specificity and nonspecificity—a major problem in biologically oriented psychopathology. *Psychopathology, 18,* 82-87.

Heinrichs, D. W., Hanlon, T. E. & Carpenter, W. T. (1984). The quality of life scale: An instrument for rating the schizophrenic deficit syndrome. *Schizophrenia Bulletin, 10*(3), 388-396.

Hemphill, R. E., Reiss, M. & Taylor, A. L. (1944). Study of histology of testis in schizophrenia and other mental disorders. *Journal of Mental Science, 90,* 681-695.

Herz, M. I. (1986). Toward an integrated approach to the treatment of schizophrenia. *Psychotherapy and Psychosomatics, 46,* 45-57.

Hildreth, A. G. (1924). Osteopathy in the cure of insanity. *The Western Osteopath, 18*(8), 7-8.

Hildreth, A. G. (1929). Fifteen years at Still-Hildreth. *The Journal of Osteopathy, 36,* 518-521.

Hildreth, A. G. (1930). *Old osteopathy for the cure of insanity.* Paper presented in Philadelphia, PA. Month and occasion of presentation unknown.

Hildreth, A. G. (1938). *The lengthening shadow of Dr. Andrew Taylor Still* (3rd ed.). Kirksville, MO: Osteopathic Enterprises, Inc.

Hoffer, A. (1976). The medical model and milieu therapy. *Orthomolecular Psychiatry, 5*(4), 246-252.

Hoffer, A. (1987). *Common questions on schizophrenia and their answers.* New Canaan, CT: Keats Publishing, Inc.

Hogarty, G. E. (1984). Depot neuroleptics: The relevance of psychosocial factors—a United States perspective. *Journal of Clinical Psychiatry, 45*(5), 36-42.

Hopkins, A. (1981). *Epilepsy, the facts.* Oxford: Oxford University Press.

Hornykiewicz, O. (1982). Brain catecholamines in schizophrenia—a good case for noradrenaline. *Nature, 299,* 484-486.

Horrobin, D. F. (1979). Schizophrenia: Reconciliation of the dopamine, prostaglandin, and opioid concepts and the role of the pineal. *The Lancet,* 529-531.

Hoskins, R. G. & Sleeper, R. G. (1933). Organic functions in schizophrenia. *Archives of Neurological Psychiatry, 30,* 123-140.

Huxley, A. (1944). *The perennial philosophy.* New York: Harper & Row.

Hyde, A. P. (1985). *Living with schizophrenia.* Chicago: Contemporary Books.

Iguchi, H., Kato, K. & Ibayashi, H. (1982). Age-dependent reduction in serum melatonin concentration in healthy human subjects. *Journal of Clinical Endocrinology and Metabolism, 55,* 27-29.

Isaac, G. (1978). Steroid hormones in schizophrenia. *Schizophrenia Bulletin, 4*(1), 19.

Jablensky, A. (1989). Epidemiology and cross-cultural aspects of schizophrenia. *Psychiatric Annals, 19*(10), 516-524.

Jacobson, B. & Kinney, D. K. (1980). Perinatal complications in adopted and non-adopted schizophrenics and their controls. *Acta Psychiatrica Scandinavica, 62* (supplement 285), 337-346.

Jahnke, R. (1986). Choosing body therapies for good health. *Venture Inward, 2*(2), 41-45.

Jahnke, R. (1990). Qigong: Awakening and mastering the profound medicine that lies within. *Newsletter of the International Society for the Study of Subtle Energies and Energy Medicine, 3,* 3-7.

Jansen, K. L. R., Dragunow, M. & Faull, R. L. M. (1990). Sigma receptors are highly concentrated in the rat pineal gland. *Brain Research, 507,* 158-160.

Johnstone, E. C., Crow, T. J, Frith, C. D., Husband, J. & Kreel, I. (1976). Cerebral ventricular size and cognitive impairment in chronic schizophrenia. *Lancet, II,* 924-926.

Josiassen, R. C., Roemer, R. A., Johnson, M. M. & Shagass, C. (1990). Are gender differences in schizophrenia reflected in brain event-related potentials? *Schizophrenia Bulletin, 16*(2), 229-246.

Judd, F. K., Burrows, G. D. & Norman, T. R. (1983). Psychosis after withdrawal of steroid therapy. *The Medical Journal of Australia,* 350-351.

Judith, A. (1987). *Wheels of life.* St. Paul, MN: Llewellyn Publications.

Kane, J. M., Rifkin, A. & Woerner, M. (1983). Low dose neuroleptic treatment of outpatient schizophrenics, I: Preliminary results for relapse rates. *Archives of General Psychiatry, 40,* 893-896.

Kane, J. M., Rifkin, A., Woerner, M., Reardon, G., Kreisman, D., Blumenthal, R. & Borenstein, M. (1985). High-dose versus low-dose strategies in the treatment of schizophrenia. *Psychopharmacology Bulletin, 21,* 533-537.

Karp, R. A. (1986). *Edgar Cayce encyclopedia of healing.* New York: Warner Books, Inc.

Kasanin, J. (1933). The acute schizoaffective psychoses. *American Journal of Psychiatry, 13,* 97-126.

Katkin, S., Ginsburg, M., Rifkin, J. J. & Scott, J. T. (1971). Effectiveness of female volunteers in the treatment of outpatients. *Journal of Counseling Psychology, 18,* 97-100.

Katkin, S., Zimmerman, U., Rosenthal, T. & Ginsburg, M. (1975). Using volunteer therapists to reduce hospital readmissions. *Hospital and Community Psychiatry, 26,* 151-153.

Keats, M. M. & Mukerjee, S. (1988). Antiaggressive effect of adjunctive clonazepam in schizophrenia associated with seizure disorder. *Journal of Clinical Psychiatry, 49*(3), 117-118.

Keefe, R. S. E., Mohs, R. C., Davidson, M., Losonczy, M. F., Silverman, J. M., Lesser, J. C., Horvath, T. B. & Davis, K. L. (1988). Kraepelinian schizophrenia: A subgroup of schizophrenia? *Psychopharmacology Bulletin, 24*(1), 56-61.

Kemali, D., Maj, M., Ariano, M. G., Arena, F. & Lovero, N. (1985). 24-hour plasma levels of prolactin, cortisol, growth hormone and catecholamines in schizophrenic patients. *Neuropsychobiology 14,* 109-114.

Kemali, D, Maj, M., Iorio, G., Marciano, G., Nolfe, S., Galderisi, S. & Salvati, A. (1985). Relationship between CSF noradrenaline levels, C-EEG indicators of activation and psychosis ratings in drug-free schizophrenic patients. *Acta Psychiatrica Scandinavica, 71,* 19-24.

Kieffer, G. (ed.). (1988). *Kundalini for the new age: Selected writings of Gopi Krishna*. New York: Bantam.

King, L. J. (1983). Occupational therapy and neuropsychiatry. *Occupational Therapy in Mental Health*, 3(1), 1-14.

Kiriike, N., Izumiya, S, Nishiwaki, S., Maeda, Y., Nagata, T. & Kawakita, Y. (1988). TRH and DST in schizoaffective mania, mania, and schizophrenia. *Biological Psychiatry*, 24, 415-422.

Kirkpatrick, B. & Buchanan, R. W. (1990). The neural basis of the deficit syndrome of schizophrenia. *The Journal of Nervous and Mental Disease*, 178(9), 545-555.

Kitay, J. I. & Altschule, M. D. (1954). *The pineal gland* (pp. 79-95). Cambridge, MA: Harvard University Press.

Klein, D. C. & Weller, J. L. (1970). Indole metabolism in the pineal gland, a circadian rhythm in N-acetyltransferase. *Science*, 169, 1093-1095.

Kolakowska, T., Williams, A. O., Ardern, M., Reveley, M. A., Jambor, K., Gelder, M. G., & Mandelbrote, B. M. (1985). Schizophrenia with good and poor outcome, I: Early clinical features, response to neuroleptics and signs of organic dysfunction. *British Journal of Psychiatry*, 146, 229-246.

Kopala, L. & Clark, C. (1990). Implications of olfactory agnosia for understanding sex differences in schizophrenia. *Schizophrenia Bulletin*, 16(2), 255-261.

Korr, I. (1947). The neural basis of the osteopathic lesion. *Journal of the American Osteopathic Association*, 47, 191-198.

Korr, I. (1948). The emerging concept of the osteopathic lesion. *Journal of the American Osteopathic Association*, 48, 127-138.

Korr, I. (1955a). Clinical significance of the facilitated state. *Journal of the American Osteopathic Association*, 54(5), 277-282.

Korr, I. (1955b). The concept of facilitation and its origin. *Journal of the American Osteopathic Association*, 55(5), 265-268.

Korr, I. (ed.). (1970). *The physiologic basis of osteopathic medicine*. The Postgraduate Institute of Osteopathic Medicine and Surgery: Kirksville, MO.

Korr, I. (1976). The spinal cord as organizer of disease processes: Some preliminary perspectives. *Journal of the American Osteopathic Association*, 76, 35-45.

Korr, I. (ed.). (1978). *The neurobiological mechanisms in manipulative therapy*. New York: Plenum Publishing.

Korr, I. M., Wilkinson, P. N. & Chornock, F. W. (1967). Axonal delivery of neuroplasmic components of muscle cells. *Science*, 155(20), 342-345.

Kraepelin, E. (1919). *Dementia praecox and paraphrenia.* Translated by R. M. Barclay. New York: Robert E. Krieger Publishing Co., Inc., 1971.

Kreamer, P. (1986). There's the rub: Massage goes hand in hand with better running. *The Runner,* p. 22.

Kripke, D. F. & Risch, S. C. (1986). Therapeutic effects of bright light in depressed patients. *Annals of the New York Academy of Science, 453,* 270-281.

Lahmeyer, H. W. & Bellur, S. N. (1987). Cardiac regulation and depression. *Journal of Psychiatric Research, 21*(1), 1-6.

Leff, J. P. (1985). Social factors and maintenance neuroleptics in schizophrenic relapse: An integrative model. *Integrative Psychiatry, 3,* 72-88.

Leff, J., Kuipers, L., Berkowitz, R., Vaughn, C. & Sturgeon, D. (1983). Life events, relatives' expressed emotion, and maintenance neuroleptics in schizophrenic relapse. *Psychological Medicine, 13,* 799-806.

Lerchl, A., Nonaka, K. O., Stokkan, K. A. & Reiter, R. J. (1990). Marked rapid alterations in nocturnal pineal serotonin metabolism in mice and rats exposed to weak intermittent magnetic fields. *Biochemical and Biophysical Research Communications, 169*(1), 102-108.

Lewine, R. J. (1986). Reply to Grau and Mueser. *Schizophrenia Bulletin, 12*(1), 9-11.

Lewine, R. J., Gulley, L. R., Risch, S. C., Jewart, R. & Houpt, J. L. (1990). Sexual dimorphism, brain morphology, and schizophrenia. *Schizophrenia Bulletin, 16*(2), 195-203.

Lewis, M. S. (1989). Age incidence and schizophrenia: Part I. The season of birth controversy. *Schizophrenia Bulletin, 15*(1), 59-73.

Lewis, S. W. & Murray, R. M. (1987). Obstetric complications, neurodevelopmental deviance, and risk of schizophrenia. *Journal of Psychiatric Research, 21*(4), 413-421.

Lewy, A. J. & Newsome, D. A. (1983). Different types of melatonin circadian secretory rhythms in some blind subjects. *Journal of Clinical Endocrinology and Metabolism, 56,* 1103-1107.

Lewy, A. J., Wehr, T. A., Gold, P. W. & Goodwin, F. K. (1979). Plasma melatonin in manic-depressive illness. In E. Usdin, I. J. Kopin & J. Barchas (eds.), *Catecholamines: Basic and clinical frontiers, Vol. II* (pp. 1173-1175), Oxford: Pergamon Press.

Lewy, A. J., Wehr, T. A., Goodwin, F. K., Newsome, D. & Rosenthal,

N. E. (1981). Manic-depressive patients may be supersensitive to light. *Lancet*, 383-384.

Li, R. K. (1981). Activity therapy and leisure counseling for the schizophrenic population. *Therapeutic Recreation Journal*, 44-49.

Licht, S. (1983). History of ultraviolet therapy. In Stillwell, G. K. (ed.), *Therapeutic electricity and ultraviolet radiation* (174-193). Baltimore, MD: Williams & Wilkins.

Licht, S. (1983). Therapeutic electricity. In Stillwell, G. K. (ed.), *Therapeutic electricity and ultraviolet radiation* (1-64). Baltimore, MD: Williams & Wilkins.

Lickey, M. E. & Gordon, B. (1983). *Drugs for mental illness.* New York: W. H. Freeman and Company.

Lieberman, C. (1979). Schizoaffective illness defies the dichotomy . . . and keeps DSM-III pondering. *Schizophrenia Bulletin, 5*(3), 436-440.

Lozovsky, D. B., Koplin, I. J. & Saller, C. F. (1985). Modulation of dopamine receptor supersensitivity by chronic insulin; Implication in schizophrenia. *Brain Research, 343,* 190-193.

Mackay, A. V. (1980). Positive and negative schizophrenic symptoms and the role of dopamine. *British Journal of Psychiatry, 137,* 379-386.

Mackota, C. & Lamb, H. R. (1989). Vocational rehabilitation. *Psychiatric Annals, 19*(10), 548-552.

MacShein, B. & Murphy, G. (1981). Effectiveness of electromyograph biofeedback training with an acute schizophrenic population. *Journal of Psychiatric Treatment and Evaluation, 3,* 475-479.

Marcus, N. & Levin, G. (1977). Clinical applications of biofeedback: Implications for psychiatry. *Hospital and Community Psychiatry, 28,* 21-25.

Marder, S. R., Van Putten, T. & Mintz, J. (1987). *Archives of General Psychiatry, 44,* 518-521.

Mason, J. W., Giller, E. L. & Kosten, T. R. (1988). Serum testosterone differences between patients with schizophrenia and those with affective disorders. *Biological Psychiatry, 23,* 357-366.

McCall, W. V. (1989). Physical treatments in psychiatry: Current and historical use in the southern United States. *Southern Medical Journal, 82*(3), 345-351.

McGarey, W. A. (1970). *Edgar Cayce and the palma christi.* Virginia Beach, VA: Edgar Cayce Foundation.

McGarey, W. A. (1974). *Acupuncture and body energies.* Phoenix, AZ: Gabriel Press.

McGarey, W. A. (1983). *The Edgar Cayce remedies.* New York: Bantam Books.

McGarey, W. A. (1983). *Physician's reference notebook.* Virginia Beach, VA: A.R.E. Press.

McGlashan, T. H. & Bardenstein, K. K. (1990). Gender differences in affective, schizoaffective, and schizophrenic disorders. *Schizophrenia Bulletin, 16*(2), 319-330.

McGowan, T. (1989). *Epilepsy.* New York: Franklin Watts.

McGue, M. & Gottesman, I. I. (1989). Genetic linkage in schizophrenia: Perspectives from genetic epidemiology. *Schizophrenia Bulletin, 15*(3), 453-464.

McKenna, P. J., Kane, J. M. & Parrish, K. (1985). Psychotic syndromes in epilepsy. *American Journal of Psychiatry, 142*(8), 895-904.

McNeil, T. F. & Kau, L. (1978). Obstetric factors in the development of schizophrenia. In *The Nature of Schizophrenia* (L. C. Wynne, R. L. Cromwell & Matthysse, S., eds.), pp. 401-429, New York: John Wiley.

Mednick, S. A. (1958). A learning theory approach to research in schizophrenia. *Psychological Bulletin, 55,* 316-327.

Mednick, S. A. (1970). Breakdown in individuals at high risk for schizophrenia: Possible predispositional perinatal factors. *Mental Hygiene, 54,* 50-63.

Mednick, S. A., Mura, E., Schulsinger, F., & Mednick, B. (1971). Perinatal conditions and infant development in children with schizophrenic parents. *Social Biology, 18,* 103-113.

Mednick, S. A. & Schulsinger, F. (1965). A longitudinal study of children with a high risk for schizophrenia: A preliminary report. In *Methods and goals in human behavior genetics* (S. Vandenberg, ed.), pp. 255-296. New York: Academic Press.

Meltzer, H. Y. (1976). Neuromuscular dysfunction in schizophrenia. *Schizophrenia Bulletin, 2*(1), 106-135.

Meltzer, H. Y. (1979). Biology of schizophrenia subtypes: A review and proposal for method of study. *Schizophrenia Bulletin, 5*(3), 460-479.

Meltzer, H. Y. (1987). Biological studies in schizophrenia. *Schizophrenia Bulletin, 13*(1), 80-111.

Meltzer, H. Y., Arora, R. C. & Metz, J. (1984). Biological studies of schizoaffective disorders. *Schizophrenia Bulletin, 10*(1), 49-64.

Miles, A. & Philbrick, D. R. (1988). Melatonin and psychiatry.

Biological Psychiatry, 23, 405-425.

Milin, J., Bajic, M. & Brakus V. (1988). Morphodynamic reactive response of the pineal gland of rats chronically exposed to stable strong magnetic field. *Neuroscience, 26*(3), 1083-1092.

Miller, B. F. & Keane, C. B. (1972). *Encyclopedia and dictionary of medicine and nursing.* London: W. B. Saunders Company.

Milsum, J. H. (1985). A model of the eustress system for health/illness. *Behavioral Science, 30,* 179-186.

Min, K., Seo, I. S. & Song, J. (1987). Postnatal evolution of the human pineal gland. *Laboratory Investigation, 57*(6), 724-728.

Mintz, E. E. (1983). *The psychic thread.* New York: Human Sciences Press.

Mohamed, S. N., Merskey, H., Kazarian, S., & Disney, T. F. (1982). An investigation of the possible inverse relationships between the occurrence of rheumatoid arthritis, osteoarthritis, and schizophrenia. *Canadian Journal of Psychiatry, 27,* 381-383.

Moszkowska, A., Kordon, C. & Ebels, I. (1971). Biochemical fractions and mechanisms involved in the pineal modulation of pituitary gonadotropin release. In G. E. W. Wolstenhome & J. Knight (eds.), *The pineal gland* (p. 241). London: Churchhill Livingstone.

Motta, M., Schiaffini, O., Piva, F. & Martini, L. (1971). Pineal principles and the control of adrenocorticotropin secretion. In G. E. W. Wolstenhome & J. Knight (eds.), *The pineal gland* (p. 279). London: Churchhill Livingstone.

Mullen, P. E., Linsell, C., Silman, R. E., Edwards, R., Carter, S., Hooper, J., Leone, R., Laude, C., Smith, I. & Towell, P. (1978). The human pineal: New approaches and prospects. *Journal of Psychosomatic Research, 22,* 357-376.

Mullen, P. E. & Silman, R. E. (1977). The pineal and psychiatry: A review. *Psychological Medicine, 7,* 407-417.

Murphy, G. & Ballou, R. O. (eds.). (1960). *William James on psychial research.* New York: The Viking Press.

Murray, R. M. & Harvey. (1989). The congenital origins of schizophrenia. *Psychiatric Annals, 19*(10), 525-529.

Naegeli-Osjord, H. (1989). Possession and exorcism in the light of my personal experience. In K. P. Freeman, M. L. Albertson, & D. S. Ward (eds.), *Proceedings of the Second International Conference on Paranormal Research* (pp. 467-479). Fort Collins, CO: Rocky Mountain Research Institute.

Nasrallah, H. A., McCalley-Whitters, M. & Jacoby, C. G. (1982). Cerebral ventricular enlargement in young manic males. *Journal of Affective Disorders, 4,* 15-19.

Nasrallah, H. A., Schwarzkopf, S. B., Olson, S. C. & Coffman, J. A. (1990). Gender differences in schizophrenia on MRI brain scans. *Schizophrenia Bulletin, 16*(2), 205-210.

Naylor, R. J. & Olley, J. E. (1959). The distribution of haloperidol in rat brain. *British Journal of Pharmacology, 36,* 208-209.

Neppe, V. M. & Tucker, G. J. (1988a). Modern perspectives on epilepsy in relation to psychiatry: Classification and evaluation. *Hospital and Community Psychiatry, 39*(3), 263-271.

Neppe, V. M. & Tucker, G. J. (1988b). Modern perspectives on epilepsy in relation to psychiatry: Behavioral disturbances of epilepsy. *Hospital and Community Psychiatry, 39*(4), 389-396.

Nielsen, B. M., Mehlsen, J. & Behnke. (1988). Altered balance in the autonomic nervous system in schizophrenic patients. *Clinical Physiology, 8,* 193-199.

Nigl, A. J., North, C. S. (1989). Current concepts of schizophrenia. *Comprehensive Therapy, 15*(3), 8-21.

North, C. S. (1989). Current concepts of schizophrenia. *Comprehensive Therapy, 15*(3), 8-21.

Nott, P. N. (1982). Psychiatric illness following childbirth in Southampton: A case register study. *Psychological Medicine, 12,* 557-561.

Noyes, R., Jr. (1985). Beta-adrenergic blocking drugs in anxiety and stress. *Psychiatric Clinics of North America, 8*(1), 119-132.

Nuechterlein, K. H. & Dawson, M. E. (1984). A heuristic vulnerability/stress model of schizophrenic episodes. *Schizophrenia Bulletin, 10*(2), 300-312.

Oesterreich, T. K. (1966). *Possession: Demonical and other among primitive races, in antiquity, the Middle Ages, and modern times.* New York: University Books.

Ohman, A. (1981). Electrodermal activity and vulnerability to schizophrenia: A review. *Biological Psychology, 12,* 87-145.

Overall, J. E. & Gorham, D. R. (1962). The brief psychiatric rating scale. *Psychiatric Reports, 10,* 799-812.

Oyebode, F. & Davison, K. (1989). Epileptic schizophrenia: Clinical features and outcome. *Acta Psychiatrica Scandinavica, 79,* 327-331.

Pagano, J. (1987). Chiropractic: Beyond back pains. *Venture Inward, 3*(4), 13-17.

Parkes, A. S. (1976). *Patterns of sexuality and reproduction.* Oxford: Oxford University Press.

Parnas, J., Mednick, S. A., Moffit T. E. & Crapuche, F. (1981). Perinatal complications and adult schizophrenia. *Trends in Neurosciences, 4*(10), 262-264.

Parnas, J., Schulsinger, F., Teasdale, T. W., Schulsinger, H., Feldman, P. M. & Mednick, S. A. (1982). Perinatal complications and clinical outcome within the schizophrenia spectrum. *British Journal of Psychiatry, 140,* 416-420.

Pasamanick, B. & Knobloch, H. (1971). Epidemiological studies on the complications of pregnancy and the birth process. In Caplan, G. (ed.), *Prevention of mental disorders in children* (pp. 74-79). New York: Basic Books.

Pavel, S. & Goldstein, R. (1981). Narcoleptic-like alterations of the sleep cycle in cats induced by a specific vasotocin antiserum. *Brain Research Bulletin, 7,* 453-454.

Pavel, S., Psatta, D. & Goldstein, R. (1977). Slow-wave sleep induced in cats by extremely small amounts of synthetic and pineal vasotocin injected into the third ventricle of the brain. *Brain Research Bulletin, 2,* 251-254.

Pearlson, G. D., Garbacz, D. J., Moberg, P. J., Ahn, H. S. & De Paulo, J. R. (1985). Symptomatic, familial, perinatal, and social correlates of CAT changes in schizophrenics and bipolars. *Journal of Nervous and Mental Disorders, 173,* 42-50.

Pearlson, G. D. & Veroff, A. E. (1981). Computerized tomographic scan changes in manic-depressive illness. *Lancet, 2,* 470.

Perez, M. M. & Trimble, M. R. (1980). Epileptic psychosis—Diagnostic comparison with process schizophrenia. *British Journal of Psychiatry, 137,* 245-249.

Peterson, B. (ed.). (1979). *The collected papers of Irvin M. Korr.* Colorado Springs, CO: American Academy of Osteopathy.

Philo, R. & Reiter, R. (1978). Characterization of pinealectomy induced convulsions in the Mongolian gerbil. *Epilepsia, 19,* 485-492.

Pollack, M., Woerner, M., Goodman, W. & Greenberg, I. (1966). Childhood development patterns of hospitalized adult schizophrenic and non-schizophrenic patients and their siblings. *American Journal of Orthopsychiatry, 36,* 510-517.

Pope, H. G. & Katz, D. L. (1987). Bodybuilder's psychosis. *The Lancet,* 863.

Pope, H. G. & Katz, D. L. (1988). Affective and psychotic symptoms associated with anabolic steroid use. *American Journal of Psychiatry, 145*(4), 487-490.

Pope, H. G. & Lipinski, J. F. (1978). Diagnosis in schizophrenia and manic-depressive illness. *Archives of General Psychiatry, 35,* 811-828.

Post, R. M. (1990). Non-lithium treatment of bipolar disorder. *Journal of Clinical Psychiatry, 51*(8), suppl., 9-16.

Prerost, F. J. (1988). Use of humor and guided imagery in therapy to alleviate stress. *Journal of Mental Health Counseling, 10*(1), 16-22.

Prien, R. F. & Gelenberg, A. J. (1989). Alternatives to lithium for preventive treatment of bipolar disorder. *American Journal Psychiatry, 146*(7), 840-848.

Pugh, C., Steinert, J. & Priest, R. Propranolol in schizophrenia: A double-blind, placebo-controlled trial of propranolol as an adjunct to neuroleptic medication. *British Journal of Psychiatry, 143,* 151-156.

Quigley, W. H. (1954). *Case histories of mental illness under chiropractic.* Davenport, Iowa: Clear View Sanitarium.

Quigley, W. H. (1958). *Case histories of mental illness under chiropractic.* Davenport, Iowa: Clear View Sanitarium.

Quigley, W. H. (1973). Physiological psychology of chiropractic. In H. S. Schwartz (ed.), *Mental health and chiropractic* (pp. 113-118). New York: Sessions Publishers.

Quigley, W. H. (1983). Pioneering mental health: Institutional psychiatric care in chiropractic. *Chiropractic History, 3*(1), 69-73.

Ralph, C. L. (1984). Pineal bodies and thermoregulation. In R. J. Reiter (ed.), *The pineal gland* (pp. 193-220). New York: Raven Press.

Reilly, H. J. & Brod, R. H. (1975). *The Edgar Cayce handbook for health through drugless therapy.* Virginia Beach, VA: A.R.E Press.

Reiter, R. J. (1977). Pineal interaction with the central nervous system. *Waking and Sleeping, 1,* 253-258.

Reiter, R. J. (ed.). (1984). *The pineal gland.* New York: Raven Press.

Reveley, A. M., Reveley, M. A. & Murray, R. M. (1984). Cerebral ventricular enlargement in non-genetic schizophrenia: A controlled twin study. *British Journal of Psychiatry, 144,* 89-93.

Rieder, R. O., Mann, L. S., Weinberger, D. R., van Kammen, D. P. & Post, R. M. (1983). Computed tomographic scans in patients with schizophrenia, schizoaffective, and bipolar affective disorder. *Archives of General Psychiatry, 40,* 735-739.

Roberts, G. W., Done, D. J., Bruton, C. & Crow, T. J. (1990). A "mock up" of schizophrenia: Temporal lobe epilepsy and schizophrenia-like psychosis. *Biological Psychiatry, 28,* 127-143.

Robinson, J. W. (1980). Helping others manage stress. *Journal of Extension*, 46-53.

Rodin, A. E. (1963). The growth and spread of Walker 256 carcinoma in pinealectomized rats. *Cancer Research, 23*, 1545.

Rogers, C. R. (1957). The necessary and sufficient conditions of therapeutic personality change. *Journal of Consulting Psychology, 21*, 95-103.

Rogo, D. S. (1987). *The infinite boundary.* New York: Dodd, Mead & Co.

Rosenthal, N. E., Sack, D. A., Gillin, J. C., Lewy, A. J., Goodwin, F. K., Davenport, Y., Mueller, P. S., Newsome, D. A. & Wehr, T. A. (1984). Seasonal affective disorder: A description of the syndrome and preliminary findings with light therapy. *Archives of General Psychiatry, 41*, 72-79.

Rubin, L. B. (1985). *Just friends.* New York: Harper & Row.

Rubin, L. S. (1976). Sympathetic-parasympathetic imbalance as a diagnostic concomitant of schizophrenia: Implications for pharmacotherapy. *Research Communications in Psychology, Psychiatry and Behavior, 1*, 73-89.

Sannella, L. (1987). *The kundalini experience: Psychosis or transcendence.* Lower Lake, CA: Integral Publishing.

Scheiber, S. C., Cohen, R., Yamamura, H., Novak, R. & Beutler, L. (1981). Dialysis for schizophrenia: An uncontrolled study of 11 patients. *American Journal of Psychiatry, 138*, 662-667.

Scheinbaum, B. W. (1979). Psychiatric diagnostic error. *Schizophrenia Bulletin, 5*(4), 560-564.

Schiffer, R. B. (1987). Epilepsy, psychosis, and forced normalization. *Archives of Neurology, 44*, 253.

Schneider, K. (1959). *Clinical Psychopathology.* New York: Grune and Stratton, Inc.

Schneider, S. J. & Pope, A. T. (1982). Neuroleptic-like electroencephalographic changes in schizophrenics through biofeedback. *Biofeedback and Self-Regulation, 7*(4), 479-490.

Schulz, S. C. & Pato, C. N. (1989). Pharmacologic treatment of schizophrenia. *Psychiatric Annals, 19*(10), 536-541.

Schwartz, H. S. (1973). *Mental health and chiropractic, a multidisciplinary approach.* New York: Sessions Publishers.

Seeman, M. V. (1983). Interaction of sex, age, and neuroleptic dose. *Comprehensive Psychiatry, 24*, 125-128.

Seeman, M. V. & Hauser, P. (1984). The influence of gender on family environment. *International Journal of Family Psychiatry, 5*, 227-232.

Seeman, M. V. & Lang, M. (1990). The role of estrogens in schizophrenia gender differences. *Schizophrenia Bulletin, 16*(2), 185-194.

Seilheimer, T. & Lee, M. (1987). Community integration through therapeutic recreation: The Scorpions' second season. *International Journal of Partial Hospitalization, 4*(3), 235-240.

Severini, V. & Vererando, A. (1967). Physiological effects of massage on the cardiovascular system. *Europa Medicophysica, 3,* 165-183.

Shepard, L. A. (1984). *Encyclopedia of occultism and parapsychology.* (2nd ed.) Detroit, MI: Book Tower.

Sheppard, G. P. (1979). High-dose propranolol in schizophrenia. *British Journal of Psychiatry, 134,* 470-476.

Singh, M. M. & Kay, S. R. (1979). Dysphoric response to neuroleptic treatment in schizophrenia: Its relationship to autonomic arousal and prognosis. *Biological Psychiatry, 14*(2), 277-295.

Slater, E. & Beard, A. W. (1963). The schizophrenia-like psychoses of epilepsy: Psychiatric aspects. *British Journal of Psychiatry, 109,* 95-129.

Slater, V., Linn, M. W., Harris, R. & Odutola, A. A. (1981). A retrospective review of relapse. *Journal of Psychiatric Treatment and Evaluation, 3,* 515-521.

Snyder, S. H. & Reivich, M. (1966). Regional localization of lysergic acid diethylamide in monkey brain. *Nature,* 1093-1095.

Souetre, E., Salvati, E., Krebs, B., Belugou, J. & Darcourt, G. (1989). Abnormal melatonin response to 5-methoxypsoralen in dementia. *American Journal of Psychiatry, 146*(8), 1037-1040.

Spitzer, R. L., Endicott, J. E. & Robins, E. (1978). Research diagnostic criteria: Rationale and reliability. *Archives of General Psychiatry, 35,* 773-782.

Spohn, H. E. & Patterson, T. (1979). Recent studies of psychophysiology in schizophrenia. *Schizophrenia Bulletin, 5*(4), 581-611.

Srinivasan, T. M. (ed.). (1988). *Energy medicine around the world.* Phoenix: Gabriel Press.

Stearn, J. (1967). *Edgar Cayce—the sleeping prophet.* New York: Bantam Books.

Stein, F. & Nikolic, S. (1989). Teaching stress management techniques to a schizophrenic patient. *The American Journal of Occupational Therapy, 43*(3), 162-169.

Sternberg, D. E., Charney, D. S., Heninger, G. R., Leckman, J. F., Hafstad, K. M. & Landis D. H. (1982). Impaired presynaptic regulation of norepinephrine in schizophrenia. *Archives of General Psychiatry, 39,* 285-289.

Stevens, J. R. (1988). Psychiatric aspects of epilepsy. *Journal of Clinical Psychiatry, 49*(4), suppl., 49-57.

Stickney, S. K., Hall, R. C. & Gardner, E. R. (1980). The effect of referral procedures on aftercare compliance. *Hospital and Community Psychiatry, 31*(8), 567-569.

Still, A. T. (1897). *Autobiography of A. T. Still.* Kirksville, MO: Published by author.

Still, F. M. (1933). *Comparison of osteopathic and medical results in dementia praecox.* Paper presented at the American Osteopathic Association Convention, Milwaukee, WI.

Straube, E. R. (1983). High and low arousability in schizophrenia: A clue to cause and development of the illness ascertained by differences in autonomic nervous system reactivity? *Advances in Biological Psychiatry, 13,* 197-114.

Straube, E. R., Schied, H. W., Rein, W. & Breyer-Pfaff, U. (1987). Autonomic nervous system differences as predictors of short-term outcome in schizophrenics. *Pharmacopsychiat. 20,* 105-110.

Strauss, J. S. (1985). Negative symptoms: Future developments of the concept. *Schizophrenia Bulletin, 11*(3), 457-461.

Strauss, J. S. & Bellak, L. (1979). Epilogue: Subtypes of the schizophrenic syndrome —their current status. *Schizophrenia Bulletin, 5*(3), 507-508.

Strauss, J. S. & Docherty, J. P. (1979). Subtypes of schizophrenia: Descriptive models. *Schizophrenia Bulletin, 5*(3), 447-452.

Strauss, M. (1985). *Recovering from the new age: Therapies for kundalini crisis.* Unpublished manuscript. There is a copy in the A.R.E. Library reference section.

Sugrue, T. (1942). *There is a river: The story of Edgar Cayce.* Virginia Beach: VA: A.R.E. Press.

Sutherland, W. L. (1976). *Osteopathy in the cranial field.* 3rd edition. H. I. Magoun (ed.). Kirksville, MO: The Journal Printing Co.

Svensson, T. H. (1987). Peripheral, autonomic regulation of locus coerueus noradrenergic neurons in brain: Putative implications for psychiatry and psychopharmacology. *Psychopharmacology, 92,* 1-7.

Tandon, R. & Greden, J. F. (1989). Cholinergic hyperactivity and negative schizophrenic symptoms. *Archives of General Psychiatry, 46,* 745-753.

Tarrier, N., Vaughn, C., Lader, M. H. & Leff, J. P. (1979). Bodily reactions to people and events in schizophrenics. *Archives of General Psychiatry, 36,* 311-315.

Thoelen, H., Stricker, E., Feer, H., Massini, M. A. & Staub, H. (1960). Ueber die anwendung der kunstlichen niere bei schizophrenie und myasthenia gravis. *Dtsch. Med.Wochenschr., 85,* 1012-1016.

Thygesen, P., Hermann, K. & Willanger, R. (1970). Concentration camp survivors in Denmark. *Danish Medical Bulletin, 17,* 65-108.

Torrey, E. F. (1988). *Surviving schizophrenia: A family manual.* New York: Harper & Row, Publishers.

Tourney, G. & Erb, J. L. (1979). Temporal variations in androgens and stress hormones in control and schizophrenic subjects. *Biological Psychiatry, 14,* 395-404.

Tourney, G. & Hatfield, L. (1972). Plasma androgens in male schizophrenics. *Archives of General Psychiatry, 27,* 753-755.

Tramer, M. (1929). Über die biologische Bedeutung des Geburtsmonates, insbesondere für die Psychoseerkrankung. *Schweizer Archiv für Neurolgie und Psychiatrie, 24,* 17-24.

Trimble, M. (1977). The relationship between epilepsy and schizophrenia: A biochemical hypothesis. *Biological Psychiatry, 12*(2), 299-303.

Tsuang, M. T. & Simpson, J. C. (1984). Schizoaffective disorder: Concept and reality. *Schizophrenia Bulletin,* 14-25.

Tsuang, M. T., Woolson, R. F., Winokur, G. & Crowe, R. R. (1981). Stability of psychiatric diagnosis. *Archives of General Psychiatry, 38,* 535-539.

Turner, C. D. & Bagnara, J. T. (1971). *General endocrinology.* Philadelphia: W. B. Saunders Co.

Turner, G. D. (1957). *Chiropractic, electrotherapy, and hydrotherapy from the Edgar Cayce records.* Presentation at the A.R.E. Congress class on physical balance. Virginia Beach,VA: unpublished.

Turner, S. W., Toone, B. K. & Brett-Jones, J. R. (1986). Computerized tomographic scan changes in early schizophrenia. *Psychological Medicine, 16,* 219-225.

Underwood, H. (1984). The pineal and circadian rhythms. In R. J. Reiter (ed.). *The pineal gland* (pp. 221-252). New York: Raven Press.

van Kammen, D. P., Schulz, S. C., Balow, J. E., Zahn, T. P., Mundinger, G., Flye, M. W. & Bunney, W. E. (1983). Failure of hemodialysis to diminish psychotic behavior in schizophrenia: Behavioral and psychophysiological evaluation. *Artificial Organs*, 7(3), 310-316.

van Kammen, D. P. & Antelman, S. (1984). Impaired noradrenergic transmission in schizophrenia? *Life Sciences, 34*, 1403-1413.

Vaughn, C. & Leff, J. P. (1976). The measurement of expressed emotion in the families of psychiatric patients. *British Journal of Social and Clinical Psychology, 15*, 157-165.

Wagemaker, H. & Cade, R. (1978). Hemodialysis in chronic schizophrenic patients. *Southern Medical Journal, 71*, 1463-1469.

Wagemaker, H. & Cade, R. (1979). The experimental use of hemodialysis in the treatment of chronic schizophrenia. *Psychopharmacology Bulletin, 15*, 13-14.

Walker, C. E. (1981). *Clinical practice of psychology*. New York: Pergamon Press.

Watson, C. G. (1990). Schizophrenic birth seasonality and the age-incidence artifact. *Schizophrenia Bulletin, 16*(1), 5-10.

Weinberg, R. & Kolodny K. (1988). The relationship of massage and exercise to mood enhancement. *The Sport Psychologist, 2*, 202-211.

Wendel, O. T., Waterbury, L. D. & Pierce L. A. (1974). Increase in monoamine concentrations in rat brain following melatonin administration. *Experentia, 30*, 1167-1168.

Wetterberg, L., Beck-Friis, J., Aperia B., Kjellman, B. F., Ljunggren, J. G., Petterson, U. & Sjolin, A. (1979). Melatonin/cortisol ratio in depression. *Lancet,* 1361.

Wetterberg, L., Aperia, B., Kjellman, B. F., Ljunggren, J. G., Petterson, U., Sjolin, A. & Tham, A. (1981). Pineal-hypothalamic-pituitary function in patients with depressive illness. In K. Fuxe, J. A. Gustafsson & L. Wetterberg (eds.), *Steroid Hormone Regulation of the Brain* (pp. 397-403). Oxford: Pergamon Press.

Wetterberg, L., Aperia, B., Beck-Friis, J., Kjellman, B. F., Ljunggren, J. G., Nilsonne, A., Patterson, U., Tham, A. & Unden, F. (1982). Melatonin and cortisol levels in psychiatric illness. *Lancet,* 100.

Wettlin, H. B. (1976). *Edgar Cayce's clairvoyance in treating mental illness.* Unpublished dissertation. Hollywood, FL: Heed University.

Whalley, L. J., Christie, J. E., Bennie, J., Dick, J., Blackburn, I. M., Blackwood, D., Watts, G. S. & Fink, G. (1985). Selective increase in plasma luteinising hormone concentrations in drug-free young men with mania. *British Medical Journal, 290*, 99-102.

Whalley, L. J., Christie, J. E., Blackwood, D. H., Bennie, J., Dick, H.,

Blackburn, I. M. & Fink, G. (1989). Disturbed endocrine function in the psychoses. *British Journal of Psychiatry, 155,* 462-467.

White, J. (1990). *Kundalini, evolution, and enlightenment.* New York: Paragon House.

Wickland, C. A. (1924). *Thirty years among the dead.* Los Angeles: National Psychological Laboratory.

Wilber, K. (1981). *Up from Eden: A transpersonal view of human evolution.* Boulder: Shambhala.

Williams, R. T. (1980). Creatively coping with stress. *Journal of Extension,* 24-30.

Wilson, B. W., Stevens, R. G. & L. E. Anderson. (1989). Neuroendocrine mediated effects of electromagnetic-field exposure: Possible role of the pineal gland. *Life Sciences, 45,* 1319-1332.

Windsor, J. C. (1969, January). *A holistic theory of mental illness.* Paper presented to the second annual symposium of the Research Division of the Edgar Cayce Foundation, Phoenix, Arizona. Included in the *Physician's reference notebook,* pp. 244-257, Virginia Beach, VA: A.R.E. Press.

Windsor, J. C. (1989). *Commentary on possession.* Available from the author: P.O. Box 557, Williamsburg, VA 23187.

Winters, W. D., Alcaraz, M., Cervantes, M. Y. & Flores-Guzman, C. (1973). The synergistic effect of reduced visual input on ketamine action—The possible role of the pineal gland. *Neuropharmacology, 12,* 407-416.

Wise, S. S. (1989). Carbamazepine: Treatment option for bipolar patients. *Hospital and Community Psychiatry, 40*(2), 123-124.

Woerner, M. G., Pollack, M. & Klein, D. F. (1973). Pregnancy and birth complications in psychiatric patients. *Acta Psychiatrica Scandinavica, 49,* 712-716.

Woody, R. H. (1979). Intimacy-related anxiety and massage. *Voices, 15*(1), 36-42.

Wyatt, R., Termini, B. A. & Davis, J. (1971). A review of the literature 1960-1970: Part II. Sleep studies. *Schizophrenia Bulletin, 4,* 45-66.

Wyatt, R. J., Alexander, F. C., Egan, M. F. & Kirch, D. G. (1988). Schizophrenia, just the facts. *Schizophrenia Research, 1,* 3-18.

Yorkston, N. J., Zaki, S. A., Pitcher, D. R., Gruzelier, J. H., Hollander, D. & Sergeant, H. G. (1977). Propranolol as an adjunct to the treatment of schizophrenia. *Lancet, II,* 575-578.

Young, I. M., Leone, P. L., Stovell, P. & Silman, R. E. (1986). Night/day urinary 6-hydroxymelatonin production as a function of age, bodymass, and urinary creatinine levels: A population study in 110 subjects aged 3-80. *Journal of Endocrinology,* Suppl. Abstract No 32, 111.

Zahn, T. P., Carpenter, W. T. & McGlashan, T. H. (1981). Autonomic nervous system activity in acute schizophrenia. *Archives of General Psychiatry, 38,* 251-258.

Zisapel, N. & Laudon, M. (1983). Inhibition by melatonin of dopamine release from rat hypothalamus. *Brain Research, 272,* 378-381.

Zubin, J. (1985). Negative symptoms: Are they indigenous to schizophrenia? *Schizophrenia Bulletin, 11*(3), 461-469.

Zubin, J. & Spring, B. (1977). Vulnerability—a new view of schizophrenia. *Journal of Abnormal Psychology, 86*(2), 103-126.

A.R.E. PRESS

T he A.R.E. Press publishes quality books, videos, and audiotapes meant to improve the quality of our readers' lives—personally, professionally, and spiritually. We hope our products support your endeavors to realize your career potential, to enhance your relationships, to improve your health, and to encourage you to make the changes necessary to live a loving, joyful, and fulfilling life.

OF RELATED INTEREST:

Also by David McMillin: A CD-ROM interactive database, *Edgar Cayce on Health and Healing* (Version 2.0), and books on *Alzheimer's Disease and the Dementias: An Alternative Perspective, Principles and Techniques of Nerve Regeneration, Case Studies in Depression, The Treatment of Depression: A Holistic Approach,* and *Case Studies in Schizophrenia.*

You may also be interested in the *Edgar Cayce Handbook for Health Through Drugless Therapy* by Harold J. Reilly & Ruth Brod
ISBN 0-87604-215-9   Paperback   Order #2073 $14.95

or

Physician's Reference Notebook by A.R.E. Associated Physicians (William McGarey, M.D., et al.)
ISBN 0-87604-175-6   Hardcover   Order #322 $24.95

To order the CD-ROM or any of these books or to receive a free catalog, call

1-800-723-1112

Or write

A.R.E. Press
P.O. Box 656
Virginia Beach, VA 23451-0656
(All prices subject to change.)

DISCOVER HOW THE EDGAR CAYCE MATERIAL CAN HELP YOU!

The Association for Research and Enlightenment, Inc. (A.R.E.®), was founded in 1931 by Edgar Cayce. Its international headquarters are in Virginia Beach, Virginia, where thousands of visitors come year round. Many more are helped and inspired by A.R.E.'s local activities in their own hometowns or by contact via mail (and now the Internet!) with A.R.E. headquarters.

People from all walks of life, all around the world, have discovered meaningful and life-transforming insights in the A.R.E. programs and materials, which focus on such areas as holistic health, dreams, family life, finding your best vocation, reincarnation, ESP, meditation, personal spirituality, and soul growth in small-group settings. Call us today on our toll-free number

1-800-333-4499

or

Explore our electronic visitor's center on the
INTERNET: http://www.are-cayce.com

We'll be happy to tell you more about how the work of the A.R.E. can help you!

A.R.E.
67th Street and Atlantic Avenue
P.O. Box 595
Virginia Beach, VA 23451-0595